Contents

D0709326

Introduction

What Does "Organic" Really Mean?

The word "organic" has many meanings. A college student struggling through the first semester of organic chemistry might be surprised to discover the class exploring synthetic plastics and petroleum products alongside the compounds used or produced by living organisms.

At the other end of the spectrum, a contemporary artist known for geometrical abstraction may turn the art world on its head by venturing into a new "organic period," trading a world of straight lines and hard edges for more lifelike, free-flowing shapes.

But in the world of food products, the word "organic" takes on a set of very specific meanings.

What Is Organic Food?

While the word "organic" is sometimes used casually to suggest an interest in a healthy, natural diet, in other contexts using the word "organic" assumes the power of law and becomes the subject of carefully defined rules and regulations.

In the broadest possible terms, organic agriculture refers to foods that are produced and brought to market without the use of man-made chemicals. More specifically, the United States Department of Agriculture (USDA) describes organic food as products grown and produced using "materials and practices that enhance the ecological balance of natural systems and that integrate the parts of the farming system into an ecological whole."

Organic farmers are dedicated to mindful use of the land. They champion the use of renewable resources, carefully preserving nutrient-rich soil and conserving water to ensure that these resources will be available for future generations. Organic farming practices aim to maintain ecological balance and biodiversity, reduce pollution, and treat animals and the land respectfully.

To be considered organic, meat, poultry, eggs, and dairy products must be from animals raised in a clean, healthy, humane environment with regular access to fresh air and pasture. They must be fed certified organic foods that contain no animal byproducts. Organic farm animals must not be given antibiotics or growth hormones.

Organic produce is grown and cultivated without the use of synthetic pesticides, chemical fertilizers, sewage sludge, bioengineering, or ionizing radiation. Similarly, organic foods cannot be processed using radiation, industrial solvents, genetically modified ingredients, or chemical food additives.

Instead of using synthetic and chemical fertilizers and pesticides, organic farmers carefully select disease-resistant crops, rely on natural fertilizers to nourish soil, and rotate crops or mulch to avoid depleting the soil and to control weeds and prevent diseases. Organic farmers combat crop-destroying pests by using predatory insects, insect traps, or beneficial microorganisms.

The Organic Movement

It's difficult for most of us to truly imagine what life was like even fifty or sixty years ago. Today, in a world where five-year-olds play around with portable electronic devices that are significantly more powerful than the computers that flew the Apollo spacecraft to the moon, it's hard to remember that until the 1960s, many households still did not even have telephones, and not long before that a large number of rural homes had no electrical service.

In a matter of decades our world has changed to a remarkable extent—and it has changed on a global scale. Technology, which can be defined as the application of scientific knowledge for practical purposes through the use of man-made inventions and specialized processes, has transformed every aspect of our existence. These changes are perhaps most readily apparent in information and communications technologies, medicine, and transportation, but they are equally momentous—if sometimes less visible—in agriculture and food production.

As a case in point, consider the fact that in 1830, it took upwards of 300 labor hours and five acres of farmland to produce 100 bushels of wheat.[1] By 1980, 150 years later, that same 100 bushels could be produced on three acres of land using only about three labor hours of effort. Reductions in land use and total labor effort have declined even more for corn, soy, and other major crops.

Beginning with the rise of the industrial age at the end of the eighteenth and beginning of the nineteenth centuries, a series of major technological innovations helped to transform agriculture from an inefficient, extremely labor-intensive process to a far more streamlined enterprise capable of feeding many more people at lower cost, with less effort and on less farmland.

---

[1] A labor hour is the equivalent of one person working for one hour. So in our example, 300 labor hours could mean one person working for 300 hours, or 300 people working for one hour, or ten people working for thirty hours, or any other combination of workers and hours whose product multiplies to 300.

Some of the major technological innovations that made these impressive efficiencies possible were:

- Mechanized farm machinery
- Hybridization techniques to create new cultivars
- Nitrogen-rich chemical fertilizers
- Chemical pesticides
- Vitamins and other nutritional isolates
- Refrigerated and containerized transportation
- Antibiotic and antifungal medications
- Bioengineering and genetic modifications

In retrospect, we now know that these technologies produced many undesirable and unintended consequences. But as they were developed and introduced, each of these innovations was seen as a boon to mankind, a way to increase the size and variety of the food supply while reducing the costs of production and distribution.

One of the key themes of the twentieth century has often been described as "better living through chemistry." Now, however, more than a century since the dawn of the technological age, we've learned that those advances in chemistry, and in time their more sophisticated offshoots in biology and bioengineering, can be double-edged swords.

The Origins of Organics—Rediscovering the Wisdom of Nature

The original impetus for what in time grew to be the organic movement wasn't so much a desire for less toxic, less chemically processed foods, but a growing realization that emerging, highly industrialized agricultural practices threatened to harm the land, leaving it less vital and resilient for future generations. At the same time, connections were being uncovered between the health of agricultural lands and human health, and they often provided a surprising validation of traditional farming practices.

A small number of visionaries intuitively understood that the emerging modern practices would not be sustainable in the long run. They rediscovered the power of natural cycles of planting, composting, harvesting, and systematic crop rotation and how these worked together to create a subtle pattern of biological renewal that kept the soil fertile—and had been doing so through all of human history. They saw that each new innovation, seemingly harmless on its own, could combine over time to radically alter the biology of the living earth, leaving us all poorer for it.

Rudolf Steiner's Biodynamic Agriculture (1924)

The first consciously crafted method of organic agriculture is usually attributed to Rudolf Steiner, the Austrian philosopher who is probably best remembered for the Waldorf system of holistic education he pioneered. Today, his somewhat esoteric approach to childhood learning is still taught in nearly 1,000 Waldorf Schools around the world, with nineteen teacher training centers located in the United States, Canada, and Mexico, and many more countries in Europe.

Agriculture was another prime interest of Steiner's, and like his other fields of endeavor, he tended to couch his deep and practical insights within a spiritual and philosophical framework. While a relatively small number of people were, and still are, attracted to Steiner's esoteric approach, a far larger number tend to be alienated by the mystical atmosphere that surrounds much of his work. Steiner's philosophies aside, the actual method of biodynamic agriculture he first presented in a series of lectures in 1924 is strikingly similar to many of the practices that have come to define organic agriculture in the present day.

Steiner believed that the fertility of the soil was inextricably linked to the growth of the plants and animals that lived on it, naturally creating a vital web of subtle ecological relationships. He held that the health and vitality of the plants and animals raised on a farm were inseparable from the health and vitality of the land itself, which was, in turn, inseparable from the health and vitality of the people who consumed the plants and animals that grazed and grew on that land.

For Steiner, this understanding was at once scientific, practical, philosophical, and spiritual. Like today's organic agriculture, Steiner's method emphasized the importance of natural compost and manure and insisted on the complete exclusion of man-made chemicals from the entire agricultural process. He promoted the use of natural herbs and minerals to charge the soil, creating the optimal characteristics for growth. He also had the foresight to understand the critical role of natural biodiversity in maintaining the integrity of an ecosystem. Under the principles of biodynamic agriculture, a minimum of ten percent of each farm was to be set aside as a "biodiversity preserve," allowing the wild, uncultivated development of ecologically necessary organisms. These biodiversity preserves could consist of forests and wetlands, but they could also include deliberately designed areas where insects critical to pollination and natural pest control could thrive.

However, unlike today's mainstream organic processes, Steiner's method also relied on astrological information and advocated the harnessing of "cosmic forces in the soil," with practices such as burying ground quartz crystals packed into a hollow cow's horn in the spring and digging it back up in the fall. It's difficult to imagine the United States Department of Agriculture (USDA) setting federal standards for the construction and management of "cosmic cow horn quartz soil amplifiers." It's likely that biodynamic agriculture did not have as broad an impact as it might otherwise have enjoyed because of some of Steiner's more mystical beliefs and the widespread perception that his approach was intrinsically pseudoscientific, despite the fact that it was based on a foundation of utterly rational premises and practices.

As untenable as some of Steiner's views might seem to us in retrospect, he did in

4

fact present and codify an otherwise rational and holistic approach to agriculture. Today, a number of farms use Steiner's principles. Of the approximately 150,000 hectares under Steiner-guided cultivation, almost half are in Germany. In recent years, many vineyards have turned to biodynamic agriculture for the production of their wines.

Demeter International (1927)—The First Organic Certification

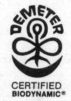

CERTIFIED
BIODYNAMIC®

In 1924, following Steiner's original lectures on biodynamic agriculture, the German agronomist Erhard Bartsch formed the Association for Research in Anthroposophical Agriculture, a group devoted to the objective, scientific study of the effects of Steiner's system. The association published a research journal called *Demeter*—in honor of the ancient Greek goddess of grain and fertility—to share their findings with the broader community.

In 1927, a cooperative for biodynamic food processing was founded in Berlin. The next year, under the auspices of Bartsch and a colleague—the German chemist Franz Dreidax—the cooperative developed the world's first certification program for ecologically produced foods and trademarked the Demeter name.

In 1928, Demeter International became the world's first ecological labeling organization. The Demeter biodynamic certification program is currently used in more than fifty countries and is considered one of the three most significant organic certification marks worldwide.

Demeter set a high bar—its biodynamic certification standards are the most stringent. Unlike other organic certification programs, Demeter-certified producers must demonstrate adherence to specific ecological practices including the maintenance of the biodiversity preserves described above. In addition, Demeter-certified producers must renew their status annually.

Sir Albert Howard (1873–1947)—The Teacher Becomes the Pupil

Sir Albert Howard is one of the true pioneers of the organic movement. In 1905, Howard traveled to India—at that time still very much a British colony—to serve as imperial economic botanist to the government of India. Essentially, he was sent from the highly developed and technologically sophisticated world of England to enlighten the benighted natives of a backward country in the proper conduct of modern agriculture.

What happened instead was that Howard found his world turned upside down in a classic case of the teacher becoming the pupil. Though he was meant to instruct the natives in the methods and benefits of the modern world, instead the natives taught him about the overwhelming benefits of the natural world.

Howard came to realize that the natives' methods of "primitive agriculture" created especially vibrant soil that supported the growth and development of remarkably healthful, life-giving produce and farm animals. Instead of forcing industrial agriculture on the people of India, Howard eventually returned to England completely convinced of the virtues of natural agriculture.

For decades he conducted exacting research and wrote passionately about the importance of natural agricultural processes and their relationship to human health. He was one of the first to recognize the complexity and interdependence between species within ecological systems, his ideas about the soil, food, and human health were similar to those of Steiner. His sentiment that "...the health of soil, plant, animal, and man is one and indivisible" could have come straight from the anthroposophical world of biodynamic agriculture.

Howard's original publications were meant for a specialized professional audience. In 1931, he published *The Waste Products of Agriculture*, which documented methods of organic composting as a natural way to maintain the vitality of soil. In 1940, he wrote his first book intended for a broader audience. *An Agricultural Testament* is regarded by many as the first volume comprehensively dedicated to organic farming, and its influence on other pioneers of the organic movement is undeniable. The eloquence and simplicity with which he wrote about the deep concept of biological interdependence in the natural terrain of the farm illustrates why his influence was so great.

In this first quote, from the preface of *An Agricultural Testament*, Howard lays out the depletion of the land sparked by the wholesale expansion of industrialized agriculture in stark terms:

> *"Since the Industrial Revolution, the processes of growth have been speeded up to produce the food and raw materials needed by the population and the factory. Nothing effective has been done to replace the loss of fertility involved in this vast increase in crop and animal production. The consequences have been disastrous. Agriculture has become unbalanced; the land is in revolt; diseases of all kinds are on the increase; in many parts of the world Nature is removing the worn-out soil by means of erosion."*

His prescription for curing the ills of toxic, industrialized farming laid out the foundation of the organic movement. Later in the text, he reminds us that:

> *"Mother earth never attempts to farm without livestock; she always raises mixed crops; great pains are taken to preserve the soil and to prevent erosion; the mixed vegetable and animal wastes are converted into humus; there is no waste; [and] the processes of growth and the processes of decay balance one another."*

The entire text of *An Agricultural Testament* is currently available online at: http://ps-urvival.com/PS/Agriculture/An_Agricultural_Testament_1943.pdf (accessed July 2014).

Lady Balfour (1889–1990) and the Haughley Experiment (1939–1980)

In 1939, inspired by Howard's research and writings, Lady Eve Balfour and several of her colleagues began an ambitious, long-term experiment to compare the effects of natural, organic farming with an essentially identical operation except for its use of man-made fertilizers and pesticides. On side-by-side farms large enough to support full farming operations including multiple life cycles of crops and livestock over many generations, they ran a remarkable forty-year-long experiment. Like any good science research project, variables were isolated and analyzed so that the only significant differences were those attributable to modern agriculture chemicals.

Years later, in 1977, Lady Balfour spoke at the International Federation of Organic Agriculture Movements conference in Switzerland (IFOAM). IFOAM is an organization founded in 1972 to provide an international focal point for the organic movement. Today, it boasts nearly 800 affiliate groups in 117 countries. At the 1977 IFOAM conference, Lady Balfour reported on what came to be known as the Haughley Experiment, named for the location of the farms in Haughley Green, Suffolk, England. She explained:

> *"Three side-by-side units of land were established, each large enough to operate a full farm rotation, so that the food chains involved—soil-plant-animal and back to the soil—could be studied as they functioned through successive rotational cycles, involving many generations of plants and animals, in order that interdependences between soil, plant, and animal, and also any cumulative effects, could manifest."*

One of the units was farmed organically, without the use of man-made chemicals. In the context of the experiment, this is often referred to as the "closed-cycle" approach because all the produce grown was fed back to the animals and returned to the soil. Although the phrase "organic farming" didn't appear until a year after the experiment began, this part of the farm in time came to be known as the "organic section."

The other unit was operated in a similar fashion, except that nitrogen-rich fertilizers, chemical herbicides, insecticides, and fungicides were used as thought to be appropriate. This part of the farm was referred to as the "mixed section" since it mixed the same principles of crop rotation and livestock management, only with the addition of the added chemicals.

The results of the Haughley Experiment were fascinating. At a gross level, the mixed

7

versus organic sections seemed to be quite similar. The differences, however, appeared in many of the more subtle details. Even though the organic section used no chemical pesticides, the plants there showed a relatively lower level of insect damage. Working animals in the organic section were found to have longer productive lives, and the richness and vitality of the soil was far greater, as shown in numerous analytical tests.

In the words of Dr. R. F. Milton, the scientist responsible for the thousands of biochemical analyses conducted on the site over many years:

> *"The analytical work carried out in connection with the Haughley Experiment has shown how wasteful of natural resources is modern commercial farming and how with a closed-cycle technique nutrients are recycled ..."*

In her 1977 report, Lady Balfour makes a far more dramatic statement, likening the use of chemical fertilizer to a drug addiction:

> *"In spite of the mixed section receiving no less organic return than its organic counterpart, it could be clearly demonstrated that its fields had become dependent on their fertilizer supplements in a manner suggestive of drug addiction. By contrast, the organic fields developed an increasing biological vigour which enabled them to be self-supporting."*

Although Lady Balfour didn't approach the spiritual aspects of organic agriculture head-on, in the manner of Steiner, she did ultimately conclude that the natural relationship between humans, food, and the earth was, ultimately, a spiritual matter. In the concluding remarks of her landmark 1977 lecture, she spoke eloquently about the larger issues of ecologically sensitive organic agriculture:

> *"There are two motivations behind an ecological approach—one is based on self-interest, however enlightened, i.e., when consideration for other species is taught solely because on that depends the survival of our own.*
>
> *The other motivation springs from a sense that the biota is a whole, of which we are a part, and that the other species which compose it and helped to create it, are entitled to existence in their own right. This is the wholeness approach, and it is my hope and belief that this is what we, as a federation, stand for.*
>
> *If I am right, this means that we cannot escape from the ethical and spiritual values of life, for they are part of wholeness."*

Throughout the history of the movement, we continually see that the pioneers of organic agriculture and animal husbandry understood their ideas in a larger context that unites human health; sustainable and ecologically balanced use of natural resources; and the ethical treatment of agricultural workers, communities, and farm animals. As individuals, we may primarily be interested in the benefits of consuming cleaner, more healthful foods, but when we choose organic, on some level we are also participating in a larger vision of the inseparable and mutually beneficial relationships between personal health, environmental health, and social justice. It's fair to say that this is precisely the vision that Lady Balfour and her colleagues in the Haughley Experiment brought so forcefully to our awareness with their rigorous and ambitious experiment.

4th Baron Northbourne Walter James (1896–1982) Coined the Term "Organic"

Lord Northbourne was an early admirer of Rudolf Steiner's biodynamic approach to agriculture. He began to apply Steiner's principles at his family's estate in Kent and in 1939 traveled to Switzerland to consult with Dr. Ehrenfried Pfeiffer, one of the world's leading authorities on biodynamic agriculture. On Northbourne's return to England, he organized and hosted the first U.K. conference on biodynamic farming methods.

In 1940, Northbourne published a book titled *Look to the Land* that is credited with introducing the term "organic farming" to the world. His choice of the word "organic" was not simply descriptive.

Through his own studies and experiences, Northbourne came to profoundly appreciate the fact that a farm wasn't just a place for things to grow—it was, in fact, a complex, living organism, as complete and integral a life form as a human being. This way of viewing living processes as not only related but also fundamentally inseparable is, of course, the very basis of Steiner's philosophy. But, as it turns out, it's also consistent with the most recent discoveries in ecological science.

For example, complex populations of bacteria work in the soil to fix nutrients and structure into the chemical compounds that allow plants and animals to best absorb and utilize them. In our own bodies, similar populations of bacteria and other microbes are not only important; they're nothing short of essential to our digestion and assimilation of nutrients and also constitute a critical part of our immune systems. Scientists are beginning to fully appreciate the pivotal role played by the human microbiome, the collection of the trillions of microbes that live in our bodies and serve essential functions. We now understand that the collective genetic contributions of these microbial communities are parallel to those managed by the extensive system of human DNA at work in our cells.

Northbourne may have been referring to the need to embrace nature in its wholeness, from our own perceived status at the top of the food chain to the lowliest, most elementary of life forms when he wrote:

"If we are to succeed in the great task before us, we must adopt a humbler attitude towards the elementary things of life than that which is implied in our frequent boasting about our so-called 'Conquest of Nature.' We have put ourselves on a pinnacle in the pride of an imagined conquest. But we cannot separate ourselves from nature if we would... There can be no quarrel between ourselves and nature any more than there can be a quarrel between a man's head and his feet."

Dr. James Lovelock later expanded Northbourne's concept of the farm as an integral, living organism. While working with NASA in the 1960s, Lovelock proposed the gaia hypothesis. Lovelock suggested that the entire earth is best understood as a single living organism. The similar notions championed by Steiner, Northbourne, and Lovelock aren't just interesting academic philosophies. They have powerful and practical applications to questions regarding atmospheric and oceanic science; global weather patterns, including anticipating and coping with pressures on the world food supply from droughts and famine; addressing the damaging impact of industrial toxins and pollutants, including radioactive wastes and, of course, enormous implications for the health and sustainability of farmlands and waterways.

Northbourne's deep insights, expressed in *Look to the Land*, brilliantly anticipated the importance of our current awareness of systems biology—the notion that in nature, nothing ever takes place in isolation.

J. I. Rodale (1898–1971)—The Great Organic Promoter

Jerome Irving Rodale (born Jerome Irving Cohen) was another vociferous proponent of the organic movement whose efforts were originally inspired by Albert Howard. In many ways, Rodale (pronounced with an emphasis on the last syllable rather than the first, as it's usually spoken) arguably became the greatest single promoter and popularizer of organic farming. His influence on the acceptance of organic agriculture and the value of consuming organic foods as part of a healthy lifestyle—especially in the United States—can hardly be overstated. In many ways, while Steiner made organic farming possible and Howard made it inevitable, Rodale made it personal. His message of "better living through nature" reached millions of people and opened the door to the eventual mainstreaming of the organic movement.

In response to his own weak and sickly childhood, Rodale became intensely interested in a broad range of choices that support a healthy life, embracing exercise, herbal therapy, and even traditional folk remedies. When exposed to Howard's book *An Agricultural Testament*, Rodale became an enthusiastic supporter. And while Howard's ideas found a strong and dedicated following in Europe, at the time Rodale first encountered them, they had made precious little impact in the United States.

Following Howard's ideas about the importance of holistic agriculture and the inevitable association between agricultural health and human health, Rodale in 1940 established an experimental organic farm in Emmaus, Pennsylvania. In 1942, he began publishing *Organic Gardening* magazine—originally under the title *Organic Farming and Gardening*. Recognizing his unique role in inspiring the effort, Rodale even reached out to Howard, who acted as associate editor for the magazine's launch. To this day, *Organic Gardening* remains the most widely read information source for the natural food movement worldwide. At its peak, the magazine had a print circulation in excess of 1,250,000. Today, with the rise of web-based information access, print circulation has diminished to about 275,000 while the online version of *Organic Gardening* has been visited by nearly 650,000 unique users worldwide.

Rodale was also interested in how a healthy lifestyle could help to prevent illness, rather than having to cure problems after they arise. In 1950, Rodale Press began to publish *Prevention* magazine, which also continues to be widely read.

Unlike Steiner, Howard, and Northbourne—great agricultural innovators whose ideas shaped the movement—Rodale did not pioneer organic agricultural techniques. Instead, he served as an exceedingly effective communicator, educator, advocate, and popularizer who brought the organic food and farming movement to the world at large.

Rachael Carson (1907–1964) and *The Silent Spring* (1962)

While Rodale and the great agricultural innovators in whose footsteps he followed were busy sharing their ideas and implementing the practical applications of organic and holistic agriculture, other voices started to sound the alarm about the dangers of man-made agricultural chemicals. As evidence mounted, scientists began to educate the general public about the hidden interconnections between living things and the ways in which damaging, man-made pollutants could enter the food chain.

Up to this point, the negative aspects of artificial nitrogen-rich fertilizers and chemical pesticides had been expressed primarily in terms of their harmful impact on the integrity of farm soil and its ultimate impact on the vitality of the foods grown in that soil. But by the 1950s and early 1960s, a wide range of toxic effects on wildlife and human health started to become evident. Until then, the "better living through chemistry" ethos of the early twentieth century continued to prevail, and few yet had reason to question it.

The first truly influential advocate decrying the human dangers of man-made chemicals was an eloquent, soft-spoken marine biologist named Rachael Carson. Her 1962 book, *The Silent Spring*, awakened a global environmental movement to the misguided use of chemicals and the dangers of synthetic pesticides. Carson was shocked to discover the indiscriminate destructive power of pesticides like DDT, lindane, and chlordane, which, along with other long-lived "persistent organic pollutants" (also known as "POPs") were finally banned in 2004 by the 151 signatory nations of the Stockholm Convention of 2001. (178 parties, plus all the nations of the European Union now participate in the ban.) In fact, Carson was inspired to write *The Silent Spring* after a friend shared with her how each year, following the spraying of the woods outside her home with DDT, she would find her property littered with the bodies of dead birds.

Carson proposed that instead of thinking of these toxic chemicals as pesticides, carefully targeted to kill crop-damaging insects and vermin, they be thought of instead as "biocides" because their effects were never just limited to the pests they were intended to kill. She brought to light how even extremely small amounts of these chemicals—perhaps harmless on their own—could gradually accumulate in the tissues of animals, including humans, and eventually reach significant levels of toxicity.

She was a particularly effective environmental advocate in part because her writing was eloquent, speaking powerfully about the dangers of a world polluted by toxic, artificial chemicals. This passage from *The Silent Spring* is an example of the evocative writing that inspired the organic movement and served as a kind of manifesto for environmental activists:

"As crude a weapon as the cave man's club, the chemical barrage has been hurled against the fabric of life—a fabric on the one hand delicate and destructible, on the other miraculously tough and resilient, and capable of striking back in unexpected ways. These extraordinary capacities of life have been ignored by the practitioners of chemical control who have brought to their task no 'high-minded orientation,' no humility before the vast forces with which they tamper."

Today, every consumer who chooses organic food options to limit his or her body's exposure to pesticides and other toxic chemicals, or expresses concern that we might not know enough yet to be sure that supposedly harmless genetic modifications are, in fact, harmless, owes a debt to Carson for sounding the alarm. In a world where banned toxins long ago trapped in Arctic ice and are now, with rising global temperatures, flooding the world's oceans, more than half a century later Carson's message is more urgent and as relevant than ever.

Organic Food Marketing—A Long and Winding Path to the Mainstream (1869–present)

Long before the emergence of biodynamic agriculture and the organic food movement, a broader "health food" movement was already in place. Some of the advocates of those early days of the movement remain household names today. Dr. John Harvey Kellogg, of Kellogg's breakfast cereal fame, invented his trademark whole grain breakfast flakes as part of the rigorous regime of healthy vegetarian eating and physical exercise he promoted at his sanitarium in Battle Creek, Michigan. Reverend

Sylvester Graham, an American dietician, lent his name to the graham cracker, originally an unsweetened biscuit made with graham flour, a special mix of unbleached wheat flour with added bran and germ. And to this day, the iconoclastic American health food advocate Paul Bragg's name remains on the shelves of virtually every health food store on the labels of Bragg's liquid amino acids and apple cider vinegar. In addition to numerous books and lectures, Bragg coached several Olympic athletes. Television health and exercise guru Jack LaLanne credited Bragg for much of his health and success, saying:

> "...Bragg saved my life at age 15 when I attended the Bragg Crusade in Oakland, California."

Kellogg, Graham, and Bragg are just three of the colorful and often larger-than-life characters of the days before the official birth of the organic movement early in the twentieth century.

The first health food store on record is the Thomas Martindale Company, opened in 1869 in Philadelphia's Old City quarter. The store is still in operation today, not far from its original location, and is now known as Martindale's Natural Market. Martindale's, and others like it, were spurred on by the early natural health and whole foods pioneers.

Until the 1970s, however, organic and natural foods were primarily local bulk offerings found at small produce markets and other specialty shops. At that point, there were few, if any, of the standardized, branded, and packaged organic food products we know today.

Against the backdrop of the increasing awareness of the benefits of a more natural lifestyle, the potential dangers of pesticides and other industrial toxins, and the broad counterculture trends of the 1960 and 1970s unfolding in the U.S. and around the world, the explosive growth of the health food market may have been driven at least in part by an act of congress.

The Proxmire Vitamin Bill of 1976 blocked an effort by the U.S. Food and Drug Administration (FDA) to control the production and sale of vitamins and other health supplements, attempting to relegate them to the status of drugs. With passage of the Proxmire bill, however, an open, highly lucrative market for vitamins and other supplements helped to push the health food store from the fringes of commerce toward the mainstream. In time, the proliferation of neighborhood health food stores inspired the next logical business move: the rise of the natural food supermarket.

With 387 stores (as of July 2014) in the United States, Canada, and the U.K. Whole Foods Markets dominate the health food supermarket sphere, with 2013 gross revenues approaching $13 billion. Structured like a modern supermarket, the typical Whole Foods store combines everyday groceries; conventional and organic produce;

environmentally sensitive household products; fresh baked items; conventional, organic, and sustainable meats and fish; a salad bar; and a deli serving sandwiches, salads, and specialty foods.

Unlike most neighborhood organic co-ops, community-sponsored agriculture (CSAs), and some farmers markets and "mom and pop" health food stores, Whole Foods is very much a profit-driven business. While the stores carry many organic offerings, from produce to packaged and branded sauces, pasta, cookies, and a plethora of other foods, the stores also, in the words of Whole Foods CEO John Mackey, "...sell a bunch of junk."

Mackey further observed that the sale of healthy bulk items including grains, seeds, nuts, and beans now accounts for only about 1% of total revenues, down from as much as 20% in the halcyon days when Whole Foods Markets functioned more as purveyors of genuinely healthy goods and less like a specialty food boutique.

In the same sense that many products identified and labeled as "natural foods" are not necessarily organic or even particularly healthful, Whole Foods Markets as well as other smaller or regional operations continue to market the promise of the organic lifestyle, but in fact have become more like conventional supermarkets, most of which now stock organic and environmentally sensitive food products.

Why Go Organic?

The early history of the biodynamic and organic movement is populated by a cast of colorful characters of remarkable insight, ingenuity, and persistence. The concepts and practices they pioneered gave birth to the modern environmental and organic food movements.

The reasons for "going organic" are the same today as they were a century ago:

- To minimize our personal exposure to toxic chemicals introduced into the food supply by industrial agriculture.
- To consume foods grown in clean, vital soil to promote our own optimal health and wellness.
- To support the sustainable and ecologically balanced management of farmlands and waterways.
- To protect our shared air, water, and land resources from the damaging runoff of agricultural chemicals.
- To encourage the just and ethical treatment of agricultural workers and the development of their communities, domestically and around the world.
- To support the humane treatment of farm animals and livestock.
- To be an informed consumer, demanding the information required to make conscious choices and tradeoffs regarding the products we purchase.

- To affirm our understanding of the complex and often subtle relationships between our human needs and desires; the earth's critical biosphere; and the plants, animals, fish, microbes, and other living things that dwell on our planet.

Any one of these is sufficient justification to prefer organic and sustainable alternatives when they're available and to seek expanded access to and availability of these alternatives in the marketplace.

Today, organic foods, fabrics, herbs, cosmetics, wine, and other products can be readily found, often in mainstream markets. In the United States, organic foods represent the fastest growing sector of the food industry, with United States sales nearly tripling between 2011 and 2013 (see the accompanying chart, below, from the U.S. Department of Agriculture).

It's often said that consumers vote with their pocketbooks. Year after year, consumers seem to be voting in support of an ever-larger role for organic products.

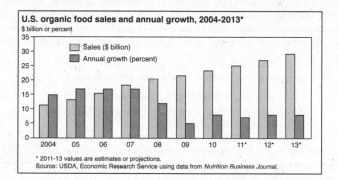

U.S. organic food sales and annual growth, 2004-2013*
$ billion or percent

* 2011-13 values are estimates or projections.
Source: USDA, Economic Research Service using data from *Nutrition Business Journal.*

Organic Food Certification and Eco-Labeling

It would be helpful if consumers could count on all organic foods being held to the same high standards. But, as is often the case, consumers, corporations, scientists, government agencies, and advocacy groups all have different and often conflicting perspectives. This has led to any number of labeling controversies and, ultimately, to the creation of different types of organic certifications and even other types of eco-labeling such as "Fair Trade Certified."

Furthermore, the rules for organic labeling vary by location. Specific practices can differ between countries or between states, provinces, or other jurisdictions within a country. If a product contains some ingredients that have been organically produced and others produced by conventional methods, there are rules governing the claims that can be made for the product as a whole and specifying how the individual ingredients may be described.

When you're shopping for the natural or organic foods you want to include in your diet, it makes sense to understand your options so that you can make informed decisions about which foods are best for you.

Do you want to try to buy only 100% certified organic foods, or are you willing to accept foods that can be legally labeled as organic but may include up to 5% of ingredients produced by conventional methods and that also may contain genetically modified organisms, known as GMOs? What are your personal tradeoffs between products that are locally sourced versus sustainably produced? Are you interested in Fair Trade Certified products or other types of certification?

Knowing your options and understanding exactly what each of the many labels means allows you to balance your concerns about issues including nutritional value, local sourcing, relative cost, and a host of social and environmental factors. Understanding these different options enables you to take charge of the quality of the food you and your family consume. It also enables you to make choices and use your purchasing power that support and reflect the social, economic, and ecological values you hold.

The USDA recognizes three distinct, legally defined levels of organic certification and an additional designation for farms aiming to gain certification:

- 100% Organic—This certification is reserved for foods that are made completely from certified organic ingredients. They are also certified to be free of GMOs.
- Organic—The term "organic" can be applied to foods that contain at least 95% certified organic ingredients. Unlike 100% organic products, the non-organic portion of these products is allowed to contain GMOs.
- Made with Organic Ingredients—This term can be used for products containing at least 70% certified organic ingredients.
- Transitional—This is a designation reserved for farms on the path to organic certification but that have recently been used for conventional agriculture. During the transitional period, producers must adhere to all organic standards for a period of time, often two to three years, and demonstrate that both the land and production practices satisfy organic requirements before they can be certified as organic.

Only organic and 100% organic products are allowed to display the USDA organic seal. Food products listed as "made with organic ingredients" may not use the seal. In addition, products that contain less than 70% certified organic ingredients may display that individual components are organic, but may not describe the overall product with any of the three organic designations or display the official seal.

Other eco-labels such as "sustainably produced," "free-range," "hormone-free," and "locally sourced" impart some additional information that may be desirable for some consumers, but by themselves do not certify or even suggest that the food products meet organic standards. Of course, some of these products may also carry an organic designation.

The National Organic Program

In the United States, the National Organic Program (NOP) regulates all organic crops, livestock, and agricultural products certified to USDA organic standards. Organic certification agencies inspect and verify that all stakeholders—organic farmers, ranchers, distributors, processors, and traders—comply with the USDA organic regulations. The USDA also acts globally, auditing organic certification agencies operating outside the United States to ensure that they are accurately certifying organic products.

The National List

The NOP compiles a National List of Allowed and Prohibited Substances that identifies substances that may and may not be used in organic crop and livestock production. It also lists the substances that may be used in or on processed and multi-ingredient organic products. Although the National List prohibits the use of most synthetic substances, there are exceptions such as a synthetic vaccine to prevent eye infections in livestock that are allowed. Similarly, the National List permits the use of most naturally occurring substances but prohibits some such as arsenic, which is a natural but toxic substance. The National List also names substances that are restricted for use in specific situations—for selected crops or in limited amounts.

The National Organic Standards Board

The National Organic Standards Board (NOSB) is a federal advisory committee composed of four farmers/growers, three environmentalists/resource conservationists, three consumer/public interest advocates, two handlers/processors, one retailer, one scientist (toxicology, ecology, or biochemistry), and one USDA-accredited certifying agent appointed by the Secretary of Agriculture. The NOSB advises the USDA about the substances that should be permitted or prohibited in organic farming and processing. The NOSB also makes recommendations about a variety of issues related to organic agriculture and certification, such as organic pet food standards and organic inspector qualifications. Recommendations made by the NOSB do not become official policy until they are approved and adopted by the USDA.

Companions to the Organic Movement

Organic food production embodies at least two different, complementary values. Consumers drawn to organic foods recognize that they offer health benefits compared to conventionally produced foods. Organically produced foods are free of man-made pesticides, fertilizers, and other alterations such as genetically modified organisms (GMOs). Some research suggests that organic foods also may contain critical nutrients in larger quantities or in more bioavailable forms than their conventional counterparts.

The second benefit of choosing organic food is less tangible but no less important because it signifies personal and social values. Opting for organically grown and produced foods reflects sensitivity to the holistic relationship between the foods we eat and the living earth that supports their growth.

These same social and ethical values can manifest in other ways. For example, in parallel with the organic food movement there is an increasing social awareness of the importance of sustainability—creating foods and other products in ways that protect the ability of the land and the sea to continue supporting us into the future. There is also an increasing social awareness about ethical issues concerning how foods and other products are made, such as the economic viability of small farms; treatment of workers, especially in developing economies; and larger environmental concerns, including the importance of sustainability and biodiversity.

While these issues are distinct from the regulations governing organic certification, they are very much a part of the larger movement that brought the desirability of organic food into a broad awareness within our culture. These other movements are only indirectly related to organic certification, but they often overlap. Today, it's not unusual to see a bag of roasted coffee beans that is both organically and sustainably produced that also bears an additional mark such as Fair Trade or Rainforest Alliance certification.

Sustainability

The sustainability movement arose in response to the fact that many conventional approaches to the production and utilization of goods take more from the land and the sea than they return. Concerns about sustainability apply to many types of food products and to fields as varied as lumber production and energy conservation as well. Conventional, nonsustainable practices may be financially profitable in the short run, but over time pose a serious risk of depleting irreplaceable natural resources.

For example, scientists have long warned that large-scale, high-tech commercial fishing is, in effect, "strip mining" the world's oceans. Removing fish from the sea faster than they can be replenished through their natural rates of reproduction may seem a distant and invisible concern, but this depletion is already threatening an important part of the world's food supply. Vulnerable populations in less economically developed economies have already been critically affected. Even in the United States, many small and often family-owned fishing operations that operate closer to shore are finding traditional fishing grounds so barren that they are no longer economically viable.

If fish were trees, the oceans would look like forests stripped nearly bare.

While sustainability marks don't carry the force of government regulation, they are associated with voluntary standards and requirements. For example, the Marine Stewardship Council (MSC) publishes a set of guidelines for the sustainable production of seafood. Fisheries that are independently certified to comply with these guidelines are granted the right to use the phrase "Certified Sustainable Seafood" and the MSC logo.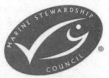

Purchasing sustainably grown organic food is an endorsement of wise stewardship of the land and affirms the relationship between the health of soil, animals, and crops, and the people who consume the foods from them.

Fair Trade Certification

Fair Trade Certified products must meet specific requirements for environmental stewardship, working conditions and labor practices, and fair economic policies. The Fair Trade certification applies to a wide and expanding set of food products including bananas, oranges, and other fresh and dried fruits, vegetables, and juices; cocoa, coffee, and tea; crops including rice, quinoa, sugar, and spices; nuts and seeds and their oils; and wine.

The Fair Trade system was originally developed in the late 1980s with the intention of economically empowering smaller producers of crops like coffee beans so that more of the economic benefit of their work could remain local, helping their economies to develop. Since that time, the Fair Trade mark has been extended to include larger producers—for example, tea plantations—while continuing to enforce safe and sustainable practices and improved worker rights.

Fair Trade products may or may not also be organically produced, but they do represent a confluence of ecological, social, economic, and human values that many drawn to the organic movement find appealing.

Rainforest Alliance Certification

The Rainforest Alliance, also founded in the late 1980s, and the Fair Trade system share similar missions and goals, but they differ in focus and strategy. Rather than emphasizing how products are traded, Rainforest Alliance certification offers a holistic approach to sustainable agriculture, focusing equally on the three pillars of sustainability—social, economic, and environmental.

The Rainforest Alliance is teaching farmers to farm efficiently and responsibly, growing their bottom line today and conserving the fertile soils and natural resources on which they and their children will depend in the future. Farmers are empowered with the knowledge and skills to negotiate for themselves in the global marketplace. Over 100 crops, as well as livestock, can be certified. The Rainforest Alliance Certified™ seal on products promotes environmental responsibility, social equity, and economic viability for farm communities.

Local Sourcing and the Farm-to-Table Movement

For most of human history a person's diet was made up almost exclusively of locally grown foods. Rare exceptions included the salt and exotic spices needed to help preserve and flavor foods in the days before refrigerators and freezers. For thousands of years, many of the world's most dramatic explorations were driven by the search for more direct and economical routes for importing spices, silk, and other desirable commodities from distant, often exotic lands.

With the advent of modern transportation, particularly refrigerated shipping by sea and air, the movement of food products over large distances became technologically and economically feasible. Previously unthinkable realities—like serving ripe tomatoes and pineapples in the dead of winter—became commonplace.

The traditional cycle of harvesting a bounty of fresh foods during the summer and autumn months and "putting them up" with home canning and tucking them away in root cellars for the colder months gave way to a new world of globally distributed agriculture. Today's consumers expect fresh fruits and vegetables to be available year-round since they're always in season somewhere in the world.

But in recent years, the hidden costs of the new global system became more apparent. With the atmospheric buildup of heat-trapping greenhouse gases—largely through the use of fossil fuels for transportation and power generation—it's become increasingly important to consider the "carbon footprint" of the products we consume.

The complete cost, in both dollars and environmental impact, of growing a tomato locally and bringing it to the consumer's kitchen is much lower than growing that tomato in South America and having to transport it. Environmental activists have long argued that the actual cost of transporting that tomato—or that pineapple or that case of Scandinavian mountain spring water—isn't actually factored into the price charged to the consumer. The direct and indirect costs of the cumulative environmental damage of greenhouse gas pollution and other toxic effects of transporting those products over long distances is a bill that will come due in the future, when we are forced to deal with the repercussions of human-induced climate change.

This is one of the most powerful motivations for those who support a shift back to consuming a larger proportion of locally produced and sourced foods. Locally sourced foods are featured prominently at farmers markets. Produce and meat sections in some grocery stores—sometimes including larger chain stores—are now touting locally sourced foods. Some orchards, ranches, and farms have made a strong move to be recognized not only as valuable contributors to the local economy but also as artisanal brands, whether organically certified or not, that promise better taste and freshness.

Many savvy chefs have learned the benefits of developing close working relationships with local farmers and ranchers. These "farm-to-table" relationships offer them access to the freshest seasonal ingredients. In many cases, farmers will grow specific varieties or unusual ingredients requested by the chef. These close working relationships also offer a deeper sense of accountability for the integrity of the foods produced, since the supplier gets direct feedback from their customer—the chef—and the customer's customers—the dining public.

The farm-to-table movement also includes the direct-to-consumer delivery of freshly grown fruits and vegetables, sometimes on a weekly or monthly subscription basis.

Wildcrafted Foods

Wildcrafting is the practice of harvesting things directly from their natural environment, collecting them in their raw, uncultivated state.

Wildcrafting usually refers to herbs, roots, and mushrooms, but can also apply to lichens, moss, and even in some cases fruits, vegetables, grains, and grasses. Wildcrafted products are often used in herbal teas, tinctures, and other herbal and medicinal preparations.

Depending on your perspective, wildcrafted products are either not organic at all—since they weren't cultivated according to the rules and regulations of organic agriculture—or they're the most organic products you can find, even if no government agency or trade organization would certify them as such.

Whatever their legal status, unless the wildcrafted product grew in a contaminated environment, it's likely to be at least as biologically complex and nutrient-dense as its best organically raised counterpart. The natural environment is far more rich and varied than any agricultural setting. Undisturbed natural soil contains an extensive spectrum of factors derived from the long-term ecological associations between compatible species ranging from invisible bacteria and indigenous insects to mushroom mycelia and to the gut bacteria of scavengers who may have eaten a parent plant and excreted a seed embedded in natural fertilizer.

Wildcrafting gathers together the unmolested products of nature, fully embodying the richness that organic agriculture practices do their best to approximate.

Other Certified Food Labels

Certified Naturally Grown

Certified Naturally Grown is a label that indicates that the food was grown in accordance with USDA organic standards but that it was grown on a farm that was not certified organic by the USDA. Certified Naturally Grown (CNG) is a nonprofit organization that independently certifies small, direct-market farmers and beekeepers that use natural methods. Like organic farmers, CNG producers do not use synthetic fertilizers, pesticides, herbicides, fungicides, antibiotics, hormones, or genetically modified seeds.

Certified Humane®

Certified Humane farm animals are reared with humane and grateful animal husbandry—sufficient space to pasture, clean and sanitary shelter, and fresh water. The feed contains no added hormones or antibiotics. Meat, poultry, egg, and dairy products may bear this label.

Food Alliance Certified

Growing from a joint project of Oregon State University, Washington State University, and the Washington State Department of Agriculture, Food Alliance is a voluntary, third-party certification granted to farms that meet specific standards of sustainable agricultural practices. Food Alliance certification has been shown to lead to better conditions for farm workers, more humane treatment of animals, decreased use of pesticides, more naturally vital soil, cleaner water, and enhanced wildlife habitats.

Non-GMO Project Verified

The Non-GMO Project is a nonprofit organization that verifies that food products are grown and processed without using genetic engineering. The Project also works with food manufacturers, distributors, growers, and seed suppliers to reduce cross-pollination or contamination risk of the non-GMO food supply with GMOs.

SCS Third-Party Certification

SCS Global Services is a third-party organization that performs independent testing and certification of foods and other products and services including validation of sustainable agriculture and forestry, carbon neutrality, responsible sourcing, and green construction materials and practices.

Their certification labels feature the company's kingfisher graphic surrounded by information specific to the certification. For example, SCS food labels include "certified organic," "certified pesticide residue free," and "certified antioxidant superfood."

All Organic Food is Natural, But Not All Natural Food Is Organic

Food producers often describe their products as "natural" or even "all natural." These terms have become buzzwords in the marketplace, but what do they mean?

Unlike organic certification, the terms "natural" or even "all natural" have no legally accepted definitions, and there are no mechanisms to regulate so-called natural food products. The term "all natural" should mean that the food does not contain artificial or synthetic ingredients, but with the exception of USDA-certified poultry and meat, there is no organization to evaluate manufacturers' claims that foods are all natural, nor is there any sort of certification. While these terms are meant to imply that foods and their ingredients are minimally processed and are therefore "closer to nature," some producers have abused the terms to the point where they are essentially meaningless.

The Food and Agriculture Organization of the United Nations does not recognize these terms in its *Codex Alimentarius*, the official "big book" of international food standards. Similarly, in the United States, the Food and Drug Administration (FDA) neither regulates nor discourages labeling products as "natural," except in cases when label claims are demonstrably false or misleading.

In a press release from March 7, 2013, Ronnie Cummins, National Director of the Organic Consumer Association, addressed the question of misleading labeling head-on:

> *"Routine mislabeling and marketing has confused millions of U.S. consumers, and enabled the so-called 'natural' foods and products sector to grow into a $60*

billion dollar a year powerhouse, garnering twice as many sales in 2012 as certified organic products."

The bottom line is that the term "natural food" is largely a marketing phrase. It expresses an appealing sentiment, but on its own it doesn't really tell you anything useful about the food product itself.

Non-Certified Food Labels

The following labels are not verified or enforced by any agency or organization. The extent to which the label claims are true depends on how closely individual farmers and producers adhere to the various standards.

Bear in mind that just because a food label makes a health or nutrition claim, it does not mean that a food is healthy and the best choice for your particular needs. You should always look at the nutrition facts and balance the claim based on the nutrition information and ingredients. A food may claim to be natural but may include ingredients you wish to avoid. Or it may say "naturally sweetened" but still contain more sugar, corn syrup, or other sweeteners than you want.

Non-GMO

One of the biggest problems with food labeling is what the labels don't tell you. For example, you won't find "Contains genetically modified organisms (GMOs)" or "genetically engineered (GE) product" on food labels, but you can find out if some of your supermarket staples contain GMOs or are genetically engineered. Here's how: look at the price lookup code (PLU) on the label affixed to produce. A four-digit code tells you the produce was grown conventionally and a five-digit code that begins with the number nine means it was grown organically. A five-digit code that begins with the number eight means the produce was genetically modified.

Many companies label their food products as GMO-Free or Non-GMO to inform consumers. Because individual companies and organizations create these labels, there is no standardization or regulation. As a result, companies vary in terms of the amount of GMOs permissible in their products from 100% GMO-Free to small amounts of GMOs allowed in products.

Hormone-Free/rBGH-Free

This label indicates that cows have not been given any artificial growth hormones, like rBGH, a genetically engineered growth hormone used to increase milk production.

Raised Without Antibiotics

This label indicated that animals were not given antibiotics, which means that the meat and dairy products derived from them do not contain antibiotics. Antibiotics are routinely added to the animal feed or drinking water of cattle, hogs, poultry, and other food-producing animals for growth enhancement—to help animals gain weight faster or use less food to gain weight.

In December 2013, the FDA issued a voluntary guidance document asking animal pharmaceutical companies to voluntarily remove growth enhancement and feed efficiency as approved indications for the use of antibiotics, and no longer make them available for over-the-counter sale. The FDA intends that antibiotics only be given to food-producing animals to treat, prevent, or control disease by prescription from a veterinarian.

100% Natural

Some labels sound good but are actually not meaningful at all. For example, the term "natural" or even "all natural" or "100% natural" may mean that a food product does not contain any artificial colors, artificial flavors, preservatives, or other artificial ingredients, but because there is no universally accepted standard or definition, it is often used to describe food products that are anything but natural. Similarly, "local," "fresh," and "green" are also poorly defined and unregulated terms, which means they can be applied to almost any product to imply that it is pure or natural.

Made with Whole Grains

Other largely unregulated labeling terms that may be misleading are "made with whole grains" and "contains whole grains"—neither of these terms ensures that the food contains any particular proportion of whole grains or even more whole grains than refined grains. The Whole Grains Council produces a set of "stamps" that tell consumers how much whole grain is contained within a single serving of a given food product and whether that product contains 100% whole grain or contains a smaller portion of added bran and germ.

Free-Range

The term "free-range," which means the animals were not confined to cages, may be misleading when it is applied to beef, pork, or dairy products since the USDA only certifies free-range poultry and eggs. Even the USDA free-range certification does not tell you whether, for example, cage-free chickens were confined to a small space or if they were only able to roam free for limited periods of time.

Cage-Free

Cage-free animals are raised with freedom to roam outside and are not confined to cages. This implies more freedom than animals that are raised free-range. This term is also frequently applied to eggs from chickens raised in cage-free environments.

Genetically Modified Foods

Many large agricultural companies genetically modify some of their crops or use genetically modified ingredients to process or produce food products. Crops and foods produced this way are often referred to as genetically modified organisms, or GMOs.

Genetically modified (GM) or genetically engineered (GE) crops contain one or more genes that have been artificially inserted instead of naturally introduced via pollination or hybridization. The inserted gene or gene sequence may be an existing plant gene, or it may come from another unrelated plant, or even from a completely different species. This type of genetic engineering—inserting a foreign gene into an organism's genome—is called transgenics.

This graphic, created by the U.S. FDA, illustrates the difference between the natural acquisition of a gene through traditional plant breeding techniques and the genetic engineering that produces a transgenic variety.

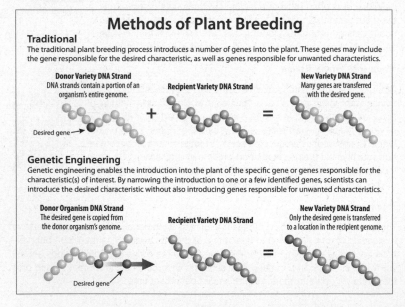

Methods of Plant Breeding

Traditional
The traditional plant breeding process introduces a number of genes into the plant. These genes may include the gene responsible for the desired characteristic, as well as genes responsible for unwanted characteristics.

Donor Variety DNA Strand
DNA strands contain a portion of an organism's entire genome.

Desired gene →

+

Recipient Variety DNA Strand

=

New Variety DNA Strand
Many genes are transferred with the desired gene.

Genetic Engineering
Genetic engineering enables the introduction into the plant of the specific gene or genes responsible for the characteristic(s) of interest. By narrowing the introduction to one or a few identified genes, scientists can introduce the desired characteristic without also introducing genes responsible for unwanted characteristics.

Donor Organism DNA Strand
The desired gene is copied from the donor organism's genome.

Desired gene →

Recipient Variety DNA Strand

=

New Variety DNA Strand
Only the desired gene is transferred to a location in the recipient genome.

Crops or plants may be genetically modified to increase their yield using the same amount of farmland, improve their quality, or enhance their resistance to pests or disease as well as their tolerance for heat, cold, or drought. Examples of transgenic crops are Bt-corn, which contains a gene from a bacterium and produces its own insecticide, and Macintosh apples, which has a gene from a moth that confers resistance to fire blight, one of the most destructive contagious diseases that can affect apple and pear trees.

Even though all crops have been genetically modified from their original wild state by domestication, selection, and controlled breeding over long periods of time, the terms transgenic crops, GM or GE crops, and biotech crops usually refer to plants with transgenes.

Along with self-generating insecticide, some of the traits that have been introduced into food crops using transgenics are enhanced flavor, slowed ripening, reduced reliance on fertilizer, and added nutrients. Examples of transgenic food crops include frost-resistant strawberries and tomatoes; slow-ripening bananas, melons, and pineapples; and insect-resistant and herbicide-tolerant corn, cotton, and soybeans. Some cooking oils, including canola oil and rapeseed oil, also have been genetically modified to reduce their bitterness and increase their resistance to herbicides. Before they were genetically modified, these oils were too bitter to be used in foods.

In the United States, nearly half of all cropland is used to grow GMOs. In terms of quantity, the largest GMO crops are alfalfa, canola, corn, cotton, papaya, soybeans, sugar beets, yellow squash, and zucchini. More than 90% of all corn, cotton, canola, sugar beets, and soybeans in the United States are grown from GE seeds.

Much of the supply of animal feed also contains GM foods. GM soybeans, corn, rapeseed oil, and food additives are commonly used in animal feed. GM-enhanced animal feed is widely used because it is cheaper than feed that does not contain GMOs.

Proponents of GM crops such as the International Service for the Acquisition of Agribiotech Applications (ISAAA), a nonprofit organization that delivers new agricultural biotechnologies to developing countries, assert that genetic modification of crops does not pose health or safety risks and offers a viable way to feed the world's growing population. The ISAAA attributes farmers' widespread adoption of GM crops to the fact that the GM crops enable farmers to save time and realize economic benefits.

The ISAAA also points to the environmental benefits of GM crops: they reduce the environmental footprint of agriculture by significantly reducing the use of pesticides, diminish carbon dioxide emissions by reducing or even eliminating plowing, and increase the efficient use of water and soil. They require less harmful chemicals to support their growth, which helps to prevent soil erosion and water contamination and reduces farmers' exposure to herbicides and pesticides. By reducing carbon dioxide emissions and pesticide use, GM crops decrease greenhouse gases and mitigate climate change.

Other advocates of GM crops point to their economic benefit in developing countries and areas where growing conditions are not ideal. They observe that crops may be modified to thrive in harsh climates or soil lacking adequate nutrients.

Despite the considerable economic advantages of GM crops, in many quarters GMOs are controversial. The controversy centers on the long-term effects of altering crop genetics. Because there has only been limited research to assess the potential harm of GMOs on human health and the environment, there is mounting concern that should GMOs pose a risk to human or ecological health, there will be no way to contain them since wind and wildlife carry seeds to other farmlands, cross-contaminating other non-GM crops.

Opposition to GM crops takes several forms. Some bioethicists contend that freedom of choice is a central tenet of ethical science and oppose what they consider to be unnatural interference with other forms of life. They also question whether there may be a conflict of interest between the companies that have invested in GM technology and anticipate profiting from it and the application of this technology to solving food shortage problems in developing countries.

Environmentalists argue that transgenic technology poses the risk of altering delicately balanced ecosystems and causing unintended harm to other organisms. They fear that transgenic crops will replace traditional crop varieties, especially in developing countries, causing the loss of biological diversity. Among the environmental concerns is the risk that pests may develop resistance to transgenics in much the same way that certain bacteria have become resistant to the antibiotics that once effectively eliminated them.

Opponents cite safety issues, such as unfavorable health consequences—including food allergies and intolerances—resulting from consumption of transgenic foods and products. They also fear that there will be unforeseen and potentially harmful long-term adverse health consequences from the consumption of foods containing foreign genes.

Activists and concerned citizens also observe that while there are no studies demonstrating specific food safety risks associated with consuming foods containing GMOs, it has not yet been established whether particular GMOs have the same nutritional value as their non-GMO counterparts, or if they may produce, as a side effect of their genetic alteration, substances that are harmful to human health.

When it comes to health and safety concerns related to consumption of GMO food, there are many questions about risks, but no conclusive answers. Animal feeding studies suggest that there may be toxic effects associated with GMO foods, and several point to specific health problems resulting from diets of GM foods.

There also are concerns about the environmental impact of GM crops. GM crops may accidentally migrate to other farmlands and even out into the wilderness. Because

GM crops are designed for cultivation in carefully controlled environments, when they are introduced into wild varieties of the same species, they may prompt a cascade of environmental problems. Among the most worrisome is that GM plants may transfer genes to natural, non-GM plants. The possibility exists that transgenic crops will infiltrate beyond their intended areas and inadvertently transfer genes to species not targeted for transgenics.

Should GMO Foods Be Labeled?

To find out how much protein or how many calories the food product you are purchasing contains, you can refer to the information on the label. You can also determine whether the food contains trans-fats, high-fructose corn syrup, or gluten. But the label will not tell you if the food is a GMO or contains GMO ingredients.

In the United States there is only one reliable way to ensure that foods do not contain GMOs. The USDA guidelines say that GMO foods or foods containing GMO ingredients cannot be labeled 100% organic, so people who wish to avoid consuming GMOs have a way to do so—they can consume only 100% organic foods that bear the USDA Organic seal.

Although choosing USDA-certified organic foods helps consumers avoid GMOs, many interest groups have asked that all foods containing GMOs be clearly labeled as such so that consumers can make informed purchasing decisions. Although the FDA published a draft guidance for labeling foods that have been bioengineered, the guidelines are voluntary; there are no federal standards or official product marks identifying bioengineered foods. In the United States in 2014, only Connecticut, Maine, and Vermont had laws requiring the labeling of GMOs.

More than sixty countries—including members of the European Union, Australia, Brazil, Turkey, South Africa, Russia, and China—require labeling of all GM food. In the United States more than sixty bills have been introduced in twenty-two states to require GE labeling or prohibit the sale of genetically engineered foods.

In recent years, GMO labeling requirements have been on the ballot in several elections. In 2012, California's Proposition 37, which required labeling of all GMO products, was very narrowly defeated. In 2013, the Washington State People's Right to Know Genetically Engineered Food Act also was defeated. In these and other state labeling initiatives, large food companies such as Dupont, Monsanto, Pepsico, Coca-Cola, and Nestlé as well as the Grocery Manufacturers Association (GMA) have effectively lobbied against labeling initiatives and financed aggressive campaigns to thwart GMO labeling legislation. Reportedly, more than $45 million was spent to defeat California's Proposition 37.

Despite GMA lobbying and the massive anti-labeling campaigns underwritten by large food companies, states continue to put GMO labeling on their ballots. These ballot measures reflect public sentiment. Public opinion polls conducted by Consumer

Reports, *The Washington Post*, Reuters/NPR, MSNBC, and *The New York Times* all find that the overwhelming majority of Americans—93% or more—favor labeling GM foods.

Are Organic Foods Better for Your Health?

As we've seen, there are many compelling reasons to choose organic foods over their conventional counterparts. In addition to any possible nutritional benefits, organic foods are produced in an ecologically friendly and environmentally sustainable fashion. Organic foods are also typically produced in a way that values ethical and social concerns, from the humane treatment of animals to the fair and equitable treatment of agricultural workers.

But it's probably safe to say that for most consumers, a key motivation for "going organic" is the desire to eat foods that are less toxic and more nutritious.

So naturally, we have to ask the question, "Are organic foods actually better for your health?"

The Infamous Stanford Study

Many scientific studies have been conducted to attempt to determine whether organic food is more nutritious or healthier than non-organic food. However, the one recent study that has arguably gained the most notoriety was conducted by Stanford University's School of Medicine and published in the September 4, 2013 issue of the *Annals of Internal Medicine*.

The Stanford study made headlines when it announced that there was no "...strong evidence that organic foods are significantly more nutritious than conventional foods."

News outlets including major TV networks, newspapers, health websites, and magazines were quick to trumpet the study's negative message, tearing down the organic movement with a vengeance. Here are just a few examples of the headlines:

- "Organic Food No More Nutritious Than Non-Organic, Study Finds" (MSNBC)
- "Researchers Find That Organic Food Offers Few Extra Health Benefits Other Than Moral Superiority" (jezebel.com)
- "Organic Food Is No Healthier Than Conventional Food" (U.S. News and World Report)
- "Stanford Scientists Cast Doubt on Advantages of Organic Meat and Produce" (The New York Times)
- "Save Your Cash? Organic Food Is Not Healthier: Stanford U." (New York Daily News)

But the media's rush to judgment isn't the whole story. It's important to understand exactly what the Stanford study actually considered, found, and concluded.

First, it's critical to understand that the researchers at Stanford didn't directly analyze any food products. Instead, they conducted what's known as a meta-analysis. The team of researchers compiled, aggregated, and analyzed the results of more than 200 studies that had already been performed. Employing the techniques of meta-analysis to bring together data from many previous studies is a well-known process and in and of itself is not controversial. However, the way the meta-analysis is conducted can have an enormous impact on the conclusions that are reached. It's possible, as we'll see, for two different meta-analyses of the same or similar data to arrive at wildly different conclusions.

Next, in this light, it's essential to review the criteria the study's authors used to analyze the data and draw their conclusions. In the Stanford study, the primary measure used to assess the nutritional value of organic foods was whether the organic foods contained more vitamins and other selected nutrients than comparable, conventionally raised non-organic products. That's fair enough. But which nutrients did they consider, and to what extent did their choices provide a valid basis for comparison?

Mark Bittman, a well known and well respected New York Times columnist and food journalist, assailed the criteria used in the Stanford study. Addressing the question of how the researchers at Stanford judged the relative nutritional value of organics, he observed that by using their criteria, a bowl of Frosted Flakes cereal would be deemed more nutritious than an apple.

Forget the "empty calories," the processed carbohydrates, and the slathering of sugar—because the ultra-sweet cereal had been artificially fortified with synthetic vitamins, it would have scored higher than the apple with its natural, metabolically beneficial fiber and wide spectrum of highly bioavailable nutrients. It's unlikely that any impartial nutritionist, dietician, or other scientific expert in the field of human nutrition would judge a bowl of artificially sweetened cereal as nutritionally superior to a fresh apple—but Bittman's observation is not a bad analogy to the conduct of the Stanford study. It's a pretty good description of how the authors actually compared organic and conventional foods.

Strangely, the study did in fact conclude that organic produce was much lower in pesticides and other toxic chemical residues than conventional produce and in general carried lower levels of potentially disease-causing, antibiotic-resistant bacteria. In fact, the second sentence of the study abstract's two-line conclusion actually states: "Consumption of organic foods may reduce exposures to pesticide residues and antibiotic-resistant bacteria."

Many critics of the Stanford study have, in various ways, asked, "If reducing the body's load of cancer-causing chemicals, crippling nerve toxins, metabolically disruptive hormones, unwanted antibiotic medications, and potentially disease-causing antibiotic resistant bacteria doesn't qualify as 'nutritionally superior,' then what does?"

However, as measured by the study's criteria for evaluating the nutritional value of organic foods, these critical factors were overshadowed by the final judgment, stated in the first sentence of the same two-line conclusion, "The published literature lacks strong evidence that organic foods are significantly more nutritious than conventional foods."

Considering that the elimination of toxic, man-made substances from the diet is the primary motivation for most consumers of organic foods, it seems unfortunate that media opted to focus so exclusively and intensely on the first conclusion so that the second conclusion was completely eclipsed.

The Newcastle Study

But that's not even the whole story. Along with several of her colleagues, Kirsten Brandt, M.D., a senior researcher at Newcastle University's School of Agriculture, Food and Rural Development in the U.K., performed a study posing the exact same question the Stanford team asked: are organically grown and produced foods more nutritious? The conclusions of the Newcastle group's meta-analysis, which was published more than a year before the Stanford report and considered many of the same research studies, were the exact opposite of those reached by the Stanford researchers.

In particular, Brandt's study found that organic produce was, in fact, generally higher in several important classes of nutrients that were not even considered in the Stanford study. Brandt noted that many of the compounds compared in organic and conventional produce in the Stanford study were ones that showed the smallest differences, while other important nutrients that showed a clear advantage for organics were excluded from the analysis.

On closer reading, Brandt also found that the Stanford study failed to make a proper distinction between two related but different classes of nutrients that share a confusingly similar spelling. Brandt's Newcastle study found that organic produce consistently contained higher levels of critically important compounds called flavanols, while the Stanford report erroneously confused flavanols with flavonols. The two are spelled exactly the same way, except for the vowel after the "v".

Flavanols—spelled with an "a" after the "v"—are powerful, highly bioavailable antioxidants with additional beneficial cell protecting abilities. Flavonols—spelled with an "o" after the "v"—also are beneficial, but as a group they generally are poorly absorbed and utilized by the body. Both types of compounds—flavanols and flavonols—belong to a larger family of plant compounds called flavonoids. By failing to distinguish properly between them, the Stanford report downplayed a key health benefit of organic produce that Dr. Brandt's team highlighted.

Why Are Flavanols So Important?

One remarkable example of the importance of flavanols (with an "a") in the diet is provided by Norman Hollenberg, M.D., Ph.D., a professor of medicine at Harvard Medical School. In his research, Hollenberg found that one particular flavanol compound—called *epicatechin*—is so important for human health that he believes it should actually be reclassified as a vitamin.

Vitamins are nutrient compounds that are recognized as indispensable to human health, and by definition, they cannot be manufactured in our own bodies. Part of the definition of a vitamin is that consuming too little of it in our diet must be associated with one or more specific diseases. According to these stringent requirements, there are currently only thirteen families of compounds recognized as vitamins. (By the way, you might be surprised to learn that by this strict, technical definition, vitamin D is actually not a vitamin at all—it's a hormone. But it has a long history of being described and treated as a vitamin in much the same way that a tomato is not actually a vegetable but a fruit.)

Hollenberg's studies clearly demonstrate that adequate levels of epicatechin can considerably reduce the risk of cancer, diabetes, heart failure, and stroke. Since these are four of the five most common killer diseases (the other being chronic obstructive pulmonary disease, or COPD, which is mainly caused by smoking, air pollution, and environmental or occupational exposures), some medical authorities think that Hollenberg makes a pretty good case.

For example, Daniel Fabricant, Ph.D., Executive Director and CEO of the not-for-profit Natural Products Association, agrees with Hollenberg's assessment. He says, "...the link between high epicatechin consumption and a decreased risk of killer disease is so striking, it should be investigated further. It may be that these diseases are the result of epicatechin deficiency."

Flavanols are found in high concentration in natural cocoa products, some teas, and a variety of fruits and vegetables. That the Newcastle research team's meta-analysis found flavanols were significantly increased in organic produce while the Stanford team—operating under different analytical criteria and, in this particular case, with a confusion between flavanols and flavonoids (including flavonols)—did not is both significant and indicative of the different approaches and emphases of the research studies.

Different Studies, Different Conclusions

How could the Stanford study, which has been so widely cited and influential, at the same time be so unbalanced in its treatment of organic foods? How could the study conclude, as news headlines were eager to point out, that organics were in effect no better than conventional foods when the study's own findings stated, at a minimum, that organics were freer from potentially toxic chemicals and antibiotic-resistant bacteria than conventional foods?

First and foremost, the analysis of complex data—like the diverse findings of the 237 separate studies considered in the Stanford review—is not an exact science. The authors chose the criteria used to analyze the data and as such, exerted enormous influence over the conclusions that were reached.

For the Newcastle study, Brandt observed that she and her colleagues considered many of the same studies the Stanford authors reviewed. The dissimilarity, however, was that they chose a different and, in many cases, more detailed set of criteria for their analysis. They considered more types of important nutrients, including those that often showed greater rather than smaller differences between organic and conventional foods. Another major difference is that rather than averaging together many different statistics, the Newcastle group chose to perform more detailed and exacting analyses. For example, if five growing seasons were analyzed in one of the underlying studies, the Stanford group averaged the results together. But because natural variations between seasons can be significant, the Newcastle study considered each of those growing seasons, with their individual differences, as five separate sets of data.

Some critics of the Stanford study have been more cynical, observing that the study was released shortly before voting on California Proposition 37—an important measure to decide whether the state government should require food producers to disclose the use of GMOs in their products. A widely cited, negative report on organic foods just prior to the vote, they suggested, would sway public sentiment in favor of the big agricultural companies and take the wind out of the sails of the GMO labeling effort. The proposition was narrowly defeated, leaving producers free to incorporate GMOs without public disclosure.

Why Might Some Organic Foods Be More Nutritious?

Natural Maturation Means Natural Yields

There are many other reasons why organic foods may be more nutritious than conventional foods. Some of the practices used in large-scale farming are meant to rapidly increase crop yields, pushing plants to grow faster and reach their mature size and weight so that a given acre of land will turn out more tonnage of a saleable product in a shorter period of time. That's a very profitable way to do business—but it may reduce the nutritional value of the foods produced.

Many researchers believe that this type of high-yield, fast-turnaround farming provides less time for plants to mature and manufacture more of the subtle micronutrients the plants need to complete their growth cycles. Of course, when the plants manufacture these compounds for their own use and we, in turn, consume them, we benefit by taking those compounds into our own bodies.

Organic Plants Need to Work Harder—And We Reap the Rewards

Another fascinating factor is that when plants are grown organically, without the use of artificial pesticides, plants have to work harder to defend themselves. To do so, they need to reach deeper into their natural, biochemical arsenals to synthesize protective compounds to ensure their own health and viability. Once again, these compounds become available to our bodies when we consume organic produce.

It's a fascinating confluence of biology and aesthetics that some of the chemical compounds that give plants their wonderful colors and unique flavors are also intimately involved in the plant's growth and self-protection. For example, chlorophyll is a green plant pigment that directs the sunlight it absorbs into the complex process of a plant's cellular energy production. In addition to color, chlorophyll is responsible for many of the grassy flavors found in vegetables. Other plant substances, including many of the most aromatic and delectable, are components of a plant's immune and endocrine systems.

Scientifically trained aroma therapists understand that in addition to evoking aesthetic and emotional responses, plant-derived fragrances also contain remarkably complex substances known as phytochemicals that can operate directly on subtle aspects of human physiology. When used to make perfumes rather than high-potency essential oils, most of the direct chemical actions are muted or lost, though the fragrances remain.

The Biological Richness of Natural Earth

The quality of the earth has a great impact on the quality of fruits, vegetables, herbs, and grains. When plants are grown in naturally enriched soil, fortified with compost made from the organic decomposition of other plants, they are able to more easily absorb minerals and other bionutrients that have already been converted into highly bioavailable forms by the living action of the plants that contributed to the compost.

This not only may result in produce with higher levels of these minerals and other nutrients, but also facilitates biological processes within the plants, contributing to their health and therefore their ultimate nutritional value. Enzymes are natural biochemical transformers that promote the formation of important nutrients. Living things, whether plants or animals, synthesize many different types of enzymes within their own cells.

We also ingest functional enzymes that are present in our foods—especially foods that are raw and minimally processed. A great many of these enzymes are only activated in the presence of certain minerals. By growing in more mineral-rich soil, plants are able to more fully activate these enzymes and more effectively produce important biological compounds. When we eat those plants, we ingest those compounds and potentially larger amounts of plant enzymes that we can directly use in our own digestion, as well as higher levels of minerals to activate the enzymes produced by our own cells. It's a win-win-win situation.

Back to Our Roots with Heritage Varieties

Finally, although it is not part of the technical definition of organic foods, many producers have returned to the use of "heritage" varieties of fruits, vegetables, and grains. These are plant species that evolved naturally and haven't been altered through bioengineering or hybridization.

For example, most supermarket tomatoes have been modified to optimize their ability to survive the trip from a distant farm to the supermarket's shelf. These industrialized tomatoes have been modified to be hard in order to help them resist being crushed under the weight of thousands of pounds of other tomatoes when they're stacked together in massive truck beds. Similarly, some fruits and vegetables have been modified to make them frost resistant, or resistant to various plant diseases.

Other modifications are meant to make a food look more desirable in the market with a larger body, richer color, or more symmetrical form—often at the expense of its genuine quality. In the process, the flavor, texture, and nutritional value of these foods often become a secondary factor, falling behind the quest to minimize the producer's potential losses or the retailer's potential gains.

But when local farmers decide to grow organic tomatoes, strawberries, or any other crop, they are typically less concerned about these factors—in part because they're not producing on as large a scale or transporting their products over such great distances. Organic farming is also very often local farming, with an eye to freshness, quality, and sustainability.

In the organic world, especially with local sourcing and heritage varieties, crops true to their original form, texture, flavor, and nutritional value once again become viable options. This may be particularly significant for the produce found at local farmers markets, food co-ops, local farm-to-table delivery services, as well as small community gardens. Larger organic food outlets may feature local producers, but frequently also include organics from large-scale producers whose products may, like most conventional options, travel longer distances. This has become more of a factor as the demand for organic produce in the United States has increased to the point where many organic crops are now grown in Central and South America.

What Actually Matters?

Although there are many unanswered questions, issues, and controversies surrounding the assessment of the relative worth of organic foods, there are some questions we can, in fact, clearly address.

Can we conclusively say that the nutritional value of organic food products is always or even often superior to that of comparable conventional products? Let's review what the research, including Stanford's, actually shows about organic food products.

Reduced Toxic Exposure

First, research consistently demonstrates that organics have lower levels of pesticides and other toxic chemical residues than conventional foods. Organic foods also have lower levels of potentially disease-causing, antibiotic-resistant microorganisms. For many people, these findings alone are enough to answer the question of the superiority of organic foods with a resounding "yes."

Freedom from Artificially Introduced Hormones

Second, organic products are free of added hormones, including those frequently used in the production of milk and other dairy products. Exposure to these unnatural hormones as well as exposure to hormone-mimicking chemicals in plastics—known as environmental endocrine disruptors—have been linked to important health risks. Some researchers point to the use of hormones in dairy production and the role of disruptive environmental toxins, particularly in packaging materials, as potentially increasing disease risk.

Protection of the Land and Water

Third, research also consistently demonstrates that organic farming and animal husbandry practices release fewer toxins into the soil and the water supply, with potentially large downstream benefits to the human population living on the land and drinking the water. These farming practices, as well as other ecologically sensitive methods, offer long-range benefits for the sustainability of our farmlands and water-ways.

Given that protecting the land from toxification by man-made chemicals was the original inspiration for the entire organic movement, this is an exceptionally important benefit. Setting aside the extent to which you, as an individual consumer, care about this aspect of the organic lifestyle, it nonetheless represents an enormous value to our local and planetary ecosystems.

Social, Ethical, and Economic Values

Fourth, the social, ethical and economic aspects of organic food production embody values that may seem at first less immediate and substantial, but have already had an enormous impact on many peoples' lives. For example, the use of chemical pesticides results in acute poisoning of between 10,000 and 20,000 agricultural workers each year in the United States alone.

It's estimated that in Mexico, upwards of 20% of the agricultural labor force suffers from chronic pesticide poisoning, with many cases resulting in acute and debilitating symptoms. Above and beyond our natural concern for our fellow human beings, this level of toxicity can strain already burdened health-care systems, result in tragic birth defects, and alter the dynamics of communities in terms of family stability and long-term economic development.

Superior Nutritional Value

The fifth and final factor—the question of whether individual organic products are more nutritious than their conventional counterparts—may be less certain.

Many people feel that in addition to the freedom from chemical toxins undoubtedly provided by organic foods, consuming them is more satisfying. Some people claim that organic foods simply taste better, perhaps because their natural growing conditions and seasonal cycles allow for the more complex development of nutritional compounds, including those that contribute to aroma and flavor.

Many people anecdotally report feeling healthier and more energized when they shift to organic products. Are these reported benefits simply wishful thinking—attributable to a placebo effect? Or are they due primarily to the documented reduction in pesticides and other toxins—differences that may affect some people more strongly than others?

Or, perhaps, as Brandt and her colleagues concluded, organic foods really do contain higher levels of critical nutrients that were selectively, and in at least one case improperly analyzed and reported in the Stanford study. Remember, the U.K.

researchers also noted that organics have been shown to be higher in many other important bionutrients that were not even considered in the Stanford study. And, of course, there may also be other nutrients in organically raised and produced foods that have not yet been identified, or have not yet been associated with particular health benefits.

Organics—A Personal Choice

There is no question that we have much more to learn about how the methods we employ in raising our food products influence their value to us—nutritionally, and in many other ways. But the advantages and benefits of organic products that have already been clearly demonstrated make a powerful and compelling case for their value.

A personal choice to prefer organic products and, when necessary, to pay a premium for them in the marketplace, can be seen as a rational expression of self-interest as well as a commendable interest in the collective health of the planet and all the creatures who inhabit it. The "moral superiority" churlishly referred to in the negative headline previously mentioned is nothing to be ashamed of. Caring about the integrity of our planetary ecosystems, the health and welfare of agricultural workers, the survival of at-risk species, and protecting ourselves from potentially cancer-causing compounds and neurotoxins from the unbridled use of man-made chemicals shouldn't be controversial.

Perhaps, in the future, the negative headlines that followed on the heels of the Stanford study will be rewritten to tell a bigger and far more nuanced story. There is no question that additional research to fully answer unresolved questions about the health benefits of an organic diet is warranted.

Are Herbicides, Pesticides, and Chemical Fertilizers Harmful to Human Health?

There is widespread agreement that exposure to certain herbicides and pesticides can be harmful to human health. Pesticides have been linked to a variety of health problems, from neurological and endocrine disorders to birth defects and even cancer. There is less agreement about how much exposure—the amount of pesticide or pesticide residue in food or food products—is actually harmful.

Many studies have raised concerns about the health risks of farmers and other agricultural workers from occupational exposure to pesticides as well as harm from non-occupational exposure the general population receives from pesticide residues found on food and in drinking water. Some research suggests that in especially susceptible or sensitive people, even very low levels of exposure may have harmful health effects, while other research indicates that for most people, routine exposure from consuming conventional, non-organic foods with slight pesticide residue is not harmful.

It is also important to bear in mind that assessing the risks of pesticides either on human health or on the environment is neither an easy nor especially accurate process because of differences in the duration and extent or levels of exposure and the types of pesticides. Furthermore, for some of these chemicals, the effects of low-dose, long-term exposure may not yet be known.

The Centers for Disease Control (CDC) conducts ongoing assessments of the levels of environmental chemicals in the U.S. population. These assessments reveal that the majority of Americans have measurable levels of a number of chemical solvents including chlorinated pesticides, organophosphate pesticides, and pyrethroid pesticides, and that many adults and children have levels of pesticides in their bodies that exceed the levels considered "acceptable" by the Environmental Protection Agency (EPA).

Children are especially susceptible to the harmful effects of pesticide residues because of their size—the same exposure or dose affects them differently—more than it would an adult because they have lower body weights and are rapidly growing and developing. Children exposed to certain food pesticide residues may suffer developmental delays; disturbances in the reproductive, endocrine, and immune systems; certain cancers; and damage to other organs. Prenatal exposure to organophosphate pesticides has been linked to abnormal changes in the developing brain.

Since organic farming does not use synthetic pesticides and food residue studies confirm that organic produce has reduced pesticide levels, it seems reasonable to assume that consuming organic food should reduce pesticide exposure. Although there is no published research confirming reduced risk of developing pesticide-related diseases or improved health as a result of consuming organic food, several studies have found that pesticide levels in children sharply decreased or were even undetectable when they consumed an organic diet. Despite the lack of conclusive research about its health benefits, "going organic" appears to be an easy, logical way to reduce pesticide exposure.

The Environmental Protection Agency (EPA) Regulates Pesticides

In the United States, the Environmental Protection Agency (EPA) evaluates the risks associated with individual active ingredients in pesticides and the cumulative risks associated with groups of pesticides that act the same way in the body.

One of the ways the EPA evaluates the health risks of pesticides is by determining that there is "reasonable certainty of no harm" posed by pesticide residues permitted to remain on food. Before approving a pesticide, the EPA sets limits that stipulate precisely how the pesticide may be used, how often it may be used, and the types of protective clothing or equipment that must be used to handle it. These limits are meant to protect public health.

The EPA also establishes maximum residue limits that determine how much pesticide food, animal feed, and other products can contain. These pesticide residue limits are termed tolerances. Tolerances are intended to protect consumers from harmful levels of pesticides on food. FDA and USDA inspectors continuously monitor food to ensure that growers and manufacturers adhere to the established limits. The EPA maintains an International Maximum Residue Limit Database that includes the United States and seventy other countries and is searchable by crop or pesticide.

The EPA also designates certain pesticides as having "reduced risk"—these are pesticides that pose less risk to human health and the environment than existing conventional alternatives. The EPA states that the goal of this designation is to "quickly register commercially viable alternatives to riskier conventional pesticides such as neurotoxins, carcinogens, reproductive and developmental toxicants, and groundwater contaminants." For example, one of the EPA's first priorities was to compile a list of reduced risk or organophosphate alternatives since organophosphates can impair functioning of the central nervous system.

Does Washing Produce Remove Pesticides?

If you are unable to purchase organic produce or you are uncertain about whether fruits and vegetables you've purchased are free of pesticides, you can take steps to remove a considerable amount, but probably not 100% of surface pesticides. A quick rinse is not sufficient—produce should be rinsed for at least thirty seconds and vegetables with nooks and crannies like broccoli, cabbage, and cauliflower should be soaked in cold water for a couple of minutes before washing.

Although some people use dishwashing detergent or special produce washes to remove pesticide residue and bacteria from produce, research suggests that they are not really necessary and that soaking and scrubbing fruits and vegetables in water cleans just as effectively. Detergent can also change the aroma and flavor of fresh produce and may even penetrate the produce during washing.

Even fruits or vegetables like oranges, cucumbers or pineapples that you plan to peel should be washed before you peel them because as you cut into the skin or peel with a knife or peeler, you can transfer pesticide residue.

Using a soft brush to gently scrub the surfaces of conventionally grown, non-organic produce can remove a substantial amount of pesticides; however, it does not eliminate pesticides incorporated into the produce during its growth. Periodically wash your soft brush in the dishwasher to eliminate any bacteria it may harbor. Dry produce thoroughly using a clean cloth or paper towel before you store or serve it.

Where Can You Purchase Organic Foods?

Supermarkets, Grocery Stores, Discount Retailers, and Club Stores

It used to be challenging to find organic food—you'd have to go to a health food store or farmers market. Today, organic food is widely available. Along with tony markets like Whole Foods and Wild Oats, practically every local supermarket has an organic section, and club stores like Costco and Sam's Club stock organic food products. Discount retailers Target and Walmart also stock organic foods—about half of Target's own Simply Balanced brand is organic, and Walmart, the nation's largest grocer and organic retailer, carries Wild Oats organic food products.

Online Sources for Organic Foods

Along with local grocery stores, supermarkets, discount retailers, and club stores, organic food products can be purchased online at a variety of websites devoted exclusively to organics like mannaharvest.com, organickingdom.com, shoporganic.com, sunfood.com; specialty food sites like azurestandard.com, kalyx.com, vitacost.com, forthegourmet.com, and AbesMarket.com; and at larger sites like amazon.com.

Community Supported Agriculture

You can also join or subscribe to a Community Supported Agriculture (CSA) program. Community Supported Agriculture consists of a group of consumers that support a farm operation so that they are stakeholders in the farm. Not all CSAs include organic farms, but many participating farms use organic or biodynamic farming methods.

Members or subscribers pay in advance for the entire growing season, essentially purchasing a "share" in the farm and providing the farmer with working capital in advance of the growing season. In return, they receive a box, bag, or basket of seasonal produce weekly during the growing season. Some CSAs include several farmers to offer a variety of farm-fresh foods to members—eggs, honey, homemade bread, meat, cheese, and other farm products along with fresh produce. Other CSAs operate "market style"—farmers present the produce available each week, and members choose the foods they want.

Members benefit from participating directly in food production—learning how their food is grown, and they reap the rewards of bountiful harvests. But CSA members also share in the risks of farming, such as poor yields or failed crops, because of bad weather or pests.

Farmers benefit from financial support that not only frees them from worrying about marketing and sales but also reduces the risk of food waste. CSA farmers also have the opportunity to get to know the consumers of their produce personally.

Local Harvest, AgMap, and the Biodynamic Farming and Gardening Association CSA listings can help you locate a CSA in your community. Find them at these web addresses:

Local Harvest	www.localharvest.org/cas/
AgMap	http://agmap.psu.edu/
Biodynamic Farming and Gardening Association	https://www.biodynamics.com/content/community-supported-agriculture-introduction-csa

Home Delivery

There also are state and local services that deliver organic produce and food products straight to your door. Many partner with smaller local and family-owned organic farms to deliver farm-fresh food to your home. Some also deliver food from organic farms in Central and South America. Because produce is often sent directly from the grower, it endures less handling than produce shipped from the grower to a distribution center and then on to a retailer.

Standard delivery is generally weekly or bimonthly, and many organic food delivery services offer subscriptions that are customized to size and preferences of your household. Some services do, however, permit customers to order periodically, choosing only the items they want. In addition to saving you time and energy, organic home delivery is often environmentally conscious—many services deliver food using biodiesel-powered vehicles or even bicycles and are committed to operations that reuse, reduce, and recycle.

There are even some companies that provide meal assembly service—delivering all of the component ingredients needed to create family-size entrees—sparing you the shopping and prep time while providing hormone- and antibiotic-free meats, sustainably fished and farmed seafoods, and local seasonal and organic produce. Others provide ready-made meals that are delivered fresh, rather than frozen, to your door. Although these services tend to be costly, they are often less expensive than dining out and more effectively ensure a steady supply of freshly prepared, nutritious meals.

Food Co-ops and Buying Clubs

Food co-ops are member-owned and -operated food stores, and many stock organic, local, and minimally processed foods that contain no additives or preservatives. They aim to serve as community resources and gathering places and to forge connections between farmers and local customers. Nearly all operate as not-for-profit organizations, are only open to members, and aim to save their members money or increase their purchasing power. Some co-ops require a fee upon joining, and practically all require members to work—investing time, effort, and energy to make the co-op run smoothly.

Buying clubs are more likely to be informal or loosely organized groups of friends, colleagues, or members of other organizations who come together and buy food together from a food co-op warehouse. They buy directly in bulk from local growers, producers, and wholesalers and are composed of households that share not only cost savings but also the responsibilities of collecting money from the members, placing the orders with the distributors, helping to unload the truck when it arrives at the drop-off site, and dividing and packaging the individual household orders.

Many buying clubs operate like online farmers markets. Unlike food co-ops and buying clubs of the 1960s and 1970s, today's clubs are high-tech. Members place their orders online; farmers, producers, and wholesalers use online ordering systems; and an ever-changing array of food product information as well as requests to split orders and recipes are posted in member forums. For example, say you wanted to buy your favorite organic, fair trade coffee beans, but the best price for them was for 100 pounds. You and nineteen other club members could join together, each buying five pounds at a wholesale price. Members would then divide the coffee into five pound bags and distribute it.

Co-op grocery stores are similar to buying clubs, except that they are usually larger and more formally organized so they may serve thousands of member-owners. Most permit non-members to shop in their stores. Most carry a wide range of products including produce, lamb, beef, pork, poultry, dairy and eggs, fish and seafood, bread and baked goods, herbs, coffee, teas, sweets, and specialty foods. Because they serve more consumers, food turns over quickly, and it is not unusual to find produce picked the day you purchase it.

Farmers Markets and Farm Stands

Farmers markets and farm stands have long been reliable places to buy fresh local, organic foods. Though most feature local growers, not all foods sold at farmers markets are organic, so it's important to ask questions to be certain the produce you are purchasing is organic or local and pesticide-free. Ask vendors where fruits or vegetables were grown and whether the farm or grower is certified organic. If it's not certified, ask how it was grown.

In the summer and early fall, farmers markets offer an abundance of seasonal, often just picked produce, and many include vendors of artisan cheeses and baked goods. Along with vine-ripened tomatoes, look for antioxidant-rich purple carrots as well as the more traditional orange and white varieties, local blueberries, raspberries and strawberries, asparagus, Brussels sprouts, and ripe peaches and nectarines.

Looking for a local farmers market or store that carries organic products? The website organic.org has an interactive store finder, http://www.organic.org/storefinder, that provides retail and farmers market information by state.

Why Do Organic Foods Cost More?

Although not all organic foods are pricier than their conventionally grown, non-organic counterparts, many do cost more. You may think that the higher prices reflect how much more labor-intensive it is to grow crops with synthetic fertilizers and without herbicides and pesticides, and you'd be partly right.

Some production costs are higher. For example, organic farmers adhere to more stringent animal welfare standards, such as using only organic, non-GMO feed, which can cost twice as much as conventional feed, and certified organic seed tends to cost more than standard seed.

Organic agricultural practices like crop rotation to prevent weeds is more costly and labor-intensive than using synthetic weed killers. Biological pesticides, which many organic farmers use, are more expensive than the chemical pesticides used by conventional farmers. In addition, organic crops require special handling after they are harvested to prevent cross-contamination with conventional crops.

It's also true that organic food and livestock grow and develop more slowly than conventional crops and animals because they are not treated with chemicals and growth hormones to accelerate production. The additional time it takes to grow, mature, and ripen organic produce and naturally process organic food products contribute to their price.

But there are other reasons organic products tend to cost more.

First and foremost are economies of scale—the reduction of per-unit costs through an increase in production volume. Small organic growers and family farms have smaller yields and cannot achieve the economies of scale available to big companies.

For example, marketing and distribution costs for organic food products are higher because of relatively small volumes. In addition, organic food product distribution must be fast and efficient since without chemical preservatives, many organic food products have a shorter shelf life than non-organic products. As big companies increase production, they can pass some of their savings along to consumers in the form of lower prices.

Another reason organic foods cost more is because the demand for organic foods currently exceeds the supply. Industry observers predict that as demand for organic food and products increases, technological innovations and economies of scale should reduce costs of production, processing, distribution, and marketing for organic produce.

In addition, the cost of non-organic food often reflects the influence subsidies or other forms of state or local support. The United States has one of the most highly subsidized agricultural systems in the world—many crops including corn, wheat, and rice are heavily subsidized, which artificially lowers their prices. Most subsidies benefit large-scale agriculture.

There are USDA conservation payment programs that can help organic farmers. For example, in some states, farmers can obtain funds to help defray some of the costs of undergoing organic transition. But in general, there are far fewer subsidies available to support organic farming than to support conventional conservation practices. In fact, until the implementation of the Organic Foods Production Act in 1990, there was no support at the federal level and exceedingly little support in the states for organic agriculture. Although some strides have been made, government support for organic agriculture remains disproportionally low.

Environmentalists have advocated endeavoring to change the structure of farm subsidies so they can support sustainable and organic agriculture. One promising program was the Conservation Security Program, a voluntary program that provided financial and technical assistance to promote the conservation and improvement of soil, water, air, energy, and plant and animal life, and provided payments based on the farm's environmental stewardship. In its first years, however, the program was not adequately funded, and it was not reauthorized in the 2008 Farm Bill, so very few areas benefitted from it.

Until organic farmers receive subsidies comparable to those conventional farmers are given, the price of organic food will reflect the actual costs associated with growing and producing it rather than the artificially lower prices that subsidies enable farmers to offer consumers. Further, the price of conventional, non-organic produce does not account for the environmental costs of conventional agriculture.

It is costly for conventional farmers to make the transition to organic farming. Acquiring USDA organic certification is an arduous and costly process. To adhere to USDA standards, farm facilities and production methods may need to be modified. Administrative requirements, such as maintaining daily records that are readily available for inspection at a moments notice, is time- and labor-intensive. There also is an annual inspection/certification fee, which may be as high as $2,000 per year, depending on the size of the farm. Unlike the United States, which to date has offered farmers nearly no incentives to practice organic agriculture, many European countries actively encourage farmers to transition to organic practices.

Eating Organic Foods on a Budget

Since organic food products often cost more than their non-organic counterparts, is it possible for cost-conscious consumers to eat organic food on a budget? Nutritionists and dieticians say it is possible to economize and eat organically.

In fact, if, along with a shift to organic food you also start to prepare more of your meals from scratch, using seasonal, fresh ingredients rather than relying on restaurant meals, convenience foods, or take-out, you may actually find that your food budget shrinks.

Ten Budget-Friendly Tips to Trim Organic Food Costs

1. If you can't afford to eat exclusively organic foods, concentrate on purchasing the organic produce the Environmental Working Group identifies as the "dirty dozen"—the fruits and vegetables most likely to contain pesticide residues: apples, celery, cherries, imported grapes, lettuce, nectarines, peaches, pears, peppers, potatoes, spinach, and strawberries.
2. Buy in bulk, especially foods that you can freeze or otherwise store. Enlist family and friends to share bulk purchases.
3. Check newspapers, circulars and online sites for money-saving coupons, and use them to stock up. Check the inside labels, packaging, and websites of your favorite organic brands for discount coupons.
4. Look for frozen organic produce, especially organic berries, corn, peas, and peaches—they are often less costly than fresh and just as tasty.
5. Consider joining a buying club, community supported agriculture program, or food co-op where you join with other members to increase your purchasing power.
6. Shop online and at club stores like Costco and Sam's Club. You may find lower prices online and at club stores, especially for packaged organic food products such as pasta, cereal, and canned tomatoes.
7. Try store brand organic food products or generic organic brands, both of which are often less costly than name brand organic products.
8. Join a community garden where you can raise organic produce on your own little plot, or participate in organic gardening.
9. Shop farmers markets. Although they're not always less pricy than grocery stores, some fresh local produce may be less expensive. Ask about "seconds"—blemished, misshapen, or nearly over-ripe produce you may be able to buy at discounted prices.
10. Grow your own. Plant organic produce in your garden, pots, or even a window box. Even city dwellers can plant rooftop gardens.

Getting Started with Organics

If you are about to embark on an organic diet, begin by considering your family's or household's current diet and think about organic versions of or alternatives to the foods you eat most often. This approach can help you to ease into an organic diet without making radical changes in how and what you eat.

Choosing organic produce and dairy is a good way to start. Opt for organic fruits and vegetables that you don't peel before eating like apples, berries, bell peppers, celery, lettuce, peaches, and potatoes, since these are more likely to harbor pesticide residues than fruits and vegetables you peel such as avocados, bananas, cucumbers, oranges, and melons.

The switch to organic dairy will help you to avoid consuming hormones including bovine growth hormone, antibiotics, herbicides, and pesticides. Then you can consider organic grains and baked goods as well as organic meat, fish, and poultry. Many people also find it easy to switch to organic oils, nuts and nut butters, coffee, tea, and spices.

Plan to shop more frequently for food since organic produce and dairy tends to have a shorter shelf life because it does not contain preservatives. Shop around to learn which stores have the best selection and prices. Ask produce managers when organic produce is delivered and when it goes on sale or is marked down.

Although most markets have organic food sections, some place organic foods next to their conventional non-organic versions. Don't see your favorite organic food brands or products at your local grocery store or supermarket? Ask the manager if the store might consider stocking them.

Storing and Cooking Organic Produce—How to Preserve Fresh Flavors and Valuable Nutrients

Many locally sourced, organic vegetables are vine-ripened instead of being picked unripe and packed and shipped to distant stores. When vegetables remain on the plant to ripen, they contain more nutrients than they do when they are picked early and ripen off the vine. They taste better, too. For example, corn is very sweet the day it's picked, but after a few days it's not sweet because its natural sugar has broken down. Other nutrients also erode over time, so it's vitally important to start with the freshest produce you can find. (Flash-frozen fruits and vegetables also retain a high proportion of key nutrients.)

Ways to Store and Preserve Organic Produce

Store fruits and vegetables in cool places. Root vegetables like onions, garlic, and potatoes do better in cool, dry environs rather than the cool, dampness of the refrigerator. Mushrooms last longer when stored in a paper bag rather than a sealed plastic bag or container. Asparagus and celery stay fresh when placed upright in a glass of water. Unripe avocados will ripen quickly in a paper bag. Greens like lettuce and arugula should be washed and spun or towel dried before they are stored in an open container and wrapped in a dry towel. Beans, broccoli, leeks, parsnips, radishes, snap peas, spinach, and turnips should be stored in open containers. Most fruits, including tomatoes, do not need to be refrigerated.

Traditional methods of "putting up" produce—like canning and making jams, preserves, sauces, and confits—can be used with organic products. However, the high heat used in these methods may sacrifice some valuable nutrients.

Drying is another traditional method of preservation that's particularly suited to most types of organic produce because, when performed at lower temperatures, it can preserve more of the subtle nutrients present in organic foods.

Food dryers can extend the shelf life of fruits, vegetables, and even fish and meats by gently extracting their natural moisture by evaporation. In most dryers, slices or small chunks of food are placed on sliding trays whose bottoms are plastic screens, allowing warm air to flow all around the food. A silicon sheet can be placed in the tray to allow drying of especially wet, loose foods.

While some dryers run at fairly high temperatures—upwards of 150 degrees fahrenheit or more—the nutritionally dense, biologically active compounds in organic products are best maintained by drying them at much lower temperatures, preferably no more than about 105 degrees fahrenheit (note that better quality food dryers usually have thermostats that allow you to set your preferred temperature).

In particular, the natural enzymes present in raw foods lose their fragile structure, and therefore much of their biological activity, when they are heated much above this 105-degree threshold. Drying at a lower temperature takes a little longer, but the result is nutritionally much closer to the food in its original, most vital raw state.

Some dried foods are exactly what you would expect—dried, chewy, or crunchy versions of the original. Grapes dried into raisins and banana slices dried into crispy chips are two familiar examples. But some foods dry in surprising and wonderful ways. Half-inch-thick slices of ripe watermelon reduce in the dryer into thin wafers with an incredibly intense, sweet flavor. Leafy vegetables, especially kale, can be turned into delicious and marvelously healthful snacks when dried with just a little hint of seasoning.

Ways to Cook Organic Produce

Once you have a bounty of fresh organic foods, how should you prepare them to maximize their flavor and nutritional value? Although it's true that exposing some vegetables to heat can deplete some of their nutrient content—as much as 20% of vitamins such as vitamin C, folate, and potassium may be lost, along with enzymes that aid in digestion—others actually become more nutritious when heated. For example, the antioxidants in asparagus, cabbage, carrots, peppers, spinach, and tomatoes become more readily available when they are cooked. This is because the heat breaks down the plants' thick cell walls, freeing the nutrients stored in and bound to the cell walls.

Cooking vegetables whole or cutting them into large pieces helps them to retain water-soluble vitamins like vitamin C and vitamin B complex and a group of nutrients called polyphenolics, which are easily destroyed during food storage and cooking. In general, shorter cooking time, lower temperatures, and the smallest possible amounts of liquid to keep nutrients from leaching out into the cooking water or broth.

Although many people think cooking vegetables in a microwave is a bad idea, microwaved vegetables often have higher concentrations of some vitamins than vegetables that have been boiled or fried. Because quick cooking preserves nutrients, cooking vegetables in a microwave is not only fast and easy but also can be a healthy cooking method.

Blanching—quickly boiling vegetables, which leaves them very crisp and helps them maintain their vibrant colors and nutrients—steaming and boiling are the best cooking methods for preserving vegetables' antioxidants, but some cooking methods are better for specific vegetables. For example, steamed broccoli retains more glucosinolates, naturally occurring sulfur-containing chemicals, than boiled or roasted broccoli. In contrast, boiling carrots increases their carotenoid content, while steaming and frying reduces it. Steaming is ideal for cooking delicate fish and vegetables like asparagus, zucchini, and green beans.

Boiling also brings out the best—in terms of nutrients—in zucchini squash compared to other cooking methods. Frying, especially deep-frying, is more likely to degrade valuable nutrients. Deep-frying poses an additional risk because heating oil continuously at high temperatures creates free radicals, compounds that damage cells, block the action of critical enzymes, and interfere with a wide variety of healthy cellular processes. Free radicals can injure cell membranes, damage DNA, interfere with the proper division and replication of cells, and block the generation of energy the body needs to run.

If you want to fry vegetables, sauté them in a little olive oil or try a quick stir fry, which uses a modest amount of oil and high heat for a very short time; this works best on thinly sliced vegetables like onions, bell peppers, cabbage, carrots, eggplant, snow peas, and mushrooms. It's also an easy way to prepare grains like rice and quinoa and bite-sized uniform pieces of meat, fish, seafood, or tofu.

To get the crisp, crunchy texture of deep-frying, try oven-frying. Coat chicken, fish, or vegetables in milk, buttermilk, or beaten eggs and then dredge them in seasoned flour or breadcrumbs (substitute almond flour or corn flour for gluten-free diets), and then spray them lightly with olive oil. Bake at 425 degrees until they are browned and crispy.

Broiling heats food from above, and because it's dry heat, it works best on vegetables, meat, and fish that have been marinated or are basted as they cook. Salmon is a good candidate for broiling because it is an oily fish and is less likely to dry out during cooking. Any vegetables you might grill such as asparagus, bell peppers, corn, green beans, eggplant, onions, potatoes, radicchio, summer squash, tomatoes, and zucchini are also delicious when broiled.

Pressure-cooking intensifies flavors by cooking food in steam created by boiling water. It preserves vitamins and minerals because it takes very little time and a small amount of water. In addition to making stews and soups, use a pressure cooker to cook beef, chicken, and lamb as well as artichokes, potatoes, and beans.

No one cooking method is best for preserving the complex array of nutrients in vegetables. Since the best vegetables are the ones you and your family eat, flavor and texture should be important considerations when deciding how to cook your vegetables.

Healthy Diets

The question of precisely what constitutes a healthy diet is as complex as it is contentious. Strict vegetarians exclude all animal products from their diet, including eggs and dairy. On the other end of the spectrum, advocates of a Paleolithic or "paleo" diet point out that our ancestors' evolved while hunting, fishing, and gathering what they could, and therefore our best choice is a diet that is rich in dense animal proteins balanced with some fresh fruits and vegetables. To make matters even more complicated, different people respond to various foods in different ways, and the diet that is optimal for one person—based on their heritage, environment, lifestyle, and health status—may be disastrous for another person.

Many other authors, notably Michael Pollan, have written interesting and helpful books on the subject of the ideal diet, including *The Omnivore's Dilemma*. What we can address in this book are some of the most general and well-accepted principles about the quality of the foods we eat. Even in this arena, thinking has changed—sometimes radically. For many years health experts advised us to scrupulously avoid fats. Today, we recognize that not all fats are created equal and that some are necessary for good health. Cholesterol, once thought to be a primary cause of heart disease, is now understood to be—in moderation—essential for the body's synthesis of vitamin D and other hormones the body needs to function properly. It's even been discovered that some of the cholesterol found in the fatty plaques blocking diseased arteries may actually have been put there naturally as part of an antibacterial healing process.

Macronutrients and Micronutrients

The foods we eat provide the body with a variety of *macronutrients*: protein, lipids (the general name for fats and oils), and carbohydrates. Macronutrients make up the bulk of our diet, providing the materials we need for energy, growth, and repair. But the foods we eat also supply us with a vast array of *micronutrients* including vitamins, minerals, hormones, and oligopeptides. Micronutrients provide us with subtle components and information linkages needed to keep all the body's systems in tune.

But even among macronutrients there are great differences. For example, carbohydrates can enter the body in the form of simple sugars that are able to directly, or with very little conversion, be converted into cellular energy. But a diet high in simple sugars, whether from natural fruits and juices or from cakes and candies, puts an enormous strain on the body and can result in weakening our insulin response, playing havoc with the subtle hormonal signals that control when we're truly hungry and when we've eaten enough.

Starches, like those from wheat and other grains, are long chains of simple sugar molecules linked together by saccharide bonds. Up to a point, the body can break these bonds more slowly and use only the sugars it needs. But artificially stripping away many of the nutrients naturally present in grains—for example, to make white flour or white rice—not only strips off a wealth of important micronutrients, it also makes these starches act more like simple sugars, which, once again, strain the body.

The Subtle Differences Between Nutrient Forms

So if you really want to pay attention to what you eat, it's not enough to distinguish between macronutrients and micronutrients. We also need to pay attention to the specific forms of a nutrient. We have observed that carbohydrates are an important source of the sugar molecules used by our cells to produce energy. But a small number of carbohydrate molecules with specific properties are also taken up by the immune system. Instead of being broken down to make energy, they are built up into the glycoproteins that communicate in a kind of chemical language, allowing the immune system to recognize our own cells and therefore not attack them as if they were foreign bodies or invading germs. This is another example of a macronutrient class behaving in a way more consistent with micronutrients.

Vitamins are probably the most familiar form of micronutrient. A vitamin is a substance required by the body for proper physiological function that the body cannot produce for itself. Serious dietary deficiencies of vitamins are associated with specific diseases. For example, British sailors are sometimes called Limeys because it was discovered that their long sea journeys without access to fresh fruits and vegetables deprived them of vitamin C and caused a serious disease called scurvy. Carrying a few limes or other citrus fruits could supply the missing vitamin C and prevent the disease. Similarly, beriberi and pellagra are diseases caused by deficiencies of vitamin B1 (thiamine) and vitamin B3 (niacin), respectively.

The U.S. Recommended Daily Allowance (USRDA, or just RDA for short) for a vitamin or other nutritional substance has historically been based on the daily dietary level necessary to prevent diseases of deficiency. Today, however, many health authorities question the RDA as a guideline for how much of any micronutrient we should consume. Their argument is that our goal shouldn't just be avoiding disease, but rather optimizing health. While it's possible to take an overdose of a vitamin, mineral, or other micronutrient—especially when consumed in the form of manufactured, concentrated supplements—there is little danger of overdosing on nutrients present in living foods.

Many processed foods contain artificially added synthetic vitamins to increase their appeal to consumers. Busy mothers, the reasoning goes, might feel better about quickly serving their children a bowl of sugary-sweet cereal if it contains a long list of vitamins. The first problem, however, is that sprinkling some vitamins onto an unhealthful food doesn't magically make it good for you. The second and more subtle problem, however, is that many of the vitamins that come from live natural sources—like organic fruits and vegetables—are in molecular forms the body can easily absorb and utilize. Some synthetic vitamins, on the other hand, are less fully utilized, or have to go through more chemical processing steps in the body before they can function properly. A third and even more subtle distinction is that vitamins naturally occur as a variety of related forms, called vitamers, that can synergize with one another for optimal function. For example, vitamin A is actually a family made up of six vitamers: a plant-based carotenoid group with four members and an animal-based retinoid group with two members. Synthetic vitamins almost always occur in a single molecular form and may provide a less complete range of activities, even when they are adequately absorbed.

Minerals are chemical elements like magnesium, sodium, potassium, and calcium that the body needs to function properly. Minerals are sometimes also called electrolytes because they increase the electrical conductivity of the body's fluids. But minerals also serve many other functions in the body, and getting enough of them in our diet is important. One potential advantage of organic farming is that it continually returns minerals to the soil through the use of natural fertilizers including compost and manure. These minerals strengthen the crops and also, of course, make more of those minerals available to our bodies when we eat the foods grown in this mineral-rich soil.

Our bodies perform an astonishing number of chemical transformations that follow specific pathways, the way cars follow streets and highways. These pathways are managed by special molecules called *enzymes*. Enzymes are frequently switched on and off when they attach or release a particular mineral ion. Mineral deficiencies or functional blockages of mineral activity caused by a toxin like mercury can suppress the proper function of one or more enzyme pathways. So it's important that we consume a diet rich in the minerals we need. The quantities we require are usually quite small, but some minerals, like the iodine necessary to create thyroid hormones, are not very common in our diets. That's why iodine is usually added to our table salt.

A *catabolic enzyme* grabs hold of a substance and splits it into simpler parts. Most of the enzymes that aid digestion—whether they are generated by our own cells or are naturally present in the foods we eat—are catabolic enzymes. Conversely, *anabolic enzymes* join simpler molecules together into larger, more complex forms. Anabolic enzymes are used by the body to build and repair tissues and to generate complex signaling chemicals. That's why you'll often hear about bodybuilders using supplements and medicines that stimulate anabolic activity—some of which are banned for athletic competition. While specific anabolic compounds are regulated or illegal, it's important to remember that the body naturally engages in anabolic processes all the time.

Like the distinction between natural vitamer families and synthetic vitamins, not all minerals are equally bioavailable. In nature, mineral ions are attached to other nutrients our bodies know how to use. As we assimilate these nutrients, the minerals attached to them are directed to different parts of the body. Again, living foods like organic fruits, grains, and vegetables naturally contain a wide variety of minerals in different forms. This is generally not the case when we buy mineral supplements at the health food store or supermarket. In fact, many sources of cheap minerals are actually "inorganic" forms that the body cannot utilize well, which is why food-based mineral complexes are therefore more desirable.

These sorts of distinctions, which have been studied in depth by researchers like the late German orthomolecular ("right molecule") physician Dr. Hans Nieper (1928–1998), could easily fill an entire book. Nieper was renown for his use of specific nutritional forms in the healing of multiple sclerosis and cancer. The Linus Pauling Institute at Oregon State University is named for the great American Nobel laureate biochemist whose pioneering work in human nutrition shed light on many of these issues. The Institute's website, http://lpi.oregonstate.edu, is an excellent source for information on micronutrients and health.

For our purposes, the bottom line is that the micronutrients naturally present in living foods are typically much better and more biologically active than the synthetic "label candy" added to processed foods to make them seem more healthful.

The Basics of a Balanced Diet

A healthy diet is varied and balanced and emphasizes foods derived from plants—fruits, vegetables, legumes, and whole grains. It also may include low-fat or fat-free dairy products and lean meats, poultry, fish, beans, eggs, and nuts. Healthy diets are low in saturated fats, trans fats, cholesterol, salt, and added sugar and limit highly processed foods. Since 2006, when a trans fat labeling law took effect, many food manufacturers have eliminated or sharply reduced trans fats in their food products. Healthy diets are rich in the unsaturated fats in nuts, avocados, and vegetable oils as well as fatty fish like salmon.

Adopting an organic diet or even incorporating organic foods in a healthy diet can help to limit exposure to hormones, antibiotics, antibiotic-resistant bacteria, herbicides, pesticides, genetically modified organisms, and other synthetic ingredients that may be harmful to your health.

USDA Dietary Guidelines

The U.S. Department of Agriculture (USDA) and the U.S. Department of Health and Human Services (HHS) update "Nutrition and Your Health: Dietary Guidelines for Americans" every five years. The 2010 guidelines encourage Americans to eat less and move more in an effort to combat the nation's obesity epidemic.

The guidelines advise Americans to reduce:

- Consumption of sodium to less than 2,300 milligrams per day and cholesterol to less than 300 milligrams per day.
- Saturated fats by replacing them with monounsaturated and polyunsaturated fats.
- Consumption of trans-fatty acids by sharply limiting the intake of partially hydrogenated oils and other solid fats.
- Intake of refined grains and refined grain products with solid fats, added sugars, and sodium.
- Alcohol consumption (one drink per day for women and two for men).

The guidelines advise Americans to increase the consumption of:

- Nutrient-dense foods (e.g., fruits, lean meats and poultry, and eggs prepared without added solid fats, sugars, starches, and sodium) that provide the full range of essential nutrients and fiber, without excessive calories.

- Vegetables (especially dark green, red, and orange vegetables), beans, peas, and fruits.
- Whole grains and fat-free or low-fat dairy or fortified soy beverages.
- Fish and other seafood.
- A variety of foods high in protein, including eggs, beans, peas, soy products, and unsalted nuts and seeds.
- Foods that are rich in potassium, dietary fiber, calcium, and vitamin D, including vegetables, fruits, whole grains, and dairy.

Read more about the 2010 US Dietary Guidelines at http://www.cnpp.usda.gov/dgas2010-policydocument.htm.

MyPlate—USDA Dietary Guidelines for Consumers

MyPlate is based on the 2010 USDA Dietary Guidelines and illustrates the five food groups that comprise a healthful meal and diet using a simple, familiar image—a place setting for a meal. MyPlate makes an effort to coax Americans to consume a diet that is more plant-based. Vegetables are the largest sector on the plate, and fruit and vegetables together consume half the plate. Learn more about MyPlate at www.choosemyplate.gov.

There are many varieties of healthy diets that incorporate natural, minimally processed and organic foods. Some of the most popular include the Mediterranean diet, the whole foods diet, vegetarian and vegan diets, and the flexitarian diet.

Mediterranean Diet

Mediterranean-style eating—more plant-based foods (fruits, vegetables, and nuts), whole grains, and fish; less red and processed meats; and moderate amounts of alcohol—has been associated with healthy aging and fewer chronic diseases. People who adopt a Mediterranean diet may reduce their blood sugar and cholesterol levels, which may lower their risk of developing heart disease and cancer. Learn more about the Mediterranean diet at http://www.heart.org/HEARTORG/GettingHealthy/NutritionCenter/Mediterranean-Diet_UCM_306004_Article.jsp.

Whole Foods (Minimally Processed) Diet

Whole food diets consist of simple, nutrient-rich, minimally processed foods like whole grains, fruits and vegetables, lean protein and "good fats" (omega-3s) from fish and plants, and monounsaturated fat from plant sources. This means eating foods in as close to their natural forms as possible—for example, choosing apples instead of applesauce or a baked potato instead of potato chips or French fries.

Whole foods retain their nutrients, including phytonutrients that are often removed during processing. Whole food diets eliminate convenience foods and processed foods because they frequently contain additives and preservatives as well as added fat, sugar, and salt.

Vegetarian/Vegan Diets

Vegetarian diets vary in in terms of the foods they include and exclude.

- Lacto-vegetarian diets exclude meat, fish, poultry, and eggs, along with foods that contain them but include dairy products
- Lacto-ovo vegetarian diets exclude meat, fish, and poultry, but include dairy products and eggs.
- Ovo-vegetarian diets exclude meat, poultry, seafood, and dairy products, but include eggs.
- Vegan diets exclude meat, poultry, fish, eggs, and dairy products and foods that contain these animal products. Although some experts worry that vegan diets may be deficient in terms of protein, most vegans who consume diets containing vegetables, beans, grains, nuts, and seeds are able to obtain adequate protein in their diets.

Learn more about vegetarian diets at http://www.nutrition.gov/smart-nutrition-101/healthy-eating/eating-vegetarian.

Flexitarian Diets

Flexitarians are flexible vegetarians. The American Dietetic Association defines flexitarians as "vegetarians who occasionally eat meat." A flexitarian diet is chiefly plant-based but also includes occasional meat, dairy, eggs, poultry, and fish. Some research suggests that flexitarians are healthier and weigh less than their meat-eating counterparts.

Proposed Revisions to the Nutrition Facts Label

The FDA plans to update the Nutrition Facts label on food packages to reflect new public health information. Proposed updates include:

- Requiring the declaration of "Added Sugars" on the label. "Sugars" include both "added sugars" and sugars that are naturally occurring in food.
- Removing the requirement for declaring "Calories from fat."
- Revising the nutrients that must be declared on the label. These are nutrients for which the U.S. population is consuming inadequate amounts and are associated with the risk of chronic disease. Calcium and iron are already required; vitamin D and potassium would be newly required. The FDA proposes that mandatory labeling no longer be required for vitamin C or vitamin A because current data indicate that deficiencies are not common; these vitamins could still be declared on labels voluntarily.
- Revised Daily Values for certain nutrients that are either mandatory or voluntary on the label. Examples include calcium, sodium, dietary fiber, and vitamin D. Some Daily Values are intended to guide consumers about maximum intake—saturated fat, for example—while

others are intended to help consumers meet a nutrient requirement—iron, for example. Daily Values are used to calculate the percent daily value (%DV) on the label, which helps consumers to understand the nutrient information on the product label in the context of the total diet. The FDA is also changing the units used to declare vitamins A, E, and D from "international units," or "I.U.," to a metric measure—milligrams or micrograms—and proposes to include the absolute amounts in milligrams or micrograms of vitamins and minerals, in addition to the %DV, on the label.

Nutrition Facts

Serving Size 1 cup (228g)
Servings Per Container About 2

Amount Per Serving

Calories 170	Calories from Fat 18

	% Daily Value*
Total Fat 2g	17%
Saturated Fat 0g	8%
Trans Fat 0g	
Cholesterol 30mg	10%
Sodium 250mg	10%
Total Carbohydrate 14g	5%
Dietary Fiber 4g	16%
Sugars 0g	
Protein 2g	

Vitamin A 12%	•	Vitamin C 10%
Calcium 20%	•	Iron 14%

* Percent Daily Values are based on a 2,000 calorie diet. Your daily values may be higher or lower depending on your calorie needs:

	Calories:	2,000	2,500
Total Fat	Less than	65g	80g
Sat Fat	Less than	20g	25g
Cholesterol	Less than	300mg	300mg
Sodium	Less than	2,400mg	2,400mg
Total Carbohydrate		300g	375g
Dietary Fiber		25g	30g

Calories per gram:
Fat 9 • Carbohydrate 4 • Protein 4

Ideal Weight Chart

Height	Ideal Male Weight	Ideal Female Weight
4'6"	63–77 lbs.	63–77 lbs.
4'7"	68–84 lbs.	68–83 lbs.
4'8"	74–90 lbs.	72–88 lbs.
4'9"	79–97 lbs.	77–94 lbs.
4'10"	85–103 lbs.	81–99 lbs.
4'11"	90–110 lbs.	86–105 lbs.
5'0"	95–117 lbs.	90–110 lbs.
5'1"	101–123 lbs.	95–116 lbs.
5'2"	106–130 lbs.	99–121 lbs.
5'3"	112–136 lbs.	104–127 lbs.
5'4"	117–143 lbs.	108–132 lbs.
5'5"	122–150 lbs.	113–138 lbs.
5'6"	128–156 lbs.	117–143 lbs.
5'7"	133–163 lbs.	122–149 lbs.
5'8"	139–169 lbs.	126–154 lbs.
5'9"	144–176 lbs.	131–160 lbs.
5'10"	149–183 lbs.	135–165 lbs.
5'11"	155–189 lbs.	140–171 lbs.
6'0"	160–196 lbs.	144–176 lbs.
6'1"	166–202 lbs.	149–182 lbs.
6'2"	171–209 lbs.	153–187 lbs.
6'3"	176–216 lbs.	158–193 lbs.
6'4"	182–222 lbs.	162–198 lbs.
6'5"	187–229 lbs.	167–204 lbs.
6'6"	193–235 lbs.	171–209 lbs.
6'7"	198–242 lbs.	176–215 lbs.
6'8"	203–249 lbs.	180–220 lbs.
6'9"	209–255 lbs.	185–226 lbs.
6'10"	214–262 lbs.	189–231 lbs.
6'11"	220–268 lbs.	194–237 lbs.
7'0"	225–275 lbs.	198–242 lbs.

Whole Grains

Whole grains contain complex carbohydrates surrounded by nutrient-rich layers of bran and germ. When natural whole grains are refined—for example, when whole wheat is used to make white flour—the bran and germ are removed. The resulting flour is softer and smoother and better for making crispy breads and fluffy cakes, but a large measure of the grain's nutritional value is lost. In particular, highly beneficial plant oils and other phytonutrients (the name given to plant-based nutritional compounds) are discarded in processing.

A variety of whole, unrefined grains are commercially available, with their bran and germ layers intact. Examples include barley, brown rice, buckwheat, bulgur, millet, oatmeal, popcorn, quinoa, whole wheat bread, crackers, pasta, and wild rice. These grains are important sources of many nutrients including dietary fiber, several B vitamins (particularly thiamin, riboflavin, niacin, and folate), and minerals (iron, magnesium, and selenium). B vitamins play several essential roles in metabolism and are vital for a healthy nervous system. Folate (folic acid), a B vitamin, is especially important before and during pregnancy because it helps prevent birth defects. In addition, whole grains are digested more slowly than refined grains, which enables better absorption of their nutrients.

Eating whole grains as part of a healthy diet may reduce the risk of heart disease and certain cancers and can help with weight management. Whole grains are high in dietary fiber, and consuming foods containing fiber helps to support gastrointestinal health by reducing constipation and diverticulitis. The fiber in whole grains also helps to slow the conversion of starches into glucose, which can help to stabilize blood sugar. Whole grains also support healthy digestion and immune system function.

When nutrient-rich bran and germ are removed from whole grains, they are sometimes sold as supplements. Wheat germ and rice bran can be purchased in bulk as food-based nutritional supplements and added back into shakes and smoothies, baked goods, and other recipes to enhance their nutritional value.

Why Eat Organic Whole Grains?

Organic whole grains are grown without synthetic fertilizers and pesticides and are not treated with radiation or irrigated with repurposed runoff water. They also are not genetically modified to resist insects and weed killers. Because organic grains are grown without pesticides, they may develop additional defense mechanisms—protective compounds that also may benefit the animals and people that consume them.

Daily Goal

The amount of grains you need to eat depends on your age, sex, and level of physical activity.

Children: 3 to 6 ounces
Adults: 6 to 8 ounces
1 ounce equivalents:

1 slice of bread	½ cup cooked cereal
1 cup cereal	1 6" tortilla
½ cup rice or pasta	

Grains are divided into two subgroups: whole grains and refined grains. Whole grains contain the entire grain kernel (bran, germ, and endosperm). Examples include whole-wheat flour, bulgur (cracked wheat), oatmeal, whole cornmeal, and brown rice.

Refined grains have been milled, which gives grains a finer texture and longer shelf life. The bran and germ are removed, and there is a loss of dietary fiber, iron, and many B vitamins. Examples include white flour, degermed cornmeal, white bread, and white rice.

Most refined grains are enriched, adding back certain B vitamins (thiamin, riboflavin, niacin, and folic acid) and iron after processing, but not fiber. Food products may be made from a mixture of whole grains and refined grains.

At least half of your grains should be whole grains (48 grams per day, or three 16 oz. servings). Examples of servings of whole grains:

- 1/2 cup cooked brown rice or other cooked grain
- 1/2 cup cooked 100% whole-grain pasta
- 1/2 cup cooked hot cereal, such as oatmeal
- 1 oz. uncooked whole-grain pasta, brown rice, or other grain
- 1 slice 100% whole-grain bread
- 1 very small (1 oz.) 100% whole-grain muffin
- 1 cup 100% whole-grain ready-to-eat cereal

Look for the Whole Grain stamp when you purchase grain products, as this will make it easy for you to meet the recommended three servings or more of whole grains each day. To do so, eat three whole grain food products with the 100% Whole Grain label or six products that have any Whole Grain stamp. Look for it on these products:

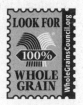

brown rice	rolled oats	whole-grain triticale
buckwheat	whole-grain barley	whole oats
bulgur	whole-grain corn	whole rye
millet	whole grain	whole wheat
oatmeal	sorghum	wild rice
quinoa		

Baking Ingredients

Arrowhead Mills, Organic Blue Corn Meal

1/3 cup

Amount per serving	Amount per serving	Amount per serving
Calories 130	**Cholesterol** 0mg	**Total Carbohydrate** 25g
Total Fat 1.5g	**Sodium** 0mg	Dietary Fiber 5g
Saturated Fat 0g	**Protein** 3g	Sugars 0g

Arrowhead Mills, Organic Yellow Corn Meal

1/3 cup

Amount per serving	Amount per serving	Amount per serving
Calories 120	**Cholesterol** 0mg	**Total Carbohydrate** 27g
Total Fat 1g	**Sodium** 0mg	Dietary Fiber 3g
Saturated Fat 0g	**Protein** 3g	Sugars 0g

Eden Foods, Kuzu Root Starch, Organic

1 tbsp

Amount per serving	Amount per serving	Amount per serving
Calories 30	**Cholesterol** 0mg	**Total Carbohydrate** 8g
Total Fat 0g	**Sodium** 0mg	Dietary Fiber NA
Saturated Fat NA	**Protein** 0g	Sugars 0g

Hodgson Mill, Certified Organic Wheat Free Yellow Corn Meal

<1/4 cup

Amount per serving	Amount per serving	Amount per serving
Calories 100	**Cholesterol** 0mg	**Total Carbohydrate** 23g
Total Fat 1g	**Sodium** 0mg	Dietary Fiber 3g
Saturated Fat 0g	**Protein** 3g	Sugars 0g

Let's Do...Organic, Organic Cornstarch

1 tbsp

Amount per serving	Amount per serving	Amount per serving
Calories 30	**Cholesterol** 0mg	**Total Carbohydrate** 7g
Total Fat 0g	**Sodium** 0mg	Dietary Fiber 0g
Saturated Fat 0g	**Protein** 1g	Sugars 0g

Bread

Garden of Eatin', Organic Bible Bread, Original Pita Breads

1 pita (57g/2 oz)

Amount per serving	Amount per serving	Amount per serving
Calories 145	**Cholesterol** 0mg	**Total Carbohydrate** 30g
Total Fat 0.5g	**Sodium** 115mg	Dietary Fiber 1g
Saturated Fat 0g	**Protein** 5g	Sugars 1g

Manna Organics, Bavarian Style Rye Sourdough Bread

50g/1.77 oz (approx. 1 slice)

Amount per serving	Amount per serving	Amount per serving
Calories 120	**Cholesterol** 0mg	**Total Carbohydrate** 25g
Total Fat 1g	**Sodium** 220mg	Dietary Fiber 8g
Saturated Fat 0g	**Protein** 5g	Sugars 0g

Manna Organics, GF Ancient Grains Bread

1 slice (28g/1 oz)

Amount per serving	Amount per serving	Amount per serving
Calories 60	**Cholesterol** 0mg	**Total Carbohydrate** 14g
Total Fat 2.5g	**Sodium** 160mg	Dietary Fiber 1g
Saturated Fat 0g	**Protein** 2g	Sugars 1g

Manna Organics, GF Ciao Chia Bread

1 slice (28g/1 oz)

Amount per serving	Amount per serving	Amount per serving
Calories 80	**Cholesterol** 0mg	**Total Carbohydrate** 14g
Total Fat 2g	**Sodium** 160mg	Dietary Fiber 1g
Saturated Fat 0g	**Protein** 1g	Sugars 1g

Manna Organics, GF Cinnamon Raisin Bread

1 slice (28g/1 oz)

Amount per serving	Amount per serving	Amount per serving
Calories 90	**Cholesterol** 0mg	**Total Carbohydrate** 17g
Total Fat 2g	**Sodium** 160mg	Dietary Fiber 1g
Saturated Fat 0g	**Protein** 1g	Sugars 5g

Manna Organics, GF Open Sesame Bread

1 slice (28g/1 oz)

Amount per serving	Amount per serving	Amount per serving
Calories 90	**Cholesterol** 0mg	**Total Carbohydrate** 15g
Total Fat 2.5g	**Sodium** 160mg	Dietary Fiber 1g
Saturated Fat 0g	**Protein** 1g	Sugars 1g

Manna Organics, GF Original Bread

1 slice (28g/1 oz)

Amount per serving	Amount per serving	Amount per serving
Calories 80	**Cholesterol** 0mg	**Total Carbohydrate** 15g
Total Fat 2g	**Sodium** 160mg	Dietary Fiber 1g
Saturated Fat 0g	**Protein** 1g	Sugars 1g

Manna Organics, Manna Bread Banana Walnut Hemp

2 oz (56g / 3/4" slice)

Amount per serving	Amount per serving	Amount per serving
Calories 140	**Cholesterol** 0mg	**Total Carbohydrate** 27g
Total Fat 3.5g	**Sodium** 5mg	Dietary Fiber 4g
Saturated Fat 0.3g	**Protein** 5g	Sugars 8g

Manna Organics, Manna Bread Carrot Raisin

2 oz (56g / 3/4" slice)

Amount per serving	Amount per serving	Amount per serving
Calories 130	**Cholesterol** 0mg	**Total Carbohydrate** 27g
Total Fat 0g	**Sodium** 6mg	Dietary Fiber 5g
Saturated Fat 0g	**Protein** 5g	Sugars 10g

Manna Organics, Manna Bread Cinnamon Date

2 oz (56g / 3/4" slice)

Amount per serving	Amount per serving	Amount per serving
Calories 150	**Cholesterol** 0mg	**Total Carbohydrate** 29g
Total Fat 0g	**Sodium** 15mg	Dietary Fiber 5g
Saturated Fat 0g	**Protein** 8g	Sugars 6g

Manna Organics, Manna Bread Fig, Fennel, and Flax

2 oz (56g / 3/4" slice)

Amount per serving	Amount per serving	Amount per serving
Calories 120	**Cholesterol** 0mg	**Total Carbohydrate** 26g
Total Fat 1.5g	**Sodium** 10mg	Dietary Fiber 5g
Saturated Fat 0g	**Protein** 4g	Sugars 8g

Manna Organics, Manna Bread Fruit and Nut

2 oz (56g / 3/4" slice)

Amount per serving	Amount per serving	Amount per serving
Calories 140	**Cholesterol** 0mg	**Total Carbohydrate** 27g
Total Fat 1g	**Sodium** 7mg	Dietary Fiber 6g
Saturated Fat 0g	**Protein** 6g	Sugars 16g

Manna Organics, Manna Bread Millet Rice

2 oz (56g / 3/4" slice)

Amount per serving	Amount per serving	Amount per serving
Calories 130	**Cholesterol** 0mg	**Total Carbohydrate** 28g
Total Fat 0g	**Sodium** 10mg	Dietary Fiber 5g
Saturated Fat 0g	**Protein** 5g	Sugars 9g

Manna Organics, Manna Bread Multigrain

2 oz (56g / 3/4" slice)

Amount per serving	Amount per serving	Amount per serving
Calories 130	**Cholesterol** 0mg	**Total Carbohydrate** 26g
Total Fat 0g	**Sodium** 10mg	Dietary Fiber 4g
Saturated Fat 0g	**Protein** 6g	Sugars 6g

Manna Organics, Manna Bread Sunseed

2 oz (56g / 3/4" slice)

Amount per serving	Amount per serving	Amount per serving
Calories 160	**Cholesterol** 0mg	**Total Carbohydrate** 29g
Total Fat 2g	**Sodium** 3mg	Dietary Fiber 7g
Saturated Fat 0g	**Protein** 6g	Sugars 11g

Manna Organics, Manna Bread Whole Rye

2 oz (56g / 3/4" slice)

Amount per serving	Amount per serving	Amount per serving
Calories 150	**Cholesterol** 0mg	**Total Carbohydrate** 32g
Total Fat 0g	**Sodium** 10mg	Dietary Fiber 5g
Saturated Fat 0g	**Protein** 6g	Sugars 7g

Manna Organics, Multigrain Flax Sourdough Bread

50g/1.77 oz (approx. 1 slice)

Amount per serving	Amount per serving	Amount per serving
Calories 140	**Cholesterol** 0mg	**Total Carbohydrate** 22g
Total Fat 4g	**Sodium** 170mg	Dietary Fiber 5g
Saturated Fat 0.5g	**Protein** 5g	Sugars 0g

Manna Organics, Sunny Sourdough Bread

50g/1.77 oz (approx. 1 slice)

Amount per serving	Amount per serving	Amount per serving
Calories 130	**Cholesterol** 0mg	**Total Carbohydrate** 24g
Total Fat 2.5g	**Sodium** 200mg	Dietary Fiber 6g
Saturated Fat 0g	**Protein** 5g	Sugars 0g

Rudi's Organic Bakery, Bagels & English Muffins, Cinnamon Raisin Bagels

1 slice = 2 oz (57g)

Amount per serving	Amount per serving	Amount per serving
Calories 130	**Cholesterol** 0mg	**Total Carbohydrate** 31g
Total Fat 1.5g	**Sodium** 240mg	Dietary Fiber 3g
Saturated Fat 0g	**Protein** 6g	Sugars 7g

Rudi's Organic Bakery, Bagels & English Muffins, Harvest Seeded English Muffins

1 slice = 2 oz (57g)

Amount per serving	Amount per serving	Amount per serving
Calories 130	**Cholesterol** 0mg	**Total Carbohydrate** 22g
Total Fat 2.5g	**Sodium** 130mg	Dietary Fiber 2g
Saturated Fat 0g	**Protein** 5g	Sugars 3g

Rudi's Organic Bakery, Bagels & English Muffins, Honey Sweet Wheat Bagels

1 slice = 2 oz (57g)

Amount per serving	Amount per serving	Amount per serving
Calories 150	**Cholesterol** 0mg	**Total Carbohydrate** 32g
Total Fat 1g	**Sodium** 250mg	Dietary Fiber 5g
Saturated Fat 0g	**Protein** 6g	Sugars 6g

Rudi's Organic Bakery, Bagels & English Muffins, Multigrain Bagels

1 slice = 2 oz (57g)

Amount per serving	Amount per serving	Amount per serving
Calories 140	**Cholesterol** 0mg	**Total Carbohydrate** 29g
Total Fat 3g	**Sodium** 230mg	Dietary Fiber 3g
Saturated Fat 0g	**Protein** 6g	Sugars 3g

Rudi's Organic Bakery, Bagels & English Muffins, Plain Bagels

1 slice = 2 oz (57g)

Amount per serving	Amount per serving	Amount per serving
Calories 120	**Cholesterol** 0mg	**Total Carbohydrate** 30g
Total Fat 1.5g	**Sodium** 270mg	Dietary Fiber 3g
Saturated Fat 0g	**Protein** 6g	Sugars 3g

Rudi's Organic Bakery, Bagels & English Muffins, Spelt English Muffins

1 slice = 2 oz (57g)

Amount per serving	Amount per serving	Amount per serving
Calories 70	**Cholesterol** 0mg	**Total Carbohydrate** 15g
Total Fat 1.5g	**Sodium** 180mg	Dietary Fiber 1g
Saturated Fat 0.5g	**Protein** 2g	Sugars 1g

Rudi's Organic Bakery, Bagels & English Muffins, White English Muffins

1 muffin (57g/2 oz)

Amount per serving	Amount per serving	Amount per serving
Calories 120	**Cholesterol** 0mg	**Total Carbohydrate** 23g
Total Fat 1.5g	**Sodium** 220mg	Dietary Fiber 1g
Saturated Fat 0g	**Protein** 4g	Sugars 2g

Rudi's Organic Bakery, Bagels & Muffins, Multigrain English Muffins with Flax

1 slice = 2 oz (57g)

Amount per serving	Amount per serving	Amount per serving
Calories 130	**Cholesterol** 0mg	**Total Carbohydrate** 25g
Total Fat 1.5g	**Sodium** 210mg	Dietary Fiber 2g
Saturated Fat 0g	**Protein** 4g	Sugars 2g

Rudi's Organic Bakery, Bagels & Muffins, Whole Grain Wheat English Muffins

1 muffin (57g/2 oz)

Amount per serving	Amount per serving	Amount per serving
Calories 130	**Cholesterol** 0mg	**Total Carbohydrate** 23g
Total Fat 1.5g	**Sodium** 220mg	Dietary Fiber 3g
Saturated Fat 0g	**Protein** 5g	Sugars 3g

Rudi's Organic Bakery, Bakery Breads 100% Whole Wheat

1 slice = 1.5 oz (43g)

Amount per serving	Amount per serving	Amount per serving
Calories 100	**Cholesterol** 0mg	**Total Carbohydrate** 18g
Total Fat 1g	**Sodium** 150mg	Dietary Fiber 3g
Saturated Fat 0g	**Protein** 4g	Sugars 2g

Rudi's Organic Bakery, Bakery Breads 14 Grain

1 slice = 1.4 oz (40g)

Amount per serving	Amount per serving	Amount per serving
Calories 90	**Cholesterol** 0mg	**Total Carbohydrate** 16g
Total Fat 1g	**Sodium** 135mg	Dietary Fiber 3g
Saturated Fat 0g	**Protein** 3g	Sugars 2g

Rudi's Organic Bakery, Bakery Breads 7 Grain with Flax

1 slice = 1.4 oz (40g)

Amount per serving	Amount per serving	Amount per serving
Calories 90	**Cholesterol** 0mg	**Total Carbohydrate** 15g
Total Fat 1.5g	**Sodium** 140mg	Dietary Fiber 3g
Saturated Fat 0g	**Protein** 4g	Sugars 2g

Rudi's Organic Bakery, Bakery Breads Colorado Cracked Wheat

1 slice = 1.5 oz (43g)

Amount per serving	Amount per serving	Amount per serving
Calories 100	**Cholesterol** 0mg	**Total Carbohydrate** 20g
Total Fat 1g	**Sodium** 170mg	Dietary Fiber 2g
Saturated Fat 0g	**Protein** 3g	Sugars 2g

Rudi's Organic Bakery, Bakery Breads Country Morning White

1 slice = 1.5 oz (43g)

Amount per serving	Amount per serving	Amount per serving
Calories 100	**Cholesterol** 0mg	**Total Carbohydrate** 20g
Total Fat 1g	**Sodium** 180mg	Dietary Fiber 1g
Saturated Fat 0g	**Protein** 3g	Sugars 2g

Rudi's Organic Bakery, Bakery Breads Double Fiber

1 slice = 1.6 oz (45g)

Amount per serving	Amount per serving	Amount per serving
Calories 90	**Cholesterol** 0mg	**Total Carbohydrate** 17g
Total Fat 1g	**Sodium** 170mg	Dietary Fiber 6g
Saturated Fat 0g	**Protein** 5g	Sugars 1g

Rudi's Organic Bakery, Bakery Breads Harvest Seeded

1 slice = 1.6 oz (45g)

Amount per serving	Amount per serving	Amount per serving
Calories 110	**Cholesterol** 0mg	**Total Carbohydrate** 19g
Total Fat 3g	**Sodium** 140mg	Dietary Fiber 2g
Saturated Fat 0g	**Protein** 4g	Sugars 3g

Rudi's Organic Bakery, Bakery Breads Honey Sweet Whole Wheat

1 slice = 1.5 oz (43g)

Amount per serving	Amount per serving	Amount per serving
Calories 100	**Cholesterol** 0mg	**Total Carbohydrate** 19g
Total Fat 1g	**Sodium** 160mg	Dietary Fiber 3g
Saturated Fat 0g	**Protein** 4g	Sugars 2g

Rudi's Organic Bakery, Bakery Breads Jewish Light Rye

1 slice = 1.5 oz (43g)

Amount per serving	Amount per serving	Amount per serving
Calories 100	**Cholesterol** 0mg	**Total Carbohydrate** 20g
Total Fat 0.5g	**Sodium** 220mg	Dietary Fiber 1g
Saturated Fat 0g	**Protein** 3g	Sugars 0g

Rudi's Organic Bakery, Bakery Breads Multigrain Oat

1 slice = 1.5 oz (43g)

Amount per serving	Amount per serving	Amount per serving
Calories 100	**Cholesterol** 0mg	**Total Carbohydrate** 20g
Total Fat 1g	**Sodium** 180mg	Dietary Fiber 2g
Saturated Fat 0g	**Protein** 3g	Sugars 2g

Rudi's Organic Bakery, Bakery Breads Nut & Oat

1 slice = 1.5 oz (43g)

Amount per serving	Amount per serving	Amount per serving
Calories 110	Cholesterol 0mg	Total Carbohydrate 20g
Total Fat 1.5g	Sodium 135mg	Dietary Fiber 2g
Saturated Fat 0g	Protein 4g	Sugars 3g

Rudi's Organic Bakery, Bakery Breads Rocky Mountain Sourdough

1 slice = 1.5 oz (43g)

Amount per serving	Amount per serving	Amount per serving
Calories 100	Cholesterol 0mg	Total Carbohydrate 20g
Total Fat 0.5g	Sodium 200mg	Dietary Fiber 1g
Saturated Fat 0g	Protein 3g	Sugars 0g

Rudi's Organic Bakery, Bakery Breads Spelt

1 slice = 1.4 oz (40g)

Amount per serving	Amount per serving	Amount per serving
Calories 80	Cholesterol 0mg	Total Carbohydrate 17g
Total Fat 1g	Sodium 180mg	Dietary Fiber 1g
Saturated Fat 0.5g	Protein 3g	Sugars 3g

Rudi's Organic Bakery, Bakery Breads, Mighty Grains Seeded

1 slice = 1.6 oz (45.4g)

Amount per serving	Amount per serving	Amount per serving
Calories 120	Cholesterol 0mg	Total Carbohydrate 21g
Total Fat 3g	Sodium 150mg	Dietary Fiber 2g
Saturated Fat 0g	Protein 4g	Sugars 3g

Rudi's Organic Bakery, Bakery Breads, Spelt Ancient Grain

1 slice = 1.4 oz (40g)

Amount per serving	Amount per serving	Amount per serving
Calories 110	Cholesterol 0mg	Total Carbohydrate 19g
Total Fat 2.5g	Sodium 170mg	Dietary Fiber 2g
Saturated Fat 0g	Protein 4g	Sugars 3g

Rudi's Organic Bakery, Bakery Breads, Sprouted Honey Wheat

2 slices = 1.8 oz (51g)

Amount per serving	Amount per serving	Amount per serving
Calories 120	Cholesterol 0mg	Total Carbohydrate 25g
Total Fat 1g	Sodium 210mg	Dietary Fiber 3g
Saturated Fat 0g	Protein 5g	Sugars 3g

Rudi's Organic Bakery, Bakery Breads, Sprouted Multigrain

2 slices = 1.8 oz (51g)

Amount per serving	Amount per serving	Amount per serving
Calories 120	**Cholesterol** 0mg	**Total Carbohydrate** 24g
Total Fat 1g	**Sodium** 200mg	Dietary Fiber 3g
Saturated Fat 0g	**Protein** 5g	Sugars 2g

Rudi's Organic Bakery, Bakery Breads, Super Seeded

1 slice = 1.6 oz (45.4g)

Amount per serving	Amount per serving	Amount per serving
Calories 120	**Cholesterol** 0mg	**Total Carbohydrate** 20g
Total Fat 3.5g	**Sodium** 150mg	Dietary Fiber 2g
Saturated Fat 0.5g	**Protein** 4g	Sugars 4g

Rudi's Organic Bakery, Buns & Rolls, Organic 100% Whole Wheat Buns

1 slice = 2.3 oz (65g)

Amount per serving	Amount per serving	Amount per serving
Calories 140	**Cholesterol** 0mg	**Total Carbohydrate** 28g
Total Fat 1.5g	**Sodium** 240mg	Dietary Fiber 5g
Saturated Fat 0g	**Protein** 6g	Sugars 3g

Rudi's Organic Bakery, Buns & Rolls, Pretzel Rolls

1 slice = 1.5 oz (43g)

Amount per serving	Amount per serving	Amount per serving
Calories 100	**Cholesterol** 0mg	**Total Carbohydrate** 51g
Total Fat 0.5g	**Sodium** 470mg	Dietary Fiber 2g
Saturated Fat 0g	**Protein** 7g	Sugars 8g

Rudi's Organic Bakery, Buns & Rolls, Wheat Hamburger Buns

1 slice = 2.3 oz (65g)

Amount per serving	Amount per serving	Amount per serving
Calories 160	**Cholesterol** 0mg	**Total Carbohydrate** 31g
Total Fat 2g	**Sodium** 290mg	Dietary Fiber 3g
Saturated Fat 0g	**Protein** 5g	Sugars 4g

Rudi's Organic Bakery, Buns & Rolls, Wheat Hot Dog Rolls

1 slice = 2 oz (57g)

Amount per serving	Amount per serving	Amount per serving
Calories 140	**Cholesterol** 0mg	**Total Carbohydrate** 27g
Total Fat 1.5g	**Sodium** 250mg	Dietary Fiber 3g
Saturated Fat 0g	**Protein** 4g	Sugars 3g

Rudi's Organic Bakery, Buns & Rolls, White Hamburger Buns

1 slice = 2.3 oz (65g)

Amount per serving	Amount per serving	Amount per serving
Calories 160	**Cholesterol** 0mg	**Total Carbohydrate** 32g
Total Fat 1.5g	**Sodium** 320mg	Dietary Fiber 1g
Saturated Fat 0g	**Protein** 4g	Sugars 4g

Rudi's Organic Bakery, Buns & Rolls, White Hot Dog Rolls

1 slice = 2 oz (57g)

Amount per serving	Amount per serving	Amount per serving
Calories 140	**Cholesterol** 0mg	**Total Carbohydrate** 28g
Total Fat 1.5g	**Sodium** 280mg	Dietary Fiber 1g
Saturated Fat 0g	**Protein** 4g	Sugars 3g

Rudi's Organic Bakery, Frozen Organic, Ancient Grains Bread

1 slice = 1.4 oz (40g)

Amount per serving	Amount per serving	Amount per serving
Calories 110	**Cholesterol** 0mg	**Total Carbohydrate** 19g
Total Fat 2.5g	**Sodium** 170mg	Dietary Fiber 2g
Saturated Fat 0.5g	**Protein** 4g	Sugars 3g

Rudi's Organic Bakery, Frozen Organic, Harvest Marvelous Multigrain

1 slice = 1.4 oz (40g)

Amount per serving	Amount per serving	Amount per serving
Calories 90	**Cholesterol** 0mg	**Total Carbohydrate** 15g
Total Fat 1.5g	**Sodium** 140mg	Dietary Fiber 3g
Saturated Fat 0g	**Protein** 4g	Sugars 2g

Rudi's Organic Bakery, Frozen Organic, Harvest Scrumptious Spelt

1 slice = 1.4 oz (40g)

Amount per serving	Amount per serving	Amount per serving
Calories 80	**Cholesterol** 0mg	**Total Carbohydrate** 17g
Total Fat 1g	**Sodium** 180mg	Dietary Fiber 1g
Saturated Fat 0.5g	**Protein** 3g	Sugars 3g

Rudi's Organic Bakery, Frozen Organic, Harvest Sunshine Seeded

1 slice = 1.6 oz (45g)

Amount per serving	Amount per serving	Amount per serving
Calories 110	**Cholesterol** 0mg	**Total Carbohydrate** 19g
Total Fat 3g	**Sodium** 140mg	Dietary Fiber 2g
Saturated Fat 0g	**Protein** 4g	Sugars 3g

Rudi's Organic Bakery, Sandwich Flatz, 100% Whole Wheat Sandwich Flatz

1 slice = 1.5 oz (43g)

Amount per serving	Amount per serving	Amount per serving
Calories 90	**Cholesterol** 0mg	**Total Carbohydrate** 20g
Total Fat 1g	**Sodium** 170mg	Dietary Fiber 5g
Saturated Fat 0g	**Protein** 4g	Sugars 2g

Rudi's Organic Bakery, Sandwich Flatz, Multigrain Sandwich Flatz

1 slice = 1.5 oz (43g)

Amount per serving	Amount per serving	Amount per serving
Calories 100	**Cholesterol** 0mg	**Total Carbohydrate** 20g
Total Fat 1.5g	**Sodium** 150mg	Dietary Fiber 5g
Saturated Fat 0g	**Protein** 4g	Sugars 1g

Vermont Bread Company, Organic Multigrain Bread

1 slice (31g/1.1 oz)

Amount per serving	Amount per serving	Amount per serving
Calories 80	**Cholesterol** 0mg	**Total Carbohydrate** 17g
Total Fat 1g	**Sodium** 135mg	Dietary Fiber 2g
Saturated Fat 0g	**Protein** 3g	Sugars 2g

Vermont Bread Company, Organic Oat Bread

1 slice (31g/1.1 oz)

Amount per serving	Amount per serving	Amount per serving
Calories 80	**Cholesterol** 0mg	**Total Carbohydrate** 17g
Total Fat 1g	**Sodium** 140mg	Dietary Fiber 2g
Saturated Fat 0g	**Protein** 2g	Sugars 2g

Vermont Bread Company, Organic Old Fashioned White Bread

1 slice (28g)

Amount per serving	Amount per serving	Amount per serving
Calories 70	**Cholesterol** 0mg	**Total Carbohydrate** 14g
Total Fat 1g	**Sodium** 120mg	Dietary Fiber 0g
Saturated Fat 0g	**Protein** 2g	Sugars 1g

Vermont Bread Company, Organic Soft Multigrain Bread

1 slice (40g/1.4 oz)

Amount per serving	Amount per serving	Amount per serving
Calories 110	**Cholesterol** 0mg	**Total Carbohydrate** 21g
Total Fat 2g	**Sodium** 170mg	Dietary Fiber 3g
Saturated Fat 0g	**Protein** 3g	Sugars 2g

Vermont Bread Company, Organic Soft Wheat Bread

1 slice (40g/1.4 oz)

Amount per serving	Amount per serving	Amount per serving
Calories 110	**Cholesterol** 0mg	**Total Carbohydrate** 21g
Total Fat 2g	**Sodium** 200mg	Dietary Fiber 2g
Saturated Fat 0g	**Protein** 3g	Sugars 2g

Vermont Bread Company, Organic Soft White Bread

1 slice (40g/1.4 oz)

Amount per serving	Amount per serving	Amount per serving
Calories 110	**Cholesterol** 0mg	**Total Carbohydrate** 21g
Total Fat 2g	**Sodium** 200mg	Dietary Fiber <1g
Saturated Fat 0g	**Protein** 3g	Sugars 2g

Vermont Bread Company, Organic Spelt Bread

1 slice (31g/1.1 oz)

Amount per serving	Amount per serving	Amount per serving
Calories 90	**Cholesterol** 0mg	**Total Carbohydrate** 17g
Total Fat 1g	**Sodium** 160mg	Dietary Fiber 2g
Saturated Fat 0g	**Protein** 3g	Sugars 2g

Vermont Bread Company, Organic Sprouted Wheat Bread

1 slice (31g)

Amount per serving	Amount per serving	Amount per serving
Calories 70	**Cholesterol** 0mg	**Total Carbohydrate** 14g
Total Fat 1g	**Sodium** 140mg	Dietary Fiber 2g
Saturated Fat 0g	**Protein** 3g	Sugars 1g

Vermont Bread Company, Organic Whole Wheat Bread

1 slice (31g/1.1 oz)

Amount per serving	Amount per serving	Amount per serving
Calories 80	**Cholesterol** 0mg	**Total Carbohydrate** 15g
Total Fat 1.5g	**Sodium** 150mg	Dietary Fiber 2g
Saturated Fat 0g	**Protein** 2g	Sugars <1g

Bread Crumbs

Mary's Gone Crackers, Caraway Crumbs

1/2 cup

Amount per serving	Amount per serving	Amount per serving
Calories 160	**Cholesterol** 0mg	**Total Carbohydrate** 28g
Total Fat 3g	**Sodium** 190mg	Dietary Fiber 3g
Saturated Fat 0g	**Protein** 3g	Sugars 0g

Mary's Gone Crackers, Original Crumbs

1/2 cup

Amount per serving	Amount per serving	Amount per serving
Calories 160	**Cholesterol** 0mg	**Total Carbohydrate** 28g
Total Fat 3g	**Sodium** 190mg	Dietary Fiber 3g
Saturated Fat 0g	**Protein** 3g	Sugars 0g

Cereal Bars

Annie's, Organic Berry Berry Granola Bars

1 bar (28g)

Amount per serving	Amount per serving	Amount per serving
Calories 120	**Cholesterol** 0mg	**Total Carbohydrate** 20g
Total Fat 3.5g	**Sodium** 5mg	Dietary Fiber 1g
Saturated Fat 1.5g	**Protein** 2g	Sugars 7g

Annie's, Organic Chocolate Chip Granola Bars

1 bar (28g)

Amount per serving	Amount per serving	Amount per serving
Calories 120	**Cholesterol** 0mg	**Total Carbohydrate** 19g
Total Fat 4g	**Sodium** 5mg	Dietary Fiber 1g
Saturated Fat 1.5g	**Protein** 2g	Sugars 7g

Annie's, Organic PB & J Granola Bars

1 bar (28g)

Amount per serving	Amount per serving	Amount per serving
Calories 120	**Cholesterol** 0mg	**Total Carbohydrate** 18g
Total Fat 4.5g	**Sodium** 30mg	Dietary Fiber 1g
Saturated Fat 1g	**Protein** 2g	Sugars 8g

Annie's, Organic Peanut Butter Chewy Granola Bars

1 bar (28g)

Amount per serving	Amount per serving	Amount per serving
Calories 120	**Cholesterol** 0mg	**Total Carbohydrate** 18g
Total Fat 4.5g	**Sodium** 30mg	Dietary Fiber 1g
Saturated Fat 1g	**Protein** 3g	Sugars 6g

Bumble Bar Organic Sesame Bar, Amazing Almond

1 bar

Amount per serving	Amount per serving	Amount per serving
Calories 210	**Cholesterol** 0mg	**Total Carbohydrate** 15g
Total Fat 15g	**Sodium** 70mg	Dietary Fiber 5g
Saturated Fat 2g	**Protein** 7g	Sugars 7g

Bumble Bar Organic Sesame Bar, Amazing Almond

1 junior bar

Amount per serving	Amount per serving	Amount per serving
Calories 100	**Cholesterol** 0mg	**Total Carbohydrate** 7g
Total Fat 7g	**Sodium** 30mg	Dietary Fiber 2g
Saturated Fat 1g	**Protein** 3g	Sugars 3g

Bumble Bar Organic Sesame Bar, Awesome Apricot

1 bar

Amount per serving	Amount per serving	Amount per serving
Calories 180	**Cholesterol** 0mg	**Total Carbohydrate** 17g
Total Fat 12g	**Sodium** 65mg	Dietary Fiber 5g
Saturated Fat 4g	**Protein** 4g	Sugars 12g

Bumble Bar Organic Sesame Bar, Chai Almond

1 bar

Amount per serving	Amount per serving	Amount per serving
Calories 200	**Cholesterol** 0mg	**Total Carbohydrate** 18g
Total Fat 12g	**Sodium** 55mg	Dietary Fiber 4g
Saturated Fat 1.5g	**Protein** 7g	Sugars 8g

Bumble Bar Organic Sesame Bar, Cherry Chocolate

1 bar

Amount per serving	Amount per serving	Amount per serving
Calories 180	**Cholesterol** 0mg	**Total Carbohydrate** 19g
Total Fat 12g	**Sodium** 75mg	Dietary Fiber 4g
Saturated Fat 4.5g	**Protein** 4g	Sugars 14g

Bumble Bar Organic Sesame Bar, Chocolate Crisp

1 bar

Amount per serving	Amount per serving	Amount per serving
Calories 190	**Cholesterol** 0mg	**Total Carbohydrate** 21g
Total Fat 11g	**Sodium** 60mg	Dietary Fiber 3g
Saturated Fat 2g	**Protein** 5g	Sugars 10g

Bumble Bar Organic Sesame Bar, Chocolate Crisp

1 junior bar

Amount per serving	Amount per serving	Amount per serving
Calories 90	**Cholesterol** 0mg	**Total Carbohydrate** 10g
Total Fat 5g	**Sodium** 25mg	Dietary Fiber 1g
Saturated Fat 1g	**Protein** 2g	Sugars 4g

Bumble Bar Organic Sesame Bar, Chunky Cherry

1 bar

Amount per serving	Amount per serving	Amount per serving
Calories 180	**Cholesterol** 0mg	**Total Carbohydrate** 18g
Total Fat 12g	**Sodium** 60mg	Dietary Fiber 4g
Saturated Fat 4g	**Protein** 5g	Sugars 13g

Bumble Bar Organic Sesame Bar, Classic Cashew

1 bar

Amount per serving	Amount per serving	Amount per serving
Calories 210	**Cholesterol** 0mg	**Total Carbohydrate** 15g
Total Fat 15g	**Sodium** 70mg	Dietary Fiber 4g
Saturated Fat 2g	**Protein** 7g	Sugars 7g

Bumble Bar Organic Sesame Bar, Harvest Hazelnut

1 bar

Amount per serving	Amount per serving	Amount per serving
Calories 210	**Cholesterol** 0mg	**Total Carbohydrate** 15g
Total Fat 15g	**Sodium** 70mg	Dietary Fiber 5g
Saturated Fat 2g	**Protein** 7g	Sugars 7g

Bumble Bar Organic Sesame Bar, Lushus Lemon

1 bar

Amount per serving	Amount per serving	Amount per serving
Calories 190	**Cholesterol** 0mg	**Total Carbohydrate** 18g
Total Fat 11g	**Sodium** 65mg	Dietary Fiber 4g
Saturated Fat 1.5g	**Protein** 6g	Sugars 8g

Bumble Bar Organic Sesame Bar, Mixed Nut Medley

1 bar

Amount per serving	Amount per serving	Amount per serving
Calories 210	**Cholesterol** 0mg	**Total Carbohydrate** 15g
Total Fat 15g	**Sodium** 70mg	Dietary Fiber 4g
Saturated Fat 2g	**Protein** 7g	Sugars 7g

Bumble Bar Organic Sesame Bar, Original Peanut

1 bar

Amount per serving	Amount per serving	Amount per serving
Calories 210	**Cholesterol** 0mg	**Total Carbohydrate** 15g
Total Fat 15g	**Sodium** 70mg	Dietary Fiber 5g
Saturated Fat 2g	**Protein** 7g	Sugars 7g

Bumble Bar Organic Sesame Bar, Original Peanut

1 junior bar

Amount per serving	Amount per serving	Amount per serving
Calories 100	**Cholesterol** 0mg	**Total Carbohydrate** 7g
Total Fat 7g	**Sodium** 30mg	Dietary Fiber 2g
Saturated Fat 1g	**Protein** 3g	Sugars 3g

Bumble Bar Organic Sesame Bar, Paradise Pineapple

1 bar

Amount per serving	Amount per serving	Amount per serving
Calories 190	**Cholesterol** 0mg	**Total Carbohydrate** 19g
Total Fat 13g	**Sodium** 65mg	Dietary Fiber 4g
Saturated Fat 4.5g	**Protein** 5g	Sugars 14g

Clif, Organic Kid Zbar, Chocolate Brownie

1 bar (36g)

Amount per serving	Amount per serving	Amount per serving
Calories 120	**Cholesterol** 0mg	**Total Carbohydrate** 22g
Total Fat 3.5g	**Sodium** 135mg	Dietary Fiber 3g
Saturated Fat 1g	**Protein** 2g	Sugars 11g

Clif, Organic Kid Zbar, Chocolate Chip

1 bar (36g)

Amount per serving	Amount per serving	Amount per serving
Calories 120	**Cholesterol** 0mg	**Total Carbohydrate** 23g
Total Fat 3g	**Sodium** 95mg	Dietary Fiber 3g
Saturated Fat 1g	**Protein** 2g	Sugars 12g

Clif, Organic Kid Zbar, Honey Graham

1 bar (36g)

Amount per serving	Amount per serving	Amount per serving
Calories 110	**Cholesterol** 0mg	**Total Carbohydrate** 23g
Total Fat 2g	**Sodium** 100mg	Dietary Fiber 3g
Saturated Fat 0g	**Protein** 2g	Sugars 11g

Clif, Organic Kid Zbar, Iced Lemon Cookie

1 bar (36g)

Amount per serving	Amount per serving	Amount per serving
Calories 140	**Cholesterol** 0mg	**Total Carbohydrate** 24g
Total Fat 4g	**Sodium** 90mg	Dietary Fiber 3g
Saturated Fat 1.5g	**Protein** 2g	Sugars 12g

Clif, Organic Kid Zbar, Iced Oatmeal Cookie

1 bar (36g)

Amount per serving	Amount per serving	Amount per serving
Calories 130	**Cholesterol** 0mg	**Total Carbohydrate** 22g
Total Fat 4g	**Sodium** 115mg	Dietary Fiber 3g
Saturated Fat 1g	**Protein** 2g	Sugars 12g

Clif, Organic Kid Zbar, Monster Chocolate Mint (Seasonal)

1 bar (36g)

Amount per serving	Amount per serving	Amount per serving
Calories 130	**Cholesterol** 0mg	**Total Carbohydrate** 23g
Total Fat 3.5g	**Sodium** 135mg	Dietary Fiber 3g
Saturated Fat 1g	**Protein** 2g	Sugars 12g

Glutino, Gluten-Free Chocolate & Banana Organic Bars

1 bar

Amount per serving	Amount per serving	Amount per serving
Calories 100	**Cholesterol** 0mg	**Total Carbohydrate** 21g
Total Fat 1.5g	**Sodium** 35mg	Dietary Fiber 1g
Saturated Fat 0g	**Protein** 1g	Sugars 9g

Glutino, Gluten-Free WildBerry Organic Bars

1 bar

Amount per serving	Amount per serving	Amount per serving
Calories 100	**Cholesterol** 0mg	**Total Carbohydrate** 21g
Total Fat 1g	**Sodium** 65mg	Dietary Fiber 1g
Saturated Fat 0g	**Protein** 1g	Sugars 8g

Go Raw, Banana Bread Flax Bar

1 bar (12g)

Amount per serving	Amount per serving	Amount per serving
Calories 70	**Cholesterol** 0mg	**Total Carbohydrate** 9g
Total Fat 3g	**Sodium** 0mg	Dietary Fiber 2g
Saturated Fat 1g	**Protein** 1g	Sugars 4g

Go Raw, Live Granola Bar

1 bar (14g)

Amount per serving	Amount per serving	Amount per serving
Calories 70	**Cholesterol** 0mg	**Total Carbohydrate** 9g
Total Fat 3g	**Sodium** 0mg	Dietary Fiber 2g
Saturated Fat 0g	**Protein** 1g	Sugars 3g

Go Raw, Live Pumpkin Bar

1 bar (13g)

Amount per serving	Amount per serving	Amount per serving
Calories 60	**Cholesterol** 0mg	**Total Carbohydrate** 4g
Total Fat 4g	**Sodium** 40mg	Dietary Fiber 1g
Saturated Fat 1g	**Protein** 2g	Sugars 3g

Go Raw, Real Live Apricot Bar, Large Bar

1 bar (51g)

Amount per serving	Amount per serving	Amount per serving
Calories 220	**Cholesterol** 0mg	**Total Carbohydrate** 36g
Total Fat 7g	**Sodium** 10mg	Dietary Fiber 7g
Saturated Fat 1g	**Protein** 5g	Sugars 24g

Go Raw, Real Live Apricot Bar, Small Bar

1 bar (12g)

Amount per serving	Amount per serving	Amount per serving
Calories 50	**Cholesterol** 0mg	**Total Carbohydrate** 8g
Total Fat 1.5g	**Sodium** 0mg	Dietary Fiber 2g
Saturated Fat 0g	**Protein** 1g	Sugars 6g

Go Raw, Spirulina Energy Bar

1 bar (14g)

Amount per serving	Amount per serving	Amount per serving
Calories 70	**Cholesterol** 0mg	**Total Carbohydrate** 7g
Total Fat 4g	**Sodium** 0mg	Dietary Fiber 1g
Saturated Fat 1g	**Protein** 1g	Sugars 4g

Health Valley, Organic Apple Cobbler Multigrain Cereal Bars

1 bar (37g)

Amount per serving	Amount per serving	Amount per serving
Calories 130	**Cholesterol** 0mg	**Total Carbohydrate** 27g
Total Fat 2.5g	**Sodium** 85mg	Dietary Fiber 3g
Saturated Fat 0g	**Protein** 2g	Sugars 16g

Health Valley, Organic Blueberry Cobbler Multigrain Cereal Bars

1 bar (37g)

Amount per serving	Amount per serving	Amount per serving
Calories 130	**Cholesterol** 0mg	**Total Carbohydrate** 27g
Total Fat 2.5g	**Sodium** 85mg	Dietary Fiber 3g
Saturated Fat 0g	**Protein** 2g	Sugars 16g

Health Valley, Organic Strawberry Cobbler Multigrain Cereal Bars

1 bar (37g)

Amount per serving	Amount per serving	Amount per serving
Calories 130	**Cholesterol** 0mg	**Total Carbohydrate** 27g
Total Fat 2.5g	**Sodium** 85mg	Dietary Fiber 3g
Saturated Fat 0g	**Protein** 2g	Sugars 16g

Health Valley, Pumpkin-N-Spice™ Flax Plus® Granola Bars

1 bar (35g)

Amount per serving	Amount per serving	Amount per serving
Calories 140	**Cholesterol** 0mg	**Total Carbohydrate** 23g
Total Fat 4g	**Sodium** 80mg	Dietary Fiber 2g
Saturated Fat 0.5g	**Protein** 3g	Sugars 10g

Nature's Path, Apple Pie Crunch Chia Plus™

2 bars (40g)

Amount per serving	Amount per serving	Amount per serving
Calories 190	**Cholesterol** 0mg	**Total Carbohydrate** 27g
Total Fat 8g	**Sodium** 120mg	Dietary Fiber 3g
Saturated Fat 1g	**Protein** 3g	Sugars 8g

Nature's Path, Berry Blast™ Crispy Rice Bars

1 bar (28g)

Amount per serving	Amount per serving	Amount per serving
Calories 110	**Cholesterol** 0mg	**Total Carbohydrate** 21g
Total Fat 3g	**Sodium** 70mg	Dietary Fiber 1g
Saturated Fat 0g	**Protein** 1g	Sugars 7g

Nature's Path, Berry Strawberry™ Flax Plus® Granola Bars

1 bar (35g)

Amount per serving	Amount per serving	Amount per serving
Calories 140	**Cholesterol** 0mg	**Total Carbohydrate** 25g
Total Fat 3.5g	**Sodium** 80mg	Dietary Fiber 2g
Saturated Fat 0.5g	**Protein** 2g	Sugars 11g

Nature's Path, Chococonut™ Granola Bars

1 bar (35g)

Amount per serving	Amount per serving	Amount per serving
Calories 140	**Cholesterol** 0mg	**Total Carbohydrate** 24g
Total Fat 4.5g	**Sodium** 35mg	Dietary Fiber 2g
Saturated Fat 1.5g	**Protein** 2g	Sugars 11g

Nature's Path, Chocolate Crispy Rice Bars

1 bar (28g)

Amount per serving	Amount per serving	Amount per serving
Calories 110	**Cholesterol** 0mg	**Total Carbohydrate** 21g
Total Fat 2.5g	**Sodium** 75mg	Dietary Fiber 1g
Saturated Fat 0.5g	**Protein** 1g	Sugars 8g

Nature's Path, Chunky Chocolate Peanut Chewy Granola Bars

1 bar (35g)

Amount per serving	Amount per serving	Amount per serving
Calories 140	**Cholesterol** 0mg	**Total Carbohydrate** 24g
Total Fat 4.5g	**Sodium** 110mg	Dietary Fiber 2g
Saturated Fat 1g	**Protein** 3g	Sugars 9g

Nature's Path, Dark Chocolate Chip Chewy Granola Bar

1 bar (35g)

Amount per serving	Amount per serving	Amount per serving
Calories 140	**Cholesterol** 0mg	**Total Carbohydrate** 26g
Total Fat 3.5g	**Sodium** 70mg	Dietary Fiber 2g
Saturated Fat 1g	**Protein** 2g	Sugars 10g

Nature's Path, Honey Oat Crunch Flax Plus®

2 bars (40g)

Amount per serving	Amount per serving	Amount per serving
Calories 190	**Cholesterol** 0mg	**Total Carbohydrate** 28g
Total Fat 7g	**Sodium** 60mg	Dietary Fiber 3g
Saturated Fat 1g	**Protein** 3g	Sugars 9g

Nature's Path, Lotta' Apricotta™ Granola Bars

1 bar (35g)

Amount per serving	Amount per serving	Amount per serving
Calories 140	**Cholesterol** 0mg	**Total Carbohydrate** 23g
Total Fat 5g	**Sodium** 70mg	Dietary Fiber 2g
Saturated Fat 1.5g	**Protein** 2g	Sugars 12g

Nature's Path, Macaroon Crunch

2 bars (40g)

Amount per serving	Amount per serving	Amount per serving
Calories 200	**Cholesterol** 0mg	**Total Carbohydrate** 27g
Total Fat 8g	**Sodium** 70mg	Dietary Fiber 3g
Saturated Fat 1.5g	**Protein** 3g	Sugars 8g

Nature's Path, Mmmaple Pecan™ Flax Plus® Granola Bars

1 bar (35g)

Amount per serving	Amount per serving	Amount per serving
Calories 150	**Cholesterol** 0mg	**Total Carbohydrate** 22g
Total Fat 6g	**Sodium** 105mg	Dietary Fiber 2g
Saturated Fat 1.5g	**Protein** 2g	Sugars 10g

Nature's Path, Peanut Buddy™ Granola Bars

1 bar (35g)

Amount per serving	Amount per serving	Amount per serving
Calories 140	**Cholesterol** 0mg	**Total Carbohydrate** 22g
Total Fat 5g	**Sodium** 135mg	Dietary Fiber 2g
Saturated Fat 0.5g	**Protein** 3g	Sugars 10g

Nature's Path, Peanut Butter Crispy Rice Bars

1 bar (28g)

Amount per serving	Amount per serving	Amount per serving
Calories 110	**Cholesterol** 0mg	**Total Carbohydrate** 20g
Total Fat 3g	**Sodium** 65mg	Dietary Fiber 1g
Saturated Fat 0g	**Protein** 2g	Sugars 7g

Nature's Path, Peanut Choco Drizzle™ Crispy Rice Bars

1 bar (28g)

Amount per serving	Amount per serving	Amount per serving
Calories 120	**Cholesterol** 0mg	**Total Carbohydrate** 18g
Total Fat 4.5g	**Sodium** 50mg	Dietary Fiber 1g
Saturated Fat 1g	**Protein** 2g	Sugars 8g

Nature's Path, Peanut Choco™ Granola Bars

1 bar (35g)

Amount per serving	Amount per serving	Amount per serving
Calories 150	**Cholesterol** 0mg	**Total Carbohydrate** 22g
Total Fat 6g	**Sodium** 125mg	Dietary Fiber 2g
Saturated Fat 1.5g	**Protein** 3g	Sugars 11g

Nature's Path, Peanut Coco™ Crunch Ancient Grains

2 bars (40g)

Amount per serving	Amount per serving	Amount per serving
Calories 190	**Cholesterol** 0mg	**Total Carbohydrate** 27g
Total Fat 8g	**Sodium** 60mg	Dietary Fiber 3g
Saturated Fat 1g	**Protein** 4g	Sugars 8g

Nature's Path, Sunny Hemp™ Hemp Plus® Granola Bars

1 bar (35g)

Amount per serving	Amount per serving	Amount per serving
Calories 140	**Cholesterol** 0mg	**Total Carbohydrate** 24g
Total Fat 3.5g	**Sodium** 90mg	Dietary Fiber 3g
Saturated Fat 0.5g	**Protein** 3g	Sugars 11g

Nature's Path, Trail Mixer Chewy Granola Bar

1 bar (35g)

Amount per serving	Amount per serving	Amount per serving
Calories 140	**Cholesterol** 0mg	**Total Carbohydrate** 23g
Total Fat 4g	**Sodium** 90mg	Dietary Fiber 3g
Saturated Fat 1g	**Protein** 3g	Sugars 9g

Cereals

Ancient Harvest, Gluten-Free Quinoa Hot Cereal Flakes

1/3 cup dry

Amount per serving	Amount per serving	Amount per serving
Calories 131	**Cholesterol** 0mg	**Total Carbohydrate** 23g
Total Fat 2g	**Sodium** 2mg	Dietary Fiber 2.4g
Saturated Fat 0g	**Protein** 4.3g	Sugars 2g

Arrowhead Mills, Organic Rice and Shine Hot Cereal

1/4 cup

Amount per serving	Amount per serving	Amount per serving
Calories 150	**Cholesterol** 0mg	**Total Carbohydrate** 32g
Total Fat 1g	**Sodium** 0mg	Dietary Fiber 2g
Saturated Fat 0g	**Protein** 3g	Sugars 0g

Barbara's Bakery, Organic Corn Flakes

1 cup (30g)

Amount per serving	Amount per serving	Amount per serving
Calories 110	**Cholesterol** 0mg	**Total Carbohydrate** 25g
Total Fat 1g	**Sodium** 80mg	Dietary Fiber 0g
Saturated Fat 0g	**Protein** 0g	Sugars 3g

Barbara's Bakery, Organic Honest O's Honey Nut

1 cup (30g)

Amount per serving	Amount per serving	Amount per serving
Calories 120	**Cholesterol** 0mg	**Total Carbohydrate** 24g
Total Fat 2g	**Sodium** 80mg	Dietary Fiber 2g
Saturated Fat 0g	**Protein** 0g	Sugars 10g

Barbara's Bakery, Organic Honest O's Multigrain

1 cup (30g)

Amount per serving	Amount per serving	Amount per serving
Calories 110	Cholesterol 0mg	Total Carbohydrate 25g
Total Fat 0.5g	Sodium 20mg	Dietary Fiber 3g
Saturated Fat 0g	Protein 0g	Sugars 5g

Barbara's Bakery, Organic Honest O's Original

1 cup (30g)

Amount per serving	Amount per serving	Amount per serving
Calories 120	Cholesterol 0mg	Total Carbohydrate 22g
Total Fat 2g	Sodium 80mg	Dietary Fiber 3g
Saturated Fat 0g	Protein 0g	Sugars 1g

Barbara's Bakery, Snackimals Chocolate Crisp Cereal

3/4 cup (30g)

Amount per serving	Amount per serving	Amount per serving
Calories 110	Cholesterol 0mg	Total Carbohydrate 25g
Total Fat 0.5g	Sodium 80mg	Dietary Fiber 0g
Saturated Fat 0g	Protein 0g	Sugars 0g

Barbara's Bakery, Snackimals Cinnamon Crunch Cereal

3/4 cup (30g)

Amount per serving	Amount per serving	Amount per serving
Calories 110	Cholesterol 0mg	Total Carbohydrate 26g
Total Fat 0.5g	Sodium 80mg	Dietary Fiber 3g
Saturated Fat 0g	Protein 0g	Sugars 7g

Barbara's Bakery, Snackimals Vanilla Blast Cereal

3/4 cup (30g)

Amount per serving	Amount per serving	Amount per serving
Calories 110	Cholesterol 0mg	Total Carbohydrate 26g
Total Fat 0.5g	Sodium 80mg	Dietary Fiber 3g
Saturated Fat 0g	Protein 0g	Sugars 7g

Bob's Red Mill, Organic Brown Rice Farina

1/4 cup

Amount per serving	Amount per serving	Amount per serving
Calories 150	Cholesterol 0mg	Total Carbohydrate 32g
Total Fat 1g	Sodium 5mg	Dietary Fiber 2g
Saturated Fat 0g	Protein 3g	Sugars 0g

Bob's Red Mill, Organic Creamy Buckwheat

1/4 cup

Amount per serving | Amount per serving | Amount per serving

Calories 140
Total Fat 1g
  Saturated Fat 0g

Cholesterol 0mg
Sodium 0mg
Protein 5g

Total Carbohydrate 30g
  Dietary Fiber 3g
  Sugars 0g

Cascadian Farm Organic, Ancient Grains Granola

2/3 cup (57g)

Amount per serving | Amount per serving | Amount per serving

Calories 230
Total Fat 5g
  Saturated Fat 1g

Cholesterol 0mg
Sodium 100mg
Protein 5g

Total Carbohydrate 43g
  Dietary Fiber 6g
  Sugars 10g

Cascadian Farm Organic, Berry Cobbler Granola

1/2 cup (47g)

Amount per serving | Amount per serving | Amount per serving

Calories 180
Total Fat 3g
  Saturated Fat 0.5g

Cholesterol 0mg
Sodium 70mg
Protein 4g

Total Carbohydrate 36g
  Dietary Fiber 3g
  Sugars 12g

Cascadian Farm Organic, Buzz Crunch Honey Almond Cereal

1 cup (60g)

Amount per serving | Amount per serving | Amount per serving

Calories 230
Total Fat 2.5g
  Saturated Fat 0g

Cholesterol 0mg
Sodium 270mg
Protein 5g

Total Carbohydrate 47g
  Dietary Fiber 3g
  Sugars 11g

Cascadian Farm Organic, Chocolate O's Cereal

3/4 cup (28g)

Amount per serving | Amount per serving | Amount per serving

Calories 100
Total Fat 0.5g
  Saturated Fat 0g

Cholesterol 0mg
Sodium 4mg
Protein 2g

Total Carbohydrate 24g
  Dietary Fiber 14g
  Sugars 8g

Cascadian Farm Organic, Cinnamon Crunch Cereal

3/4 cup (27g)

Amount per serving | Amount per serving | Amount per serving

Calories 110
Total Fat 2.5g
  Saturated Fat 0g

Cholesterol 0mg
Sodium 105mg
Protein 1g

Total Carbohydrate 22g
  Dietary Fiber 3g
  Sugars 8g

Cascadian Farm Organic, Cinnamon Raisin Granola

2/3 cup (60g)

Amount per serving	Amount per serving	Amount per serving
Calories 230	**Cholesterol** 0mg	**Total Carbohydrate** 46g
Total Fat 3g	**Sodium** 230mg	Dietary Fiber 3g
Saturated Fat 0.5g	**Protein** 5g	Sugars 18g

Cascadian Farm Organic, Dark Chocolate Almond Granola

2/3 cup (60g)

Amount per serving	Amount per serving	Amount per serving
Calories 250	**Cholesterol** 0mg	**Total Carbohydrate** 45g
Total Fat 5g	**Sodium** 180mg	Dietary Fiber 5g
Saturated Fat 1g	**Protein** 5g	Sugars 16g

Cascadian Farm Organic, French Vanilla Almond Granola

2/3 cup (58g)

Amount per serving	Amount per serving	Amount per serving
Calories 240	**Cholesterol** 0mg	**Total Carbohydrate** 43g
Total Fat 6g	**Sodium** 100mg	Dietary Fiber 3g
Saturated Fat 1g	**Protein** 5g	Sugars 15g

Cascadian Farm Organic, Fruit & Nut Granola

2/3 cup (59g)

Amount per serving	Amount per serving	Amount per serving
Calories 230	**Cholesterol** 0mg	**Total Carbohydrate** 43g
Total Fat 5g	**Sodium** 95mg	Dietary Fiber 3g
Saturated Fat 1g	**Protein** 5g	Sugars 17g

Cascadian Farm Organic, Fruitful O's Cereal

3/4 cup (28g)

Amount per serving	Amount per serving	Amount per serving
Calories 100	**Cholesterol** 0mg	**Total Carbohydrate** 8g
Total Fat 1g	**Sodium** 130mg	Dietary Fiber 3g
Saturated Fat 0g	**Protein** 2g	Sugars 8g

Cascadian Farm Organic, Graham Crunch Cereal

3/4 cup (28g)

Amount per serving	Amount per serving	Amount per serving
Calories 110	**Cholesterol** 0mg	**Total Carbohydrate** 23g
Total Fat 2g	**Sodium** 140mg	Dietary Fiber 3g
Saturated Fat 0g	**Protein** 2g	Sugars 8g

Cascadian Farm Organic, Hearty Morning® Cereal

3/4 cup (48g)

Amount per serving	Amount per serving	Amount per serving
Calories 170	**Cholesterol** 0mg	**Total Carbohydrate** 38g
Total Fat 2g	**Sodium** 150mg	Dietary Fiber 8g
Saturated Fat 0.5g	**Protein** 4g	Sugars 8g

Cascadian Farm Organic, Honey Nut O's Cereal

1 cup (30g)

Amount per serving	Amount per serving	Amount per serving
Calories 110	**Cholesterol** 0mg	**Total Carbohydrate** 25g
Total Fat 1g	**Sodium** 170mg	Dietary Fiber 3g
Saturated Fat 0g	**Protein** 2g	Sugars 7g

Cascadian Farm Organic, Maple Brown Sugar Granola

2/3 cup (57g)

Amount per serving	Amount per serving	Amount per serving
Calories 220	**Cholesterol** 0mg	**Total Carbohydrate** 44g
Total Fat 4g	**Sodium** 130mg	Dietary Fiber 3g
Saturated Fat 1g	**Protein** 5g	Sugars 15g

Cascadian Farm Organic, Multi Grain Squares Cereal

1 cup (53g)

Amount per serving	Amount per serving	Amount per serving
Calories 210	**Cholesterol** 0mg	**Total Carbohydrate** 44g
Total Fat 1g	**Sodium** 190mg	Dietary Fiber 4g
Saturated Fat 0g	**Protein** 5g	Sugars 7g

Cascadian Farm Organic, Oats & Honey Granola

2/3 cup (55g)

Amount per serving	Amount per serving	Amount per serving
Calories 230	**Cholesterol** 0mg	**Total Carbohydrate** 42g
Total Fat 6g	**Sodium** 110mg	Dietary Fiber 3g
Saturated Fat 1g	**Protein** 5g	Sugars 14g

Cascadian Farm Organic, Protein Granola, Apple Crisp

3/4 cup (56g)

Amount per serving	Amount per serving	Amount per serving
Calories 230	**Cholesterol** 0mg	**Total Carbohydrate** 38g
Total Fat 5g	**Sodium** 105mg	Dietary Fiber 4g
Saturated Fat 0.5g	**Protein** 10g	Sugars 13g

Cascadian Farm Organic, Protein Granola, Dark Chocolate Coconut

3/4 cup (57g)

Amount per serving	Amount per serving	Amount per serving
Calories 250	**Cholesterol** 0mg	**Total Carbohydrate** 36g
Total Fat 8g	**Sodium** 105mg	Dietary Fiber 4g
Saturated Fat 3g	**Protein** 10g	Sugars 12g

Cascadian Farm Organic, Purely O's® Cereal

1 1/4 cup (32g)

Amount per serving	Amount per serving	Amount per serving
Calories 120	**Cholesterol** 0mg	**Total Carbohydrate** 25g
Total Fat 1.5g	**Sodium** 200mg	Dietary Fiber 3g
Saturated Fat 0g	**Protein** 3g	Sugars 1g

Cascadian Farm Organic, Raisin Bran Cereal

1 cup (51g)

Amount per serving	Amount per serving	Amount per serving
Calories 180	**Cholesterol** 0mg	**Total Carbohydrate** 41g
Total Fat 1g	**Sodium** 240mg	Dietary Fiber 6g
Saturated Fat 0g	**Protein** 4g	Sugars 12g

Country Choice Organic, Fit Kids Instant Oatmeal, Berry Blast

1 pouch (36g)

Amount per serving	Amount per serving	Amount per serving
Calories 130	**Cholesterol** 0mg	**Total Carbohydrate** 26g
Total Fat 1.5g	**Sodium** 100mg	Dietary Fiber 3g
Saturated Fat 0g	**Protein** 4g	Sugars 9g

Country Choice Organic, Fit Kids Instant Oatmeal, Caramel Apple

1 pouch (36g)

Amount per serving	Amount per serving	Amount per serving
Calories 130	**Cholesterol** 0mg	**Total Carbohydrate** 26g
Total Fat 1.5g	**Sodium** 100mg	Dietary Fiber 1g
Saturated Fat 0g	**Protein** 4g	Sugars 9g

Country Choice Organic, Fit Kids Instant Oatmeal, Chocolate Chip

1 pouch (37g)

Amount per serving	Amount per serving	Amount per serving
Calories 140	**Cholesterol** 0mg	**Total Carbohydrate** 27g
Total Fat 2.5g	**Sodium** 100mg	Dietary Fiber 3g
Saturated Fat 0.5g	**Protein** 4g	Sugars 10g

Country Choice Organic, Fit Kids Instant Oatmeal, Cinnamon Toast

1 pouch (34g)

Amount per serving	Amount per serving	Amount per serving
Calories 130	**Cholesterol** 0mg	**Total Carbohydrate** 25g
Total Fat 1.5g	**Sodium** 100mg	Dietary Fiber 3g
Saturated Fat 0g	**Protein** 4g	Sugars 9g

Country Choice Organic, Instant Oatmeal, Apple Cinnamon

1 packet (36g)

Amount per serving	Amount per serving	Amount per serving
Calories 130	**Cholesterol** 0mg	**Total Carbohydrate** 27g
Total Fat 1.5g	**Sodium** 130mg	Dietary Fiber 3g
Saturated Fat 0g	**Protein** 4g	Sugars 11g

Country Choice Organic, Instant Oatmeal, Maple

1 packet (43g)

Amount per serving	Amount per serving	Amount per serving
Calories 170	**Cholesterol** 135mg	**Total Carbohydrate** 32g
Total Fat 2g	**Sodium** 135mg	Dietary Fiber 3g
Saturated Fat 0g	**Protein** 4g	Sugars 9g

Country Choice Organic, Instant Oatmeal, Original with Flax

1 packet (29g)

Amount per serving	Amount per serving	Amount per serving
Calories 110	**Cholesterol** 0mg	**Total Carbohydrate** 19g
Total Fat 2g	**Sodium** 0mg	Dietary Fiber 3g
Saturated Fat 0g	**Protein** 4g	Sugars 1g

Country Choice Organic, Multigrain Hot Cereal

1/2 cup dry (40g)

Amount per serving	Amount per serving	Amount per serving
Calories 130	**Cholesterol** 0mg	**Total Carbohydrate** 29g
Total Fat 1g	**Sodium** 0mg	Dietary Fiber 5g
Saturated Fat 0g	**Protein** 5g	Sugars 0g

Country Choice Organic, Multigrain Oatmeal, Cranberry Apple

1 packet (45g)

Amount per serving	Amount per serving	Amount per serving
Calories 170	**Cholesterol** 0mg	**Total Carbohydrate** 35g
Total Fat 2g	**Sodium** 140mg	Dietary Fiber 4g
Saturated Fat 0g	**Protein** 4g	Sugars 12g

Country Choice Organic, Multigrain Oatmeal, Maple Spice with Raisins

1 packet (45g)

Amount per serving	Amount per serving	Amount per serving
Calories 160	**Cholesterol** 0mg	**Total Carbohydrate** 34g
Total Fat 2g	**Sodium** 140mg	Dietary Fiber 4g
Saturated Fat 0g	**Protein** 4g	Sugars 13g

Country Choice Organic, Old Fashioned Oats

1/2 cup dry (40g)

Amount per serving	Amount per serving	Amount per serving
Calories 150	**Cholesterol** 0mg	**Total Carbohydrate** 27g
Total Fat 3g	**Sodium** 0mg	Dietary Fiber 4g
Saturated Fat 0.5g	**Protein** 5g	Sugars 1g

Country Choice Organic, Quick Cook Steel Cut Instant Oats

1 packet (40g)

Amount per serving	Amount per serving	Amount per serving
Calories 150	**Cholesterol** 0mg	**Total Carbohydrate** 27g
Total Fat 3g	**Sodium** 0mg	Dietary Fiber 4g
Saturated Fat 0g	**Protein** 5g	Sugars 1g

Country Choice Organic, Quick Oats

1/2 cup dry (40g)

Amount per serving	Amount per serving	Amount per serving
Calories 150	**Cholesterol** 0mg	**Total Carbohydrate** 27g
Total Fat 3g	**Sodium** 0mg	Dietary Fiber 4g
Saturated Fat 0.5g	**Protein** 5g	Sugars 1g

Country Choice Organic, Steel Cut Oats

1/4 cup dry (40g)

Amount per serving	Amount per serving	Amount per serving
Calories 150	**Cholesterol** 0mg	**Total Carbohydrate** 27g
Total Fat 3g	**Sodium** 0mg	Dietary Fiber 4g
Saturated Fat 0g	**Protein** 5g	Sugars 1g

Country Choice Organic, Whole Grain Steel Cut Oats

1/4 cup dry (40g)

Amount per serving	Amount per serving	Amount per serving
Calories 150	**Cholesterol** 0mg	**Total Carbohydrate** 27g
Total Fat 3g	**Sodium** 0mg	Dietary Fiber 4g
Saturated Fat 0g	**Protein** 5g	Sugars 1g

Dr. McDougall's Right Foods, Apple Flax Oatmeal

3/4 cup prepared (64g)

Amount per serving	Amount per serving	Amount per serving
Calories 250	Cholesterol 0mg	Total Carbohydrate 48g
Total Fat 3.5g	Sodium 270mg	Dietary Fiber 7g
Saturated Fat 0.5g	Protein 6g	Sugars 18g

Dr. McDougall's Right Foods, Cranberry Almond Oatmeal

3/4 cup prepared (87g)

Amount per serving	Amount per serving	Amount per serving
Calories 330	Cholesterol 0mg	Total Carbohydrate 64g
Total Fat 4g	Sodium 200mg	Dietary Fiber 6g
Saturated Fat 1g	Protein 9g	Sugars 20g

Dr. McDougall's Right Foods, Fruit, Flax & Nuts Oatmeal Made with Organic Oats

3/4 cup prepared (70g)

Amount per serving	Amount per serving	Amount per serving
Calories 310	Cholesterol 0mg	Total Carbohydrate 59g
Total Fat 4.5g	Sodium 330mg	Dietary Fiber 8g
Saturated Fat 1g	Protein 7g	Sugars 21g

Dr. McDougall's Right Foods, Hemp Peach Oatmeal

3/4 cup prepared (84g)

Amount per serving	Amount per serving	Amount per serving
Calories 330	Cholesterol 0mg	Total Carbohydrate 63g
Total Fat 5g	Sodium 200mg	Dietary Fiber 8g
Saturated Fat 1g	Protein 8g	Sugars 28g

Dr. McDougall's Right Foods, Organic Instant Oatmeal, Original

1 packet (28g)

Amount per serving	Amount per serving	Amount per serving
Calories 120	Cholesterol 0mg	Total Carbohydrate 21g
Total Fat 2g	Sodium 40mg	Dietary Fiber 3g
Saturated Fat 0g	Protein 4g	Sugars 0g

Dr. McDougall's Right Foods, Organic Light Oatmeal, Apple Cinnamon

1 packet (30g)

Amount per serving	Amount per serving	Amount per serving
Calories 120	Cholesterol 0mg	Total Carbohydrate 22g
Total Fat 1.5g	Sodium 110mg	Dietary Fiber 3g
Saturated Fat 0g	Protein 3g	Sugars 6g

Dr. McDougall's Right Foods, Organic Light Oatmeal, Maple Brown Sugar

1 packet (38g)

Amount per serving	Amount per serving	Amount per serving
Calories 150	**Cholesterol** 0mg	**Total Carbohydrate** 28g
Total Fat 2g	**Sodium** 180mg	Dietary Fiber 4g
Saturated Fat 0g	**Protein** 5g	Sugars 6g

Dr. McDougall's Right Foods, Organic Maple Oatmeal

3/4 cup prepared (70g)

Amount per serving	Amount per serving	Amount per serving
Calories 270	**Cholesterol** 0mg	**Total Carbohydrate** 55g
Total Fat 3.5g	**Sodium** 290mg	Dietary Fiber 7g
Saturated Fat 0.5g	**Protein** 6g	Sugars 18g

Eden Foods, Buckwheat, 100% Whole Grain, Organic, Uncooked

1/4 cup

Amount per serving	Amount per serving	Amount per serving
Calories 160	**Cholesterol** 0mg	**Total Carbohydrate** 31g
Total Fat 1g	**Sodium** 0mg	Dietary Fiber 5g
Saturated Fat 0g	**Protein** 5g	Sugars 0g

Erewhon, Buckwheat & Hemp

3/4 cup

Amount per serving	Amount per serving	Amount per serving
Calories 220	**Cholesterol** 0mg	**Total Carbohydrate** 42g
Total Fat 3g	**Sodium** 210mg	Dietary Fiber 5g
Saturated Fat 1g	**Protein** 6g	Sugars 6g

Erewhon, Cocoa Crispy Brown Rice Cereal

1 cup

Amount per serving	Amount per serving	Amount per serving
Calories 200	**Cholesterol** 0mg	**Total Carbohydrate** 44g
Total Fat 1.5g	**Sodium** 190mg	Dietary Fiber 1g
Saturated Fat 0g	**Protein** 3g	Sugars 11g

Erewhon, Corn Flakes

1 cup

Amount per serving	Amount per serving	Amount per serving
Calories 130	**Cholesterol** 0mg	**Total Carbohydrate** 30g
Total Fat 0g	**Sodium** 60mg	Dietary Fiber 1g
Saturated Fat 0g	**Protein** 3g	Sugars 0g

Erewhon, Crispy Brown Rice Gluten Free Cereal

1 cup

Amount per serving	Amount per serving	Amount per serving
Calories 110	**Cholesterol** 0mg	**Total Carbohydrate** 25g
Total Fat 0.5g	**Sodium** 160mg	Dietary Fiber 0g
Saturated Fat 0g	**Protein** 2g	Sugars <1g

Erewhon, Crispy Brown Rice No Salt Added Cereal

1 cup

Amount per serving	Amount per serving	Amount per serving
Calories 110	**Cholesterol** 0mg	**Total Carbohydrate** 25g
Total Fat 0.5g	**Sodium** 10mg	Dietary Fiber 0g
Saturated Fat 0g	**Protein** 2g	Sugars <1g

Erewhon, Crispy Brown Rice with Mixed Berries Cereal

1 cup

Amount per serving	Amount per serving	Amount per serving
Calories 120	**Cholesterol** 0mg	**Total Carbohydrate** 27g
Total Fat 0.5g	**Sodium** 100mg	Dietary Fiber 1g
Saturated Fat 0g	**Protein** 2g	Sugars 6g

Erewhon, Quinoa & Chia

3/4 cup

Amount per serving	Amount per serving	Amount per serving
Calories 230	**Cholesterol** 0mg	**Total Carbohydrate** 43g
Total Fat 3.5g	**Sodium** 190mg	Dietary Fiber 5g
Saturated Fat 0g	**Protein** 6g	Sugars <1g

Erewhon, Raisin Bran

1 cup

Amount per serving	Amount per serving	Amount per serving
Calories 180	**Cholesterol** 0mg	**Total Carbohydrate** 40g
Total Fat 1g	**Sodium** 115mg	Dietary Fiber 6g
Saturated Fat 0g	**Protein** 6g	Sugars 8g

Erewhon, Rice Twice Cereal

3/4 cup

Amount per serving	Amount per serving	Amount per serving
Calories 120	**Cholesterol** 0mg	**Total Carbohydrate** 26g
Total Fat 0g	**Sodium** 60mg	Dietary Fiber 0g
Saturated Fat 0g	**Protein** 2g	Sugars 8g

Erewhon, Strawberry Crisp

3/4 cup

Amount per serving	Amount per serving	Amount per serving
Calories 120	Cholesterol 0mg	Total Carbohydrate 28g
Total Fat 0.5g	Sodium 125mg	Dietary Fiber 1g
Saturated Fat 0g	Protein 2g	Sugars 6g

Health Valley Organic, Fiber 7 Flakes Baked Multigrain Cereal

1 cup (53g)

Amount per serving	Amount per serving	Amount per serving
Calories 200	Cholesterol 0mg	Total Carbohydrate 43g
Total Fat 1.5g	Sodium 160mg	Dietary Fiber 4g
Saturated Fat 0g	Protein 5g	Sugars 18g

Health Valley Organic, Oat Bran Flakes Baked Multigrain Cereal

1 cup (50g)

Amount per serving	Amount per serving	Amount per serving
Calories 190	Cholesterol 0mg	Total Carbohydrate 39g
Total Fat 1.5g	Sodium 190mg	Dietary Fiber 4g
Saturated Fat 0.5g	Protein 5g	Sugars 11g

Health Valley Organic, Organic Sprouted Amaranth Flakes Baked Multigrain Cereal

1 1/4 cup (55g)

Amount per serving	Amount per serving	Amount per serving
Calories 210	Cholesterol 0mg	Total Carbohydrate 43g
Total Fat 2g	Sodium 190mg	Dietary Fiber 5g
Saturated Fat 0.5g	Protein 6g	Sugars 11g

Kashi®, Kashi Organic Corn Flakes, Indigo Morning Cereal

3/4 cup (27g)

Amount per serving	Amount per serving	Amount per serving
Calories 100	Cholesterol 0mg	Total Carbohydrate 22g
Total Fat 1g	Sodium 125mg	Dietary Fiber 2g
Saturated Fat 0g	Protein 2g	Sugars 6g

Kashi®, Kashi Organic Corn Flakes, Simply Maize Cereal

3/4 cup (27g)

Amount per serving	Amount per serving	Amount per serving
Calories 100	Cholesterol 0mg	Total Carbohydrate 23g
Total Fat 1g	Sodium 110mg	Dietary Fiber 2g
Saturated Fat 0g	Protein 2g	Sugars 6g

Kirkland Signature by Nature's Path, Organic Ancient Grains Granola with Almonds

3/4 cup (55g)

Amount per serving	Amount per serving	Amount per serving
Calories 250	**Cholesterol** 0mg	**Total Carbohydrate** 39g
Total Fat 9g	**Sodium** 135mg	Dietary Fiber 6g
Saturated Fat 1.5g	**Protein** 5g	Sugars 9g

Manna Organics, Organic Steel Cut Oats

1 oz (28g)

Amount per serving	Amount per serving	Amount per serving
Calories 110	**Cholesterol** 0mg	**Total Carbohydrate** 19g
Total Fat 2g	**Sodium** 0mg	Dietary Fiber 3g
Saturated Fat 0g	**Protein** 5g	Sugars 0g

Nature's Path, Amazon® Frosted Flakes

2/3 cup (30g)

Amount per serving	Amount per serving	Amount per serving
Calories 120	**Cholesterol** 0mg	**Total Carbohydrate** 26g
Total Fat 0g	**Sodium** 115mg	Dietary Fiber 2g
Saturated Fat 0g	**Protein** 2g	Sugars 6g

Nature's Path, Apple Cinnamon Hot Oatmeal

1 packet (50g)

Amount per serving	Amount per serving	Amount per serving
Calories 210	**Cholesterol** 0mg	**Total Carbohydrate** 40g
Total Fat 2.5g	**Sodium** 100mg	Dietary Fiber 4g
Saturated Fat 0g	**Protein** 5g	Sugars 14g

Nature's Path, Chia Plus™ Coconut Chia Granola

3/4 cup (55g)

Amount per serving	Amount per serving	Amount per serving
Calories 270	**Cholesterol** 0mg	**Total Carbohydrate** 36g
Total Fat 11g	**Sodium** 50mg	Dietary Fiber 6g
Saturated Fat 4g	**Protein** 5g	Sugars 9g

Nature's Path, Corn Puffs

1 cup (16g)

Amount per serving	Amount per serving	Amount per serving
Calories 60	**Cholesterol** 0mg	**Total Carbohydrate** 12g
Total Fat 0g	**Sodium** 0mg	Dietary Fiber 1g
Saturated Fat 0g	**Protein** 2g	Sugars 0g

Nature's Path, Crispy Rice Cereal

3/4 cup (30g)

Amount per serving	Amount per serving	Amount per serving
Calories 110	**Cholesterol** 0mg	**Total Carbohydrate** 24g
Total Fat 1.5g	**Sodium** 160mg	Dietary Fiber 2g
Saturated Fat 0g	**Protein** 2g	Sugars 2g

Nature's Path, Flax Plus® Cinnamon

3/4 cup (30g)

Amount per serving	Amount per serving	Amount per serving
Calories 120	**Cholesterol** 0mg	**Total Carbohydrate** 24g
Total Fat 1g	**Sodium** 140mg	Dietary Fiber 4g
Saturated Fat 0g	**Protein** 3g	Sugars 5g

Nature's Path, Flax Plus® Flakes

3/4 cup (30g)

Amount per serving	Amount per serving	Amount per serving
Calories 110	**Cholesterol** 0mg	**Total Carbohydrate** 23g
Total Fat 1.5g	**Sodium** 135mg	Dietary Fiber 5g
Saturated Fat 0g	**Protein** 4g	Sugars 4g

Nature's Path, Flax Plus® Hot Oatmeal

1 packet (50g)

Amount per serving	Amount per serving	Amount per serving
Calories 210	**Cholesterol** 0mg	**Total Carbohydrate** 38g
Total Fat 3g	**Sodium** 140mg	Dietary Fiber 5g
Saturated Fat 0.5g	**Protein** 6g	Sugars 10g

Nature's Path, Flax Plus® Maple Pecan Crunch

3/4 cup (55g)

Amount per serving	Amount per serving	Amount per serving
Calories 220	**Cholesterol** 0mg	**Total Carbohydrate** 38g
Total Fat 7g	**Sodium** 190mg	Dietary Fiber 5g
Saturated Fat 1g	**Protein** 6g	Sugars 10g

Nature's Path, Flax Plus® Pumpkin Raisin Crunch

3/4 cup (55g)

Amount per serving	Amount per serving	Amount per serving
Calories 210	**Cholesterol** 0mg	**Total Carbohydrate** 40g
Total Fat 4.5g	**Sodium** 150mg	Dietary Fiber 7g
Saturated Fat 0.5g	**Protein** 6g	Sugars 13g

Nature's Path, Flax Plus® Raisin Bran Flakes

3/4 cup (55g)

Amount per serving	Amount per serving	Amount per serving
Calories 190	**Cholesterol** 0mg	**Total Carbohydrate** 41g
Total Fat 2.5g	**Sodium** 190mg	Dietary Fiber 8g
Saturated Fat 0g	**Protein** 6g	Sugars 12g

Nature's Path, Flax Plus® Red Berry Crunch

3/4 cup (55g)

Amount per serving	Amount per serving	Amount per serving
Calories 210	**Cholesterol** 0mg	**Total Carbohydrate** 39g
Total Fat 3.5g	**Sodium** 160mg	Dietary Fiber 5g
Saturated Fat 0.5g	**Protein** 6g	Sugars 10g

Nature's Path, Fruit Juice Sweetened Corn Flakes

3/4 cup (30g)

Amount per serving	Amount per serving	Amount per serving
Calories 120	**Cholesterol** 0mg	**Total Carbohydrate** 27g
Total Fat 0g	**Sodium** 125mg	Dietary Fiber 1g
Saturated Fat 0g	**Protein** 2g	Sugars 3g

Nature's Path, Gluten Free Hot Oatmeal Homestyle

1 packet (40g)

Amount per serving	Amount per serving	Amount per serving
Calories 170	**Cholesterol** 0mg	**Total Carbohydrate** 30g
Total Fat 2.5g	**Sodium** 0mg	Dietary Fiber 4g
Saturated Fat 0.5g	**Protein** 6g	Sugars 0g

Nature's Path, Gluten Free Selections Brown Sugar Maple with Ancient Grains

1 packet (40g)

Amount per serving	Amount per serving	Amount per serving
Calories 160	**Cholesterol** 0mg	**Total Carbohydrate** 31g
Total Fat 2g	**Sodium** 80mg	Dietary Fiber 3g
Saturated Fat 0g	**Protein** 4g	Sugars 8g

Nature's Path, Gluten Free Selections Fruit & Nut Granola

1/4 cup (30g)

Amount per serving	Amount per serving	Amount per serving
Calories 140	**Cholesterol** 0mg	**Total Carbohydrate** 20g
Total Fat 5g	**Sodium** 0mg	Dietary Fiber 2g
Saturated Fat 1g	**Protein** 3g	Sugars 8g

Nature's Path, Gluten Free Selections Honey Almond Granola

1/4 cup (30g)

Amount per serving	Amount per serving	Amount per serving
Calories 140	**Cholesterol** 0mg	**Total Carbohydrate** 21g
Total Fat 4.5g	**Sodium** 65mg	Dietary Fiber 2g
Saturated Fat 0.5g	**Protein** 3g	Sugars 7g

Nature's Path, Gluten Free Selections Spiced Apple with Flax

1 packet (40g)

Amount per serving	Amount per serving	Amount per serving
Calories 170	**Cholesterol** 0mg	**Total Carbohydrate** 31g
Total Fat 2.5g	**Sodium** 90mg	Dietary Fiber 4g
Saturated Fat 0g	**Protein** 4g	Sugars 9g

Nature's Path, Gluten Free Selections Summer Berries Granola

1/4 cup (30g)

Amount per serving	Amount per serving	Amount per serving
Calories 140	**Cholesterol** 0mg	**Total Carbohydrate** 22g
Total Fat 4g	**Sodium** 55mg	Dietary Fiber 2g
Saturated Fat 0.5g	**Protein** 3g	Sugars 8g

Nature's Path, Gluten Free Selections Vanilla Cranberry Granola

1/4 cup (30g)

Amount per serving	Amount per serving	Amount per serving
Calories 140	**Cholesterol** 0mg	**Total Carbohydrate** 21g
Total Fat 5g	**Sodium** 50mg	Dietary Fiber 2g
Saturated Fat 1g	**Protein** 3g	Sugars 7g

Nature's Path, Gorilla Munch® Cereal

3/4 cup (30g)

Amount per serving	Amount per serving	Amount per serving
Calories 120	**Cholesterol** 0mg	**Total Carbohydrate** 26g
Total Fat 1g	**Sodium** 80mg	Dietary Fiber 2g
Saturated Fat 0.2g	**Protein** 2g	Sugars 8g

Nature's Path, Hemp Plus® Granola

3/4 cup (55g)

Amount per serving	Amount per serving	Amount per serving
Calories 260	**Cholesterol** 0mg	**Total Carbohydrate** 36g
Total Fat 10g	**Sodium** 45mg	Dietary Fiber 5g
Saturated Fat 1.5g	**Protein** 6g	Sugars 10g

Nature's Path, Hemp Plus® Hot Oatmeal

1 packet (40g)

Amount per serving	Amount per serving	Amount per serving
Calories 160	**Cholesterol** 0mg	**Total Carbohydrate** 30g
Total Fat 2.5g	**Sodium** 105mg	Dietary Fiber 4g
Saturated Fat 0g	**Protein** 5g	Sugars 6g

Nature's Path, Heritage Bites®

3/4 cup (30g)

Amount per serving	Amount per serving	Amount per serving
Calories 110	**Cholesterol** 0mg	**Total Carbohydrate** 24g
Total Fat 0.5g	**Sodium** 150mg	Dietary Fiber 5g
Saturated Fat 0g	**Protein** 3g	Sugars 3g

Nature's Path, Heritage Crunch®

3/4 cup (55g)

Amount per serving	Amount per serving	Amount per serving
Calories 230	**Cholesterol** 0mg	**Total Carbohydrate** 44g
Total Fat 3g	**Sodium** 210mg	Dietary Fiber 6g
Saturated Fat 0.5g	**Protein** 6g	Sugars 6g

Nature's Path, Heritage® Flakes

3/4 cup (30g)

Amount per serving	Amount per serving	Amount per serving
Calories 120	**Cholesterol** 0mg	**Total Carbohydrate** 24g
Total Fat 1g	**Sodium** 130mg	Dietary Fiber 5g
Saturated Fat 0g	**Protein** 4g	Sugars 4g

Nature's Path, Heritage® Muesli - Raspberry Hazelnut & Ancient Grains

3/4 cup (55g)

Amount per serving	Amount per serving	Amount per serving
Calories 210	**Cholesterol** 0mg	**Total Carbohydrate** 41g
Total Fat 3.5g	**Sodium** 105mg	Dietary Fiber 6g
Saturated Fat 0g	**Protein** 6g	Sugars 9g

Nature's Path, Heritage® Muesli - Wild Blueberry Almond & Ancient Grains

3/4 cup (55g)

Amount per serving	Amount per serving	Amount per serving
Calories 210	**Cholesterol** 0mg	**Total Carbohydrate** 41g
Total Fat 3g	**Sodium** 130mg	Dietary Fiber 7g
Saturated Fat 0g	**Protein** 6g	Sugars 9g

Nature's Path, Heritage® O's

3/4 cup (30g)

Amount per serving	Amount per serving	Amount per serving
Calories 120	**Cholesterol** 0mg	**Total Carbohydrate** 23g
Total Fat 1g	**Sodium** 115mg	Dietary Fiber 3g
Saturated Fat 0g	**Protein** 4g	Sugars 3g

Nature's Path, Honey'd® Corn Flakes

3/4 cup (30g)

Amount per serving	Amount per serving	Amount per serving
Calories 120	**Cholesterol** 0mg	**Total Carbohydrate** 27g
Total Fat 0g	**Sodium** 105mg	Dietary Fiber 1g
Saturated Fat 0g	**Protein** 2g	Sugars 4g

Nature's Path, Jungle Munch

3/4 cup (30g)

Amount per serving	Amount per serving	Amount per serving
Calories 120	**Cholesterol** 0mg	**Total Carbohydrate** 26g
Total Fat 0.5g	**Sodium** 80mg	Dietary Fiber 2g
Saturated Fat 0.1g	**Protein** 2g	Sugars 9g

Nature's Path, KAMUT® Puffs

1 cup (16g)

Amount per serving	Amount per serving	Amount per serving
Calories 50	**Cholesterol** 0mg	**Total Carbohydrate** 11g
Total Fat 0g	**Sodium** 0mg	Dietary Fiber 2g
Saturated Fat 0g	**Protein** 2g	Sugars 0g

Nature's Path, Koala Crisp Cereal

3/4 cup (30g)

Amount per serving	Amount per serving	Amount per serving
Calories 110	**Cholesterol** 0mg	**Total Carbohydrate** 25g
Total Fat 1g	**Sodium** 100mg	Dietary Fiber 2g
Saturated Fat 0.3g	**Protein** 2g	Sugars 11g

Nature's Path, Leapin Lemurs Cereal

3/4 cup (30g)

Amount per serving	Amount per serving	Amount per serving
Calories 120	**Cholesterol** 0mg	**Total Carbohydrate** 25g
Total Fat 1.5g	**Sodium** 115mg	Dietary Fiber 2g
Saturated Fat 1.5g	**Protein** 2g	Sugars 8g

Nature's Path, Love Crunch® Aloha Blend

1/4 cup (30g)

Amount per serving	Amount per serving	Amount per serving
Calories 150	**Cholesterol** 0mg	**Total Carbohydrate** 20g
Total Fat 7g	**Sodium** 55mg	Dietary Fiber 2g
Saturated Fat 7g	**Protein** 2g	Sugars 6g

Nature's Path, Love Crunch® Apple Crumble

1/4 cup (30g)

Amount per serving	Amount per serving	Amount per serving
Calories 140	**Cholesterol** 0mg	**Total Carbohydrate** 22g
Total Fat 4g	**Sodium** 50mg	Dietary Fiber 2g
Saturated Fat 0.5g	**Protein** 3g	Sugars 6g

Nature's Path, Love Crunch® Carrot Cake

1/4 cup (30g)

Amount per serving	Amount per serving	Amount per serving
Calories 130	**Cholesterol** 0mg	**Total Carbohydrate** 23g
Total Fat 4g	**Sodium** 45mg	Dietary Fiber 2g
Saturated Fat 1g	**Protein** 2g	Sugars 8g

Nature's Path, Love Crunch® Dark Chocolate & Red Berries

1/4 cup (30 g)

Amount per serving	Amount per serving	Amount per serving
Calories 140	**Cholesterol** 0mg	**Total Carbohydrate** 20g
Total Fat 6g	**Sodium** 55mg	Dietary Fiber 2g
Saturated Fat 1g	**Protein** 2g	Sugars 6g

Nature's Path, Love Crunch® Dark Chocolate Macaroon

1/4 cup (30g)

Amount per serving	Amount per serving	Amount per serving
Calories 150	**Cholesterol** 0mg	**Total Carbohydrate** 20g
Total Fat 6g	**Sodium** 50mg	Dietary Fiber 2g
Saturated Fat 2.5g	**Protein** 2g	Sugars 7g

Nature's Path, Love Crunch® Gingerbread

1/4 cup (30g)

Amount per serving	Amount per serving	Amount per serving
Calories 130	**Cholesterol** 0mg	**Total Carbohydrate** 22g
Total Fat 4g	**Sodium** 50mg	Dietary Fiber 2g
Saturated Fat 0.5g	**Protein** 2g	Sugars 9g

Nature's Path, Maple Nut Hot Oatmeal

1 packet (50g)

Amount per serving	Amount per serving	Amount per serving
Calories 210	**Cholesterol** 0mg	**Total Carbohydrate** 38g
Total Fat 4g	**Sodium** 100mg	Dietary Fiber 4g
Saturated Fat 0.5g	**Protein** 5g	Sugars 11g

Nature's Path, Mesa Sunrise® Flakes

3/4 cup (30g)

Amount per serving	Amount per serving	Amount per serving
Calories 120	**Cholesterol** 0mg	**Total Carbohydrate** 24g
Total Fat 1g	**Sodium** 125mg	Dietary Fiber 3g
Saturated Fat 0g	**Protein** 3g	Sugars 4g

Nature's Path, Mesa Sunrise® Flakes with Raisins

1 cup (55g)

Amount per serving	Amount per serving	Amount per serving
Calories 210	**Cholesterol** 0mg	**Total Carbohydrate** 47g
Total Fat 1g	**Sodium** 200mg	Dietary Fiber 2g
Saturated Fat 0g	**Protein** 3g	Sugars 12g

Nature's Path, Millet Puffs

1 cup (16g)

Amount per serving	Amount per serving	Amount per serving
Calories 50	**Cholesterol** 0mg	**Total Carbohydrate** 14g
Total Fat 0g	**Sodium** 0mg	Dietary Fiber 1g
Saturated Fat 0g	**Protein** 2g	Sugars 0g

Nature's Path, Millet Rice™ Fruit Juice Sweetened

3/4 cup (30g)

Amount per serving	Amount per serving	Amount per serving
Calories 120	**Cholesterol** 0mg	**Total Carbohydrate** 22g
Total Fat 2g	**Sodium** 115mg	Dietary Fiber 3g
Saturated Fat 0g	**Protein** 4g	Sugars 4g

Nature's Path, Multigrain Oatbran Cereal

3/4 cup (30g)

Amount per serving	Amount per serving	Amount per serving
Calories 110	**Cholesterol** 0mg	**Total Carbohydrate** 24g
Total Fat 1g	**Sodium** 110mg	Dietary Fiber 5g
Saturated Fat 0g	**Protein** 3g	Sugars 4g

Nature's Path, MultiGrain Raisin Spice Hot Oatmeal

1 packet (50g)

Amount per serving	Amount per serving	Amount per serving
Calories 180	**Cholesterol** 0mg	**Total Carbohydrate** 39g
Total Fat 1g	**Sodium** 100mg	Dietary Fiber 4g
Saturated Fat 0g	**Protein** 4g	Sugars 18g

Nature's Path, Oaty Bites®

3/4 cup (30g)

Amount per serving	Amount per serving	Amount per serving
Calories 110	**Cholesterol** 0mg	**Total Carbohydrate** 23g
Total Fat 1.5g	**Sodium** 115mg	Dietary Fiber 2g
Saturated Fat 0g	**Protein** 3g	Sugars 5g

Nature's Path, Optimum Power® Blueberry Cinnamon Flax Cereal

3/4 cup (55g)

Amount per serving	Amount per serving	Amount per serving
Calories 200	**Cholesterol** 0mg	**Total Carbohydrate** 38g
Total Fat 3g	**Sodium** 230mg	Dietary Fiber 9g
Saturated Fat 0g	**Protein** 9g	Sugars 9g

Nature's Path, Optimum Power® Blueberry Cinnamon Flax Hot Oatmeal

1 packet (40g)

Amount per serving	Amount per serving	Amount per serving
Calories 160	**Cholesterol** 0mg	**Total Carbohydrate** 30g
Total Fat 2.5g	**Sodium** 120mg	Dietary Fiber 3g
Saturated Fat 0g	**Protein** 5g	Sugars 8g

Nature's Path, Optimum Slim® Low Fat Vanilla Cereal

1 cup (55g)

Amount per serving	Amount per serving	Amount per serving
Calories 200	**Cholesterol** 0mg	**Total Carbohydrate** 40g
Total Fat 2g	**Sodium** 9mg	Dietary Fiber 9g
Saturated Fat 0g	**Protein** 9g	Sugars 6g

Nature's Path, Optimum® Cranberry Ginger Hot Oatmeal

1 packet (40g)

Amount per serving	Amount per serving	Amount per serving
Calories 150	**Cholesterol** 0mg	**Total Carbohydrate** 31g
Total Fat 2g	**Sodium** 160mg	Dietary Fiber 3g
Saturated Fat 0g	**Protein** 4g	Sugars 11g

Nature's Path, Original Hot Oatmeal

1 packet (50g)

Amount per serving	Amount per serving	Amount per serving
Calories 190	**Cholesterol** 0mg	**Total Carbohydrate** 34g
Total Fat 3g	**Sodium** 0mg	Dietary Fiber 6g
Saturated Fat 0.5g	**Protein** 8g	Sugars 1g

Nature's Path, Panda Puffs™ Cereal

3/4 cup (30g)

Amount per serving	Amount per serving	Amount per serving
Calories 130	**Cholesterol** 0mg	**Total Carbohydrate** 23g
Total Fat 3.5g	**Sodium** 125mg	Dietary Fiber 2g
Saturated Fat 1g	**Protein** 2g	Sugars 7g

Nature's Path, Peanut Butter Granola

3/4 cup (55g)

Amount per serving	Amount per serving	Amount per serving
Calories 260	**Cholesterol** 0mg	**Total Carbohydrate** 35g
Total Fat 11g	**Sodium** 75mg	Dietary Fiber 4g
Saturated Fat 1.5g	**Protein** 7g	Sugars 9g

Nature's Path, Pomegran Cherry Granola

3/4 cup (55g)

Amount per serving	Amount per serving	Amount per serving
Calories 250	**Cholesterol** 0mg	**Total Carbohydrate** 38g
Total Fat 9g	**Sodium** 60mg	Dietary Fiber 4g
Saturated Fat 2.5g	**Protein** 5g	Sugars 13g

Nature's Path, Pumpkin Flax Plus® Granola

3/4 cup (55g)

Amount per serving	Amount per serving	Amount per serving
Calories 260	**Cholesterol** 0mg	**Total Carbohydrate** 37g
Total Fat 10g	**Sodium** 45mg	Dietary Fiber 5g
Saturated Fat 1.6g	**Protein** 6g	Sugars 10g

Nature's Path, Qi'a™ Superfood - Chia, Buckwheat & Hemp Cereal Apple Cinnamon

2 tbsp (30g)

Amount per serving	Amount per serving	Amount per serving
Calories 130	**Cholesterol** 0mg	**Total Carbohydrate** 15g
Total Fat 6g	**Sodium** 0mg	Dietary Fiber 4g
Saturated Fat 0.5g	**Protein** 6g	Sugars 3g

Nature's Path, Qi'a™ Superfood - Chia, Buckwheat & Hemp Cereal Cranberry Vanilla

2 tbsp (30g)

Amount per serving

Calories 140
Total Fat 6g
  Saturated Fat 0.5g

Cholesterol 0mg
Sodium 0mg
Protein 6g

Total Carbohydrate 14g
  Dietary Fiber 4g
  Sugars 3g

Nature's Path, Qi'a™ Superfood - Chia, Buckwheat & Hemp Cereal Original Flavor

2 tbsp (30g)

Amount per serving

Calories 140
Total Fat 7g
  Saturated Fat 0.5g

Cholesterol 0mg
Sodium 0mg
Protein 6g

Total Carbohydrate 13g
  Dietary Fiber 4g
  Sugars 0g

Nature's Path, Rice Puffs

1 cup (16g)

Amount per serving

Calories 50
Total Fat 0g
  Saturated Fat 0g

Cholesterol 0mg
Sodium 0mg
Protein 1g

Total Carbohydrate 14g
  Dietary Fiber 1g
  Sugars 0g

Nature's Path, SmartBran™ Cereal

1/2 cup (30g)

Amount per serving

Calories 80
Total Fat 1g
  Saturated Fat 0g

Cholesterol 0mg
Sodium 130mg
Protein 3g

Total Carbohydrate 24g
  Dietary Fiber 13g
  Sugars 6g

Nature's Path, Sunrise® Crunchy Cinnamon

2/3 cup (30g)

Amount per serving

Calories 120
Total Fat 1g
  Saturated Fat 0.2g

Cholesterol 0mg
Sodium 130mg
Protein 2g

Total Carbohydrate 26g
  Dietary Fiber 3g
  Sugars 7g

Nature's Path, Sunrise® Crunchy Honey

2/3 cup (30g)

Amount per serving

Calories 120
Total Fat 1g
  Saturated Fat 0.2g

Cholesterol 0mg
Sodium 160mg
Protein 2g

Total Carbohydrate 26g
  Dietary Fiber 3g
  Sugars 8g

Nature's Path, Sunrise® Crunchy Maple

2/3 cup (30g)

Amount per serving	Amount per serving	Amount per serving
Calories 110	**Cholesterol** 0mg	**Total Carbohydrate** 25g
Total Fat 1g	**Sodium** 130mg	Dietary Fiber 3g
Saturated Fat 0g	**Protein** 2g	Sugars 7g

Nature's Path, Sunrise® Crunchy Vanilla

2/3 cup (30g)

Amount per serving	Amount per serving	Amount per serving
Calories 110	**Cholesterol** 0mg	**Total Carbohydrate** 25g
Total Fat 1g	**Sodium** 135mg	Dietary Fiber 3g
Saturated Fat 0g	**Protein** 2g	Sugars 6g

Nature's Path, Vanilla Almond Flax Plus™ Granola

3/4 cup (55g)

Amount per serving	Amount per serving	Amount per serving
Calories 250	**Cholesterol** 0mg	**Total Carbohydrate** 36g
Total Fat 9g	**Sodium** 80mg	Dietary Fiber 5g
Saturated Fat 1.5g	**Protein** 6g	Sugars 10g

Nature's Path, Variety Pack Hot Oatmeal, Apple Cinnamon

1 packet

Amount per serving	Amount per serving	Amount per serving
Calories 210	**Cholesterol** 0mg	**Total Carbohydrate** 40g
Total Fat 2.5g	**Sodium** 100mg	Dietary Fiber 4g
Saturated Fat 0g	**Protein** 5g	Sugars 100g

Nature's Path, Variety Pack Hot Oatmeal, Flax Plus

1 packet

Amount per serving	Amount per serving	Amount per serving
Calories 210	**Cholesterol** 0mg	**Total Carbohydrate** 38g
Total Fat 3g	**Sodium** 140mg	Dietary Fiber 5g
Saturated Fat 0.5g	**Protein** 6g	Sugars 10g

Nature's Path, Variety Pack Hot Oatmeal, Maple Nut

1 packet

Amount per serving	Amount per serving	Amount per serving
Calories 210	**Cholesterol** 0mg	**Total Carbohydrate** 38g
Total Fat 4g	**Sodium** 100mg	Dietary Fiber 4g
Saturated Fat 0.5g	**Protein** 5g	Sugars 11g

Nature's Path, Variety Pack Hot Oatmeal, Raisin Spice

1 packet

Amount per serving	Amount per serving	Amount per serving
Calories 180	**Cholesterol** 0mg	**Total Carbohydrate** 39g
Total Fat 1g	**Sodium** 100mg	Dietary Fiber 4g
Saturated Fat 0g	**Protein** 4g	Sugars 18g

Nature's Path, Whole O's™ Cereal

2/3 cup (30g)

Amount per serving	Amount per serving	Amount per serving
Calories 120	**Cholesterol** 0mg	**Total Carbohydrate** 25g
Total Fat 1.5g	**Sodium** 115mg	Dietary Fiber 3g
Saturated Fat 0g	**Protein** 2g	Sugars 4g

Quaker Oats, Organic Instant Oatmeal, Maple and Brown Sugar

1 packet (41g)

Amount per serving	Amount per serving	Amount per serving
Calories 150	**Cholesterol** 0mg	**Total Carbohydrate** 31g
Total Fat 2g	**Sodium** 95mg	Dietary Fiber 3g
Saturated Fat 0g	**Protein** 4g	Sugars 12g

Quaker Oats, Organic Instant Oatmeal, Regular Flavor

1 packet (28g)

Amount per serving	Amount per serving	Amount per serving
Calories 100	**Cholesterol** 0mg	**Total Carbohydrate** 19g
Total Fat 2g	**Sodium** 0mg	Dietary Fiber 3g
Saturated Fat 0g	**Protein** 4g	Sugars 0g

Flours

Ancient Harvest, Gluten-Free Quinoa Flour 100% Whole Grain

1/4 cup dry

Amount per serving	Amount per serving	Amount per serving
Calories 132	**Cholesterol** 0mg	**Total Carbohydrate** 23g
Total Fat 2g	**Sodium** 3mg	Dietary Fiber 2.2g
Saturated Fat 0g	**Protein** 4g	Sugars 1g

Arrowhead Mills, Organic Brown Rice Flour

1/3 cup

Amount per serving	Amount per serving	Amount per serving
Calories 130	**Cholesterol** 0mg	**Total Carbohydrate** 27g
Total Fat 1g	**Sodium** 0mg	Dietary Fiber 2g
Saturated Fat 0g	**Protein** 3g	Sugars 0g

Arrowhead Mills, Organic Buckwheat Flour

1/3 cup

Amount per serving	Amount per serving	Amount per serving
Calories 115	Cholesterol 0mg	Total Carbohydrate 20g
Total Fat 1.5g	Sodium 0mg	Dietary Fiber 6g
Saturated Fat 0g	Protein 5g	Sugars <1g

Arrowhead Mills, Organic Millet Flour

1/3 cup

Amount per serving	Amount per serving	Amount per serving
Calories 130	Cholesterol 0mg	Total Carbohydrate 26g
Total Fat 1.5g	Sodium 0mg	Dietary Fiber 3g
Saturated Fat 0g	Protein 4g	Sugars 0g

Arrowhead Mills, Organic Soy Flour

1/4 cup

Amount per serving	Amount per serving	Amount per serving
Calories 100	Cholesterol 0mg	Total Carbohydrate 9g
Total Fat 4.5g	Sodium 0mg	Dietary Fiber 4g
Saturated Fat 1g	Protein 7g	Sugars 0g

Arrowhead Mills, Organic White Rice Flour

1/3 cup

Amount per serving	Amount per serving	Amount per serving
Calories 120	Cholesterol 0mg	Total Carbohydrate 28g
Total Fat 0g	Sodium 0mg	Dietary Fiber <1g
Saturated Fat 0g	Protein 2g	Sugars 0g

Bob's Red Mill, Organic Amaranth Flour

1/4 cup dry

Amount per serving	Amount per serving	Amount per serving
Calories 110	Cholesterol 0mg	Total Carbohydrate 20g
Total Fat 2g	Sodium 6mg	Dietary Fiber 3g
Saturated Fat 0.5g	Protein 4g	Sugars 0g

Bob's Red Mill, Organic Brown Rice Flour

1/4 cup

Amount per serving	Amount per serving	Amount per serving
Calories 140	Cholesterol 0mg	Total Carbohydrate 31g
Total Fat 1g	Sodium 5mg	Dietary Fiber 1g
Saturated Fat 0g	Protein 3g	Sugars 0g

Bob's Red Mill, Organic Coconut Flour

2 tbsp

Amount per serving	Amount per serving	Amount per serving
Calories 60	**Cholesterol** 0mg	**Total Carbohydrate** 10g
Total Fat 1.5g	**Sodium** 0mg	Dietary Fiber 6g
Saturated Fat 1g	**Protein** 2g	Sugars 0g

Bob's Red Mill, Organic Quinoa Flour

1/4 cup dry

Amount per serving	Amount per serving	Amount per serving
Calories 120	**Cholesterol** 0mg	**Total Carbohydrate** 21g
Total Fat 2g	**Sodium** 8mg	Dietary Fiber 4g
Saturated Fat 0g	**Protein** 4g	Sugars 0g

Bob's Red Mill, Organic White Rice Flour

1/4 cup

Amount per serving	Amount per serving	Amount per serving
Calories 150	**Cholesterol** 0mg	**Total Carbohydrate** 32g
Total Fat 0.5g	**Sodium** 0mg	Dietary Fiber 1g
Saturated Fat 0g	**Protein** 2g	Sugars 0g

Eden Foods, Short Grain Brown Rice Flour, 100% Whole Grain, Organic

1/4 cup

Amount per serving	Amount per serving	Amount per serving
Calories 150	**Cholesterol** 0mg	**Total Carbohydrate** 35g
Total Fat 1.5g	**Sodium** 0mg	Dietary Fiber 3g
Saturated Fat 0g	**Protein** 3g	Sugars 1g

Hodgson Mill, Certified Organic Oat Bran Flour

1/4 cup

Amount per serving	Amount per serving	Amount per serving
Calories 125	**Cholesterol** 0mg	**Total Carbohydrate** 22g
Total Fat 2g	**Sodium** 0mg	Dietary Fiber 3g
Saturated Fat 0g	**Protein** 4g	Sugars 0g

Hodgson Mill, Certified Organic Stone Ground Whole Wheat Pastry Flour

<1/4 cup

Amount per serving	Amount per serving	Amount per serving
Calories 100	**Cholesterol** 0mg	**Total Carbohydrate** 22g
Total Fat 0.5g	**Sodium** 0mg	Dietary Fiber 4g
Saturated Fat 0g	**Protein** 3g	Sugars 0g

Hodgson Mill, Certified Organic Unbleached All Purpose Naturally White Flour

1/4 cup

Amount per serving	Amount per serving	Amount per serving
Calories 100	**Cholesterol** 0mg	**Total Carbohydrate** 23g
Total Fat 0g	**Sodium** 0mg	Dietary Fiber 1g
Saturated Fat 0g	**Protein** 3g	Sugars 0g

Hodgson Mill, Organic Whole Wheat Flour

<1/4 cup

Amount per serving	Amount per serving	Amount per serving
Calories 100	**Cholesterol** 0mg	**Total Carbohydrate** 22g
Total Fat 1g	**Sodium** 0mg	Dietary Fiber 4g
Saturated Fat 0g	**Protein** 4g	Sugars 0g

Hodgson Mill, Wheat Free Organic Rye Flour

1/4 cup

Amount per serving	Amount per serving	Amount per serving
Calories 110	**Cholesterol** 0mg	**Total Carbohydrate** 23g
Total Fat 0.5g	**Sodium** 0mg	Dietary Fiber NA
Saturated Fat 0g	**Protein** 3g	Sugars 0g

Hodgson Mill, Wheat Free Organic Soy Flour

1/4 cup

Amount per serving	Amount per serving	Amount per serving
Calories 120	**Cholesterol** 0mg	**Total Carbohydrate** 10g
Total Fat 6g	**Sodium** 0mg	Dietary Fiber 6g
Saturated Fat 1g	**Protein** 10g	Sugars 2g

Jovial Foods, Jovial Organic Einkorn Flour

1/4 cup (30g)

Amount per serving	Amount per serving	Amount per serving
Calories 100	**Cholesterol** 0mg	**Total Carbohydrate** 20g
Total Fat 0.5g	**Sodium** 0mg	Dietary Fiber 2g
Saturated Fat 0g	**Protein** 4g	Sugars 0g

Lundberg Family Farms, Organic Brown Rice Flour, Dry

1/4 cup dry (40g)

Amount per serving	Amount per serving	Amount per serving
Calories 140	**Cholesterol** 0mg	**Total Carbohydrate** 29g
Total Fat 2g	**Sodium** 0mg	Dietary Fiber 3g
Saturated Fat 0g	**Protein** 3g	Sugars 1g

Grain Products

Ancient Harvest, Gluten-Free Polenta Heirloom Red & Black

2 1/2" slices (100g)

Amount per serving	Amount per serving	Amount per serving
Calories 80	**Cholesterol** 0mg	**Total Carbohydrate** 16g
Total Fat 0g	**Sodium** 270mg	Dietary Fiber 1g
Saturated Fat 0g	**Protein** 2g	Sugars 0g

Ancient Harvest, Gluten-Free Polenta Organic Basil Garlic

2 1/2" slices (100g)

Amount per serving	Amount per serving	Amount per serving
Calories 71	**Cholesterol** 0mg	**Total Carbohydrate** 15g
Total Fat 0g	**Sodium** 310mg	Dietary Fiber 1g
Saturated Fat 0g	**Protein** 2g	Sugars 1g

Ancient Harvest, Gluten-Free Polenta Organic Groon Chile & Cilantro

2 1/2" slices (100g)

Amount per serving	Amount per serving	Amount per serving
Calories 75	**Cholesterol** 0mg	**Total Carbohydrate** 16g
Total Fat 0g	**Sodium** 268mg	Dietary Fiber 1g
Saturated Fat 0g	**Protein** 2g	Sugars 1g

Ancient Harvest, Gluten-Free Polenta Organic Sun Dried Tomato & Garlic

2 1/2" slices (100g)

Amount per serving	Amount per serving	Amount per serving
Calories 74	**Cholesterol** 0mg	**Total Carbohydrate** 16g
Total Fat 0g	**Sodium** 310mg	Dietary Fiber 1g
Saturated Fat 0g	**Protein** 2g	Sugars 1g

Ancient Harvest, Gluten-Free Polenta Organic Traditional Italian

2 1/2" slices (100g)

Amount per serving	Amount per serving	Amount per serving
Calories 70	**Cholesterol** 0mg	**Total Carbohydrate** 15g
Total Fat 0g	**Sodium** 310mg	Dietary Fiber 1g
Saturated Fat 0g	**Protein** 2g	Sugars 1g

Ancient Harvest, Gluten-Free Quinoa Organic Tri-Color Grains Harmony Blend

1/4 cup dry

Amount per serving	Amount per serving	Amount per serving
Calories 170	**Cholesterol** 0mg	**Total Carbohydrate** 30g
Total Fat 2.5g	**Sodium** 2.5mg	Dietary Fiber 2g
Saturated Fat 0g	**Protein** 5g	Sugars 3g

Ancient Harvest, Gluten-Free Quinoa Organic White Grains Traditional

1/4 cup dry

Amount per serving	Amount per serving	Amount per serving
Calories 172	Cholesterol 0mg	Total Carbohydrate 31g
Total Fat 2.8g	Sodium 1mg	Dietary Fiber 3g
Saturated Fat 0g	Protein 6g	Sugars 3g

Ancient Harvest, Gluten-Free Quinoa Red Grains Inca Red

1/4 cup dry

Amount per serving	Amount per serving	Amount per serving
Calories 180	Cholesterol 0mg	Total Carbohydrate 33g
Total Fat 2.5g	Sodium 2mg	Dietary Fiber 4g
Saturated Fat 0g	Protein 6g	Sugars 6g

Frieda's, Organic Polenta (Basil & Garlic)

1/4 tube (113g)

Amount per serving	Amount per serving	Amount per serving
Calories 90	Cholesterol 0mg	Total Carbohydrate 19g
Total Fat 0g	Sodium 300mg	Dietary Fiber 0g
Saturated Fat 0g	Protein 2g	Sugars 0g

Frieda's, Organic Polenta (Green Chile & Cilantro)

1/4 tube (113g)

Amount per serving	Amount per serving	Amount per serving
Calories 90	Cholesterol 0mg	Total Carbohydrate 18g
Total Fat 0g	Sodium 300mg	Dietary Fiber 0g
Saturated Fat 0g	Protein 2g	Sugars 0g

Frieda's, Organic Polenta (Mushroom & Onion)

1/4 tube (113g)

Amount per serving	Amount per serving	Amount per serving
Calories 90	Cholesterol 0mg	Total Carbohydrate 19g
Total Fat 0g	Sodium 300mg	Dietary Fiber <1g
Saturated Fat 0g	Protein 2g	Sugars 0g

Frieda's, Organic Polenta (Sun Dried Tomato & Garlic)

1/4 tube (113g)

Amount per serving	Amount per serving	Amount per serving
Calories 90	Cholesterol 0mg	Total Carbohydrate 19g
Total Fat 0g	Sodium 310mg	Dietary Fiber <1g
Saturated Fat 0g	Protein 2g	Sugars 0g

Frieda's, Organic Polenta (Traditional)

1/4 tube (113g)

Amount per serving	Amount per serving	Amount per serving
Calories 90	**Cholesterol** 0mg	**Total Carbohydrate** 18g
Total Fat 0g	**Sodium** 290mg	Dietary Fiber 0g
Saturated Fat 0g	**Protein** 2g	Sugars 0g

Nature's Path, Ancient Grains Frozen Waffle

2 waffles (70g)

Amount per serving	Amount per serving	Amount per serving
Calories 180	**Cholesterol** 0mg	**Total Carbohydrate** 30g
Total Fat 6g	**Sodium** 330mg	Dietary Fiber 5g
Saturated Fat 1g	**Protein** 4g	Sugars 2g

Nature's Path, Buckwheat Wildberry Frozen Waffle

2 waffles (70g)

Amount per serving	Amount per serving	Amount per serving
Calories 190	**Cholesterol** 0mg	**Total Carbohydrate** 33g
Total Fat 7g	**Sodium** 330mg	Dietary Fiber 1g
Saturated Fat 1g	**Protein** 2g	Sugars 5g

Nature's Path, Flax Plus® Fig & Flax Frozen Waffle

2 waffles (70g)

Amount per serving	Amount per serving	Amount per serving
Calories 200	**Cholesterol** 0mg	**Total Carbohydrate** 27g
Total Fat 9g	**Sodium** 390mg	Dietary Fiber 5g
Saturated Fat 1.5g	**Protein** 4g	Sugars 6g

Nature's Path, Flax Plus® Frozen Waffle

2 waffles (70g)

Amount per serving	Amount per serving	Amount per serving
Calories 200	**Cholesterol** 0mg	**Total Carbohydrate** 30g
Total Fat 8g	**Sodium** 330mg	Dietary Fiber 5g
Saturated Fat 1g	**Protein** 4g	Sugars 5g

Nature's Path, Frosted Berry Strawberry™ Toaster Pastries

1 pastry (52g)

Amount per serving	Amount per serving	Amount per serving
Calories 210	**Cholesterol** 0mg	**Total Carbohydrate** 40g
Total Fat 4g	**Sodium** 140mg	Dietary Fiber 1g
Saturated Fat 2g	**Protein** 3g	Sugars 19g

Nature's Path, Frosted Buncha Blueberries Toaster Pastries

1 pastry (52g)

Amount per serving	Amount per serving	Amount per serving
Calories 200	**Cholesterol** 0mg	**Total Carbohydrate** 38g
Total Fat 4g	**Sodium** 125mg	Dietary Fiber 1g
Saturated Fat 2g	**Protein** 2g	Sugars 20g

Nature's Path, Frosted Cherry Pomegranate Toaster Pastries

1 pastry (52g)

Amount per serving	Amount per serving	Amount per serving
Calories 200	**Cholesterol** 0mg	**Total Carbohydrate** 37g
Total Fat 4.5g	**Sodium** 150mg	Dietary Fiber 1g
Saturated Fat 3g	**Protein** 3g	Sugars 17g

Nature's Path, Frosted Granny's Apple Pie Toaster Pastries

1 pastry (52g)

Amount per serving	Amount per serving	Amount per serving
Calories 210	**Cholesterol** 0mg	**Total Carbohydrate** 39g
Total Fat 4.5g	**Sodium** 130mg	Dietary Fiber 1g
Saturated Fat 2g	**Protein** 2g	Sugars 21g

Nature's Path, Frosted Lotta Chocolatta Toaster Pastries

1 pastry (52g)

Amount per serving	Amount per serving	Amount per serving
Calories 210	**Cholesterol** 0mg	**Total Carbohydrate** 38g
Total Fat 5g	**Sodium** 130mg	Dietary Fiber 1g
Saturated Fat 3g	**Protein** 3g	Sugars 18g

Nature's Path, Frosted Mmmaple Brown Sugar Toaster Pastries

1 pastry (52g)

Amount per serving	Amount per serving	Amount per serving
Calories 210	**Cholesterol** 0mg	**Total Carbohydrate** 39g
Total Fat 4.5g	**Sodium** 125mg	Dietary Fiber 1g
Saturated Fat 3g	**Protein** 3g	Sugars 20g

Nature's Path, Frosted Wildberry Acai Toaster Pastries

1 pastry (52g)

Amount per serving	Amount per serving	Amount per serving
Calories 210	**Cholesterol** 0mg	**Total Carbohydrate** 38g
Total Fat 5g	**Sodium** 130mg	Dietary Fiber 1g
Saturated Fat 3g	**Protein** 3g	Sugars 18g

Nature's Path, Hemp Plus® Frozen Waffle

2 waffles (70g)

Amount per serving	Amount per serving	Amount per serving
Calories 200	**Cholesterol** 0mg	**Total Carbohydrate** 30g
Total Fat 8g	**Sodium** 290mg	Dietary Fiber 5g
Saturated Fat 1g	**Protein** 4g	Sugars 5g

Nature's Path, Homestyle Frozen Waffle

2 waffles (70g)

Amount per serving	Amount per serving	Amount per serving
Calories 210	**Cholesterol** 0mg	**Total Carbohydrate** 34g
Total Fat 7g	**Sodium** 460mg	Dietary Fiber 1g
Saturated Fat 1.5g	**Protein** 1g	Sugars 4g

Nature's Path, Maple Cinnamon Frozen Waffle

2 waffles (70g)

Amount per serving	Amount per serving	Amount per serving
Calories 180	**Cholesterol** 0mg	**Total Carbohydrate** 28g
Total Fat 6g	**Sodium** 230mg	Dietary Fiber 4g
Saturated Fat 1g	**Protein** 4g	Sugars 6g

Nature's Path, Pumpkin Spice Waffle

2 waffles (70g)

Amount per serving	Amount per serving	Amount per serving
Calories 210	**Cholesterol** 0mg	**Total Carbohydrate** 35g
Total Fat 7g	**Sodium** 385mg	Dietary Fiber 2g
Saturated Fat 1g	**Protein** 2g	Sugars 6g

Nature's Path, Unfrosted Berry Strawberry Toaster Pastries

1 pastry (52g)

Amount per serving	Amount per serving	Amount per serving
Calories 210	**Cholesterol** 0mg	**Total Carbohydrate** 40g
Total Fat 4.5g	**Sodium** 150mg	Dietary Fiber 1g
Saturated Fat 2g	**Protein** 3g	Sugars 18g

Nature's Path, Unfrosted Buncha Blueberries Toaster Pastries

1 pastry (52g)

Amount per serving	Amount per serving	Amount per serving
Calories 210	**Cholesterol** 0mg	**Total Carbohydrate** 40g
Total Fat 4.5g	**Sodium** 150mg	Dietary Fiber 1g
Saturated Fat 2g	**Protein** 3g	Sugars 18g

Nature's Path, Unfrosted Granny's Apple Pie™ Toaster Pastries

1 pastry (52g)

Amount per serving	Amount per serving	Amount per serving
Calories 210	**Cholesterol** 0mg	**Total Carbohydrate** 40g
Total Fat 4.5g	**Sodium** 150mg	Dietary Fiber 1g
Saturated Fat 2g	**Protein** 3g	Sugars 18g

Grains

Bob's Red Mill, Organic Amaranth Grain

1/4 cup

Amount per serving	Amount per serving	Amount per serving
Calories 190	**Cholesterol** 0mg	**Total Carbohydrate** 34g
Total Fat 3.5g	**Sodium** 10mg	Dietary Fiber 7g
Saturated Fat 1g	**Protein** 8g	Sugars 1g

Bob's Red Mill, Organic Buckwheat Groats

1/4 cup

Amount per serving	Amount per serving	Amount per serving
Calories 150	**Cholesterol** 0mg	**Total Carbohydrate** 32g
Total Fat 1.5g	**Sodium** 0mg	Dietary Fiber 5g
Saturated Fat 0g	**Protein** 6g	Sugars 1g

Eden Foods, Millet, 100% Whole Grain, Organic, Uncooked

1/4 cup

Amount per serving	Amount per serving	Amount per serving
Calories 160	**Cholesterol** 0mg	**Total Carbohydrate** 30g
Total Fat 2g	**Sodium** 5mg	Dietary Fiber 4g
Saturated Fat 0g	**Protein** 5g	Sugars 0g

Eden Foods, Quinoa, 100% Whole Grain, Organic

1/4 cup

Amount per serving	Amount per serving	Amount per serving
Calories 170	**Cholesterol** 0mg	**Total Carbohydrate** 31g
Total Fat 2.5g	**Sodium** 0mg	Dietary Fiber 4g
Saturated Fat 0g	**Protein** 5g	Sugars 1g

Eden Foods, Red Quinoa, 100% Whole Grain, Organic, Uncooked

1/4 cup

Amount per serving	Amount per serving	Amount per serving
Calories 170	**Cholesterol** 0mg	**Total Carbohydrate** 32g
Total Fat 2g	**Sodium** 5mg	Dietary Fiber 5g
Saturated Fat 0g	**Protein** 6g	Sugars 2g

Eden Foods, Short Grain Brown Rice, 100% Whole Grain, Organic

1/4 cup

Amount per serving	Amount per serving	Amount per serving
Calories 150	**Cholesterol** 0mg	**Total Carbohydrate** 35g
Total Fat 1.5g	**Sodium** 0mg	Dietary Fiber 3g
Saturated Fat 0g	**Protein** 3g	Sugars 1g

Jovial Foods, Jovial Organic Einkorn Wheat Berries

1/4 cup (50g)

Amount per serving	Amount per serving	Amount per serving
Calories 180	**Cholesterol** 0mg	**Total Carbohydrate** 33g
Total Fat 1.5g	**Sodium** 0mg	Dietary Fiber 4g
Saturated Fat 0g	**Protein** 9g	Sugars 0g

Mixes

Nature's Path, Buttermilk Pancake Mix

40g

Amount per serving	Amount per serving	Amount per serving
Calories 140	**Cholesterol** 0mg	**Total Carbohydrate** 27g
Total Fat 0.5g	**Sodium** 270mg	Dietary Fiber 2g
Saturated Fat 0g	**Protein** 7g	Sugars 5g

Nature's Path, Flax Plus® Multigrain Pancake Mix

40g

Amount per serving	Amount per serving	Amount per serving
Calories 140	**Cholesterol** 0mg	**Total Carbohydrate** 27g
Total Fat 1g	**Sodium** 240mg	Dietary Fiber 2g
Saturated Fat 0g	**Protein** 6g	Sugars 5g

Simply Organic Foods, Banana Bread Mix, Dry

2 tbsp dry mix

Amount per serving	Amount per serving	Amount per serving
Calories 90	**Cholesterol** 0mg	**Total Carbohydrate** 21g
Total Fat 0g	**Sodium** 200mg	Dietary Fiber 1g
Saturated Fat 0g	**Protein** 1g	Sugars 8g

Simply Organic Foods, Pizza Crust Mix, Dry

1/4 cup dry mix

Amount per serving	Amount per serving	Amount per serving
Calories 130	**Cholesterol** 0mg	**Total Carbohydrate** 28g
Total Fat 0.5g	**Sodium** 125mg	Dietary Fiber 1g
Saturated Fat 0g	**Protein** 1g	Sugars 0g

Pastas

Ancient Harvest, Supergrain Pasta® Elbows

57g

Amount per serving	Amount per serving	Amount per serving
Calories 205	**Cholesterol** 0mg	**Total Carbohydrate** 46g
Total Fat 1g	**Sodium** 4mg	Dietary Fiber 4g
Saturated Fat 0g	**Protein** 4g	Sugars <1g

Ancient Harvest, Supergrain Pasta® Garden Pagodas

57g

Amount per serving	Amount per serving	Amount per serving
Calories 205	**Cholesterol** 0mg	**Total Carbohydrate** 46g
Total Fat 1g	**Sodium** 4mg	Dietary Fiber 4g
Saturated Fat 0g	**Protein** 4g	Sugars <1g

Ancient Harvest, Supergrain Pasta® Linguine

57g

Amount per serving	Amount per serving	Amount per serving
Calories 205	**Cholesterol** 0mg	**Total Carbohydrate** 46g
Total Fat 1g	**Sodium** 4mg	Dietary Fiber 4g
Saturated Fat 0g	**Protein** 4g	Sugars <1g

Ancient Harvest, Supergrain Pasta® Penne

57g

Amount per serving	Amount per serving	Amount per serving
Calories 205	**Cholesterol** 0mg	**Total Carbohydrate** 46g
Total Fat 1g	**Sodium** 4mg	Dietary Fiber 4g
Saturated Fat 0g	**Protein** 4g	Sugars <1g

Ancient Harvest, Supergrain Pasta® Rotelle

57g

Amount per serving	Amount per serving	Amount per serving
Calories 205	**Cholesterol** 0mg	**Total Carbohydrate** 46g
Total Fat 1g	**Sodium** 4mg	Dietary Fiber 4g
Saturated Fat 0g	**Protein** 4g	Sugars <1g

Ancient Harvest, Supergrain Pasta® Shells

57g

Amount per serving	Amount per serving	Amount per serving
Calories 205	**Cholesterol** 0mg	**Total Carbohydrate** 46g
Total Fat 1g	**Sodium** 4mg	Dietary Fiber 4g
Saturated Fat 0g	**Protein** 4g	Sugars <1g

Ancient Harvest, Supergrain Pasta® Spaghetti

57g

Amount per serving	Amount per serving	Amount per serving
Calories 205	**Cholesterol** 0mg	**Total Carbohydrate** 46g
Total Fat 1g	**Sodium** 4mg	Dietary Fiber 4g
Saturated Fat 0g	**Protein** 4g	Sugars <1g

Ancient Harvest, Supergrain Pasta® Veggie Curls

57g

Amount per serving	Amount per serving	Amount per serving
Calories 205	**Cholesterol** 0mg	**Total Carbohydrate** 46g
Total Fat 1g	**Sodium** 4mg	Dietary Fiber 4g
Saturated Fat 0g	**Protein** 4g	Sugars <1g

Andean Dream, Quinoa & Corn Free Fusilli

1/4 cup

Amount per serving	Amount per serving	Amount per serving
Calories 207	**Cholesterol** 0mg	**Total Carbohydrate** 42g
Total Fat 1g	**Sodium** 0mg	Dietary Fiber 3g
Saturated Fat 0g	**Protein** 6g	Sugars 3g

Andean Dream, Quinoa Pasta & Corn Free Spaghetti

1/4 cup

Amount per serving	Amount per serving	Amount per serving
Calories 207	**Cholesterol** 0mg	**Total Carbohydrate** 42g
Total Fat 1g	**Sodium** 0mg	Dietary Fiber 3g
Saturated Fat 0g	**Protein** 6g	Sugars 3g

Andean Dream, Quinoa Pasta Gluten & Corn Free Macaroni

1/4 cup

Amount per serving	Amount per serving	Amount per serving
Calories 207	**Cholesterol** 0mg	**Total Carbohydrate** 42g
Total Fat 1g	**Sodium** 0mg	Dietary Fiber 3g
Saturated Fat 0g	**Protein** 6g	Sugars 3g

Andean Dream, Quinoa Pasta Gluten & Corn Free Shells

1/4 cup

Amount per serving	Amount per serving	Amount per serving
Calories 207	**Cholesterol** 0mg	**Total Carbohydrate** 42g
Total Fat 1g	**Sodium** 0mg	Dietary Fiber 3g
Saturated Fat 0g	**Protein** 6g	Sugars 3g

Annie Chun's, Organic Buckwheat Soba FreshPak Noodles

1 serving / 2 servings per package

Amount per serving	Amount per serving	Amount per serving
Calories 250	**Cholesterol** 0mg	**Total Carbohydrate** 52g
Total Fat 1g	**Sodium** 460mg	Dietary Fiber 2g
Saturated Fat 0g	**Protein** 8g	Sugars 1g

Annie Chun's, Organic Chow Mein FreshPak Noodles

1 serving / 2 servings per package

Amount per serving	Amount per serving	Amount per serving
Calories 250	**Cholesterol** 0mg	**Total Carbohydrate** 53g
Total Fat 0.5g	**Sodium** 460mg	Dietary Fiber 2g
Saturated Fat 0g	**Protein** 7g	Sugars 0g

Annie Chun's, Organic Japanese-Style Udon FreshPak Noodles

1 serving / 2 servings per package

Amount per serving	Amount per serving	Amount per serving
Calories 240	**Cholesterol** 0mg	**Total Carbohydrate** 51g
Total Fat 0.5g	**Sodium** 470mg	Dietary Fiber 2g
Saturated Fat 0g	**Protein** 6g	Sugars 0g

DeBoles, Organic Angel Hair Pasta

56g/ 1/4 of package

Amount per serving	Amount per serving	Amount per serving
Calories 210	**Cholesterol** 0mg	**Total Carbohydrate** 43g
Total Fat 1g	**Sodium** 5mg	Dietary Fiber 1g
Saturated Fat 0g	**Protein** 7g	Sugars 2g

DeBoles, Organic Angel Hair with Whole Wheat and Flax

56g/ 3/4 cup

Amount per serving	Amount per serving	Amount per serving
Calories 190	**Cholesterol** 0mg	**Total Carbohydrate** 38g
Total Fat 1.5g	**Sodium** 10mg	Dietary Fiber 6g
Saturated Fat 0g	**Protein** 6g	Sugars 0g

DeBoles, Organic Elbow Style Pasta

56g/ 1/4 of package

Amount per serving	Amount per serving	Amount per serving
Calories 210	**Cholesterol** 0mg	**Total Carbohydrate** 43g
Total Fat 1g	**Sodium** 5mg	Dietary Fiber 1g
Saturated Fat 0g	**Protein** 7g	Sugars 2g

DeBoles, Organic Fettuccini

56g/ 1/4 of package

Amount per serving	Amount per serving	Amount per serving
Calories 210	**Cholesterol** 0mg	**Total Carbohydrate** 43g
Total Fat 1g	**Sodium** 5mg	Dietary Fiber 1g
Saturated Fat 0g	**Protein** 7g	Sugars 2g

DeBoles, Organic Lasagna

70g/ 1/4 package

Amount per serving	Amount per serving	Amount per serving
Calories 260	**Cholesterol** 0mg	**Total Carbohydrate** 54g
Total Fat 1g	**Sodium** 5mg	Dietary Fiber 1g
Saturated Fat 0g	**Protein** 9g	Sugars 2g

DeBoles, Organic Linguini

56g/ 1/4 of package

Amount per serving	Amount per serving	Amount per serving
Calories 210	**Cholesterol** 0mg	**Total Carbohydrate** 43g
Total Fat 1g	**Sodium** 5mg	Dietary Fiber 1g
Saturated Fat 0g	**Protein** 7g	Sugars 2g

DeBoles, Organic Penne Pasta

57g/ 1/4 of package

Amount per serving	Amount per serving	Amount per serving
Calories 210	**Cholesterol** 0mg	**Total Carbohydrate** 41g
Total Fat 1g	**Sodium** 0mg	Dietary Fiber 1g
Saturated Fat 0g	**Protein** 7g	Sugars 2g

DeBoles, Organic Spaghetti Style Pasta

56g/ 1/4 of package

Amount per serving	Amount per serving	Amount per serving
Calories 210	**Cholesterol** 0mg	**Total Carbohydrate** 43g
Total Fat 1g	**Sodium** 5mg	Dietary Fiber 1g
Saturated Fat 0g	**Protein** 7g	Sugars 2g

DeBoles, Organic Spinach Fettuccine

56g/ 1/4 of package

Amount per serving	Amount per serving	Amount per serving
Calories 210	**Cholesterol** 0mg	**Total Carbohydrate** 43g
Total Fat 1g	**Sodium** 20mg	Dietary Fiber 3g
Saturated Fat 0g	**Protein** 7g	Sugars 1g

DeBoles, Organic Spinach Spaghetti Style Pasta

56g/ 1/4 of package

Amount per serving	Amount per serving	Amount per serving
Calories 210	**Cholesterol** 0mg	**Total Carbohydrate** 43g
Total Fat 1g	**Sodium** 20mg	Dietary Fiber 3g
Saturated Fat 0g	**Protein** 7g	Sugars 1g

DeBoles, Organic Whole Wheat Angel Hair Pasta

56g/ 1/4 of package

Amount per serving	Amount per serving	Amount per serving
Calories 210	**Cholesterol** 0mg	**Total Carbohydrate** 42g
Total Fat 1.5g	**Sodium** 10mg	Dietary Fiber 5g
Saturated Fat 0g	**Protein** 7g	Sugars 2g

DeBoles, Organic Whole Wheat Penne

56g/ 1/4 of package

Amount per serving	Amount per serving	Amount per serving
Calories 210	**Cholesterol** 0mg	**Total Carbohydrate** 42g
Total Fat 1.5g	**Sodium** 10mg	Dietary Fiber 5g
Saturated Fat 0g	**Protein** 7g	Sugars 2g

DeBoles, Organic Whole Wheat Rigatoni

56g/ about 1 cup

Amount per serving	Amount per serving	Amount per serving
Calories 210	**Cholesterol** 0mg	**Total Carbohydrate** 42g
Total Fat 1.5g	**Sodium** 10mg	Dietary Fiber 5g
Saturated Fat 0g	**Protein** 7g	Sugars 2g

DeBoles, Organic Whole Wheat Spaghetti Style Pasta

56g/ 1/4 of package

Amount per serving	Amount per serving	Amount per serving
Calories 210	**Cholesterol** 0mg	**Total Carbohydrate** 42g
Total Fat 1.5g	**Sodium** 10mg	Dietary Fiber 5g
Saturated Fat 0g	**Protein** 7g	Sugars 2g

Hodgson Mill, Certified Organic Angel Hair Whole Wheat Gourmet Pasta

2 oz dry

Amount per serving	Amount per serving	Amount per serving
Calories 215	**Cholesterol** 0mg	**Total Carbohydrate** 40g
Total Fat 2.5g	**Sodium** 0mg	Dietary Fiber 6g
Saturated Fat 0g	**Protein** 8g	Sugars 1g

Hodgson Mill, Certified Organic Fettuccine Whole Wheat Gourmet Pasta

2 oz dry

Amount per serving	Amount per serving	Amount per serving
Calories 215	**Cholesterol** 0mg	**Total Carbohydrate** 40g
Total Fat 2.5g	**Sodium** 0mg	Dietary Fiber 6g
Saturated Fat 0g	**Protein** 8g	Sugars 1g

Hodgson Mill, Certified Organic Lasagna Whole Wheat Gourmet Pasta

2 oz dry

Amount per serving	Amount per serving	Amount per serving
Calories 215	**Cholesterol** 0mg	**Total Carbohydrate** 40g
Total Fat 2.5g	**Sodium** 0mg	Dietary Fiber 6g
Saturated Fat 0g	**Protein** 8g	Sugars 1g

Hodgson Mill, Certified Organic Penne Whole Wheat Gourmet Pasta

2 oz dry

Amount per serving	Amount per serving	Amount per serving
Calories 215	**Cholesterol** 0mg	**Total Carbohydrate** 40g
Total Fat 2.5g	**Sodium** 0mg	Dietary Fiber 6g
Saturated Fat 0g	**Protein** 8g	Sugars 1g

Hodgson Mill, Certified Organic Spaghetti Whole Wheat Gourmet Pasta

2 oz dry

Amount per serving	Amount per serving	Amount per serving
Calories 215	**Cholesterol** 0mg	**Total Carbohydrate** 40g
Total Fat 2.5g	**Sodium** 0mg	Dietary Fiber 6g
Saturated Fat 0g	**Protein** 8g	Sugars 1g

Hodgson Mill, Certified Organic Spirals Whole Wheat Gourmet Pasta

2 oz dry

Amount per serving	Amount per serving	Amount per serving
Calories 215	**Cholesterol** 0mg	**Total Carbohydrate** 40g
Total Fat 2.5g	**Sodium** 0mg	Dietary Fiber 6g
Saturated Fat 0g	**Protein** 8g	Sugars 1g

Jovial Foods, Jovial 100% Organic Einkorn, Whole Wheat Fusilli Pasta

2 oz (57g)

Amount per serving	Amount per serving	Amount per serving
Calories 200	**Cholesterol** 0mg	**Total Carbohydrate** 40g
Total Fat 1.5g	**Sodium** 0mg	Dietary Fiber 2g
Saturated Fat 0g	**Protein** 8g	Sugars 1g

Jovial Foods, Jovial 100% Organic Einkorn, Whole Wheat Linguine Pasta

2 oz (57g)

Amount per serving	Amount per serving	Amount per serving
Calories 200	**Cholesterol** 0mg	**Total Carbohydrate** 35g
Total Fat 1.5g	**Sodium** 0mg	Dietary Fiber 4g
Saturated Fat 0g	**Protein** 9g	Sugars 1g

Jovial Foods, Jovial 100% Organic Einkorn, Whole Wheat Penne Rigate Pasta

2 oz (57g)

Amount per serving	Amount per serving	Amount per serving
Calories 200	**Cholesterol** 0mg	**Total Carbohydrate** 35g
Total Fat 1.5g	**Sodium** 0mg	Dietary Fiber 4g
Saturated Fat 0g	**Protein** 9g	Sugars 1g

Jovial Foods, Jovial 100% Organic Einkorn, Whole Wheat Rigatoni Pasta

2 oz (57g)

Amount per serving	Amount per serving	Amount per serving
Calories 200	**Cholesterol** 0mg	**Total Carbohydrate** 35g
Total Fat 1.5g	**Sodium** 0mg	Dietary Fiber 4g
Saturated Fat 0g	**Protein** 9g	Sugars 1g

Jovial Foods, Jovial 100% Organic Einkorn, Whole Wheat Spaghetti Pasta

2 oz (57g)

Amount per serving	Amount per serving	Amount per serving
Calories 200	**Cholesterol** 0mg	**Total Carbohydrate** 35g
Total Fat 1.5g	**Sodium** 0mg	Dietary Fiber 4g
Saturated Fat 0g	**Protein** 9g	Sugars 1g

Jovial Foods, Jovial 100% Organic White Einkorn, Fusilli Pasta

2 oz (57g)

Amount per serving	Amount per serving	Amount per serving
Calories 200	**Cholesterol** 0mg	**Total Carbohydrate** 40g
Total Fat 1.5g	**Sodium** 0mg	Dietary Fiber 2g
Saturated Fat 0g	**Protein** 8g	Sugars 1g

Jovial Foods, Jovial 100% Organic White Einkorn, Penne Rigate Pasta

2 oz (57g)

Amount per serving	Amount per serving	Amount per serving
Calories 200	**Cholesterol** 0mg	**Total Carbohydrate** 40g
Total Fat 1.5g	**Sodium** 0mg	Dietary Fiber 2g
Saturated Fat 0g	**Protein** 8g	Sugars 1g

Jovial Foods, Jovial 100% Organic White Einkorn, Spaghetti Pasta

2 oz (57g)

Amount per serving	Amount per serving	Amount per serving
Calories 200	**Cholesterol** 0mg	**Total Carbohydrate** 40g
Total Fat 1.5g	**Sodium** 0mg	Dietary Fiber 2g
Saturated Fat 0g	**Protein** 8g	Sugars 1g

Jovial Foods, Jovial Gluten Free Brown Rice Capellini Pasta

2 oz (57g)

Amount per serving	Amount per serving	Amount per serving
Calories 210	**Cholesterol** 0mg	**Total Carbohydrate** 43g
Total Fat 2g	**Sodium** 0mg	Dietary Fiber 2g
Saturated Fat 0g	**Protein** 5g	Sugars 0g

Jovial Foods, Jovial Gluten Free Brown Rice Caserecce Pasta

2 oz (57g)

Amount per serving	Amount per serving	Amount per serving
Calories 210	**Cholesterol** 0mg	**Total Carbohydrate** 43g
Total Fat 2g	**Sodium** 0mg	Dietary Fiber 2g
Saturated Fat 0g	**Protein** 5g	Sugars 0g

Jovial Foods, Jovial Gluten Free Brown Rice Fusilli Pasta

2 oz (57g)

Amount per serving	Amount per serving	Amount per serving
Calories 210	**Cholesterol** 0mg	**Total Carbohydrate** 43g
Total Fat 2g	**Sodium** 0mg	Dietary Fiber 2g
Saturated Fat 0g	**Protein** 5g	Sugars 0g

Jovial Foods, Jovial Gluten Free Brown Rice Lasagna

2 oz (57g)

Amount per serving	Amount per serving	Amount per serving
Calories 210	**Cholesterol** 0mg	**Total Carbohydrate** 43g
Total Fat 2g	**Sodium** 0mg	Dietary Fiber 2g
Saturated Fat 0g	**Protein** 5g	Sugars 0g

Jovial Foods, Jovial Gluten Free Brown Rice Penne Rigate Pasta

2 oz (57g)

Amount per serving	Amount per serving	Amount per serving
Calories 210	**Cholesterol** 0mg	**Total Carbohydrate** 43g
Total Fat 2g	**Sodium** 0mg	Dietary Fiber 2g
Saturated Fat 0g	**Protein** 5g	Sugars 0g

Jovial Foods, Jovial Gluten Free Brown Rice Spaghetti Pasta

2 oz (57g)

Amount per serving	Amount per serving	Amount per serving
Calories 210	**Cholesterol** 0mg	**Total Carbohydrate** 43g
Total Fat 2g	**Sodium** 0mg	Dietary Fiber 2g
Saturated Fat 0g	**Protein** 5g	Sugars 0g

Jovial Foods, Jovial Gluten Free Traditional Egg Tagliatelle Pasta

2 oz (57g)

Amount per serving	Amount per serving	Amount per serving
Calories 210	**Cholesterol** 40mg	**Total Carbohydrate** 40g
Total Fat 3g	**Sodium** 15mg	Dietary Fiber 2g
Saturated Fat 0g	**Protein** 5g	Sugars 0g

KOYO, Organic Fine Udon Pasta - 8 oz

1 bundle (76g)

Amount per serving	Amount per serving	Amount per serving
Calories 270	**Cholesterol** 0mg	**Total Carbohydrate** 57g
Total Fat 1g	**Sodium** 300mg	Dietary Fiber 2g
Saturated Fat 0g	**Protein** 9g	Sugars >1g

KOYO, Organic Round Udon Pasta - 8 oz

1 bundle (76g)

Amount per serving	Amount per serving	Amount per serving
Calories 270	**Cholesterol** 0mg	**Total Carbohydrate** 57g
Total Fat 1g	**Sodium** 300mg	Dietary Fiber 2g
Saturated Fat 0g	**Protein** 9g	Sugars <1g

KOYO, Organic Soba Pasta - 10 lb

1 bundle (76g)

Amount per serving	Amount per serving	Amount per serving
Calories 260	**Cholesterol** 0mg	**Total Carbohydrate** 54g
Total Fat 1.5g	**Sodium** 300mg	Dietary Fiber 2g
Saturated Fat 0g	**Protein** 9g	Sugars >1g

KOYO, Organic Soba Pasta - 8 oz

1 bundle (76g)

Amount per serving	Amount per serving	Amount per serving
Calories 260	**Cholesterol** 0mg	**Total Carbohydrate** 54g
Total Fat 1.5g	**Sodium** 300mg	Dietary Fiber 2g
Saturated Fat 0g	**Protein** 8g	Sugars 3g

KOYO, Organic Somen Pasta - 8 oz

1 bundle (76g)

Amount per serving	Amount per serving	Amount per serving
Calories 270	**Cholesterol** 0mg	**Total Carbohydrate** 57g
Total Fat 1g	**Sodium** 300mg	Dietary Fiber 2g
Saturated Fat 0g	**Protein** 9g	Sugars <1g

KOYO, Organic Udon Pasta - 10 lb

1 bundle (76g)

Amount per serving	Amount per serving	Amount per serving
Calories 270	**Cholesterol** 0mg	**Total Carbohydrate** 57g
Total Fat 1g	**Sodium** 300mg	Dietary Fiber 2g
Saturated Fat 0g	**Protein** 9g	Sugars >1g

KOYO, Organic Udon Pasta - 8 oz

1 bundlo (76g)

Amount per serving	Amount per serving	Amount per serving
Calories 270	**Cholesterol** 0mg	**Total Carbohydrate** 57g
Total Fat 1g	**Sodium** 300mg	Dietary Fiber 2g
Saturated Fat 0g	**Protein** 9g	Sugars >1g

KOYO, Organic Wide Udon Pasta - 8 oz

76g

Amount per serving	Amount per serving	Amount per serving
Calories 270	**Cholesterol** 0mg	**Total Carbohydrate** 27g
Total Fat 1g	**Sodium** 300mg	Dietary Fiber 2g
Saturated Fat 0g	**Protein** 9g	Sugars <1g

Lundberg Family Farms, Organic Brown Rice Elbow Pasta

2 oz (56g/about 1/6 of pkg)

Amount per serving	Amount per serving	Amount per serving
Calories 190	**Cholesterol** 0mg	**Total Carbohydrate** 41g
Total Fat 3g	**Sodium** 0mg	Dietary Fiber 4g
Saturated Fat 0.5g	**Protein** 4g	Sugars 1g

Lundberg Family Farms, Organic Brown Rice Penne Pasta

2 oz (56g/about 1/6 of pkg)

Amount per serving	Amount per serving	Amount per serving
Calories 190	**Cholesterol** 0mg	**Total Carbohydrate** 41g
Total Fat 3g	**Sodium** 0mg	Dietary Fiber 4g
Saturated Fat 0.5g	**Protein** 4g	Sugars 1g

Lundberg Family Farms, Organic Brown Rice Rotini Pasta

2 oz (56g/about 1/6 of pkg)

Amount per serving	Amount per serving	Amount per serving
Calories 190	**Cholesterol** 0mg	**Total Carbohydrate** 41g
Total Fat 3g	**Sodium** 0mg	Dietary Fiber 4g
Saturated Fat 0.5g	**Protein** 4g	Sugars 1g

Lundberg Family Farms, Organic Brown Rice Spaghetti Pasta

2 oz (56g/about 1/6 of pkg)

Amount per serving	Amount per serving	Amount per serving
Calories 190	**Cholesterol** 0mg	**Total Carbohydrate** 41g
Total Fat 3g	**Sodium** 0mg	Dietary Fiber 4g
Saturated Fat 0.5g	**Protein** 4g	Sugars 1g

Lundberg Family Farms, Organic Plain Original Couscous

1/4 cup dry (45g) (1 cup prepared)

Amount per serving	Amount per serving	Amount per serving
Calories 160	**Cholesterol** 0mg	**Total Carbohydrate** 37g
Total Fat 1.5g	**Sodium** 0mg	Dietary Fiber 3g
Saturated Fat 0g	**Protein** 3g	Sugars 1g

Pastariso Organic, Organic Angel Hair

2 oz (56g)

Amount per serving	Amount per serving	Amount per serving
Calories 190	**Cholesterol** 0mg	**Total Carbohydrate** 42g
Total Fat 0.6g	**Sodium** 5mg	Dietary Fiber 3g
Saturated Fat 0g	**Protein** 4g	Sugars 3g

Pastariso Organic, Organic Brown Rice Pasta, Fettucine

2 oz (56g)

Amount per serving	Amount per serving	Amount per serving
Calories 190	**Cholesterol** 0mg	**Total Carbohydrate** 42g
Total Fat 0.6g	**Sodium** 5mg	Dietary Fiber 3g
Saturated Fat 0g	**Protein** 4g	Sugars 3g

Pastariso Organic, Organic Brown Rice Pasta, Lasagna

2 oz (56g)

Amount per serving	Amount per serving	Amount per serving
Calories 190	**Cholesterol** 0mg	**Total Carbohydrate** 42g
Total Fat 0.6g	**Sodium** 5mg	Dietary Fiber 3g
Saturated Fat 0g	**Protein** 4g	Sugars 3g

Pastariso Organic, Organic Brown Rice Pasta, Linguine

2 oz (56g)

Amount per serving	Amount per serving	Amount per serving
Calories 190	**Cholesterol** 0mg	**Total Carbohydrate** 42g
Total Fat 0.6g	**Sodium** 5mg	Dietary Fiber 3g
Saturated Fat 0g	**Protein** 4g	Sugars 3g

Pastariso Organic, Organic Brown Rice Pasta, Rotini

2 oz (56g)

Amount per serving	Amount per serving	Amount per serving
Calories 190	**Cholesterol** 0mg	**Total Carbohydrate** 42g
Total Fat 0.6g	**Sodium** 5mg	Dietary Fiber 3g
Saturated Fat 0g	**Protein** 4g	Sugars 3g

Pastariso Organic, Organic Brown Rice Pasta, Spaghetti Style

2 oz (56g)

Amount per serving	Amount per serving	Amount per serving
Calories 190	**Cholesterol** 0mg	**Total Carbohydrate** 42g
Total Fat 0.6g	**Sodium** 5mg	Dietary Fiber 3g
Saturated Fat 0g	**Protein** 4g	Sugars 3g

Pastariso Organic, Organic Brown Rice Pasta, Spinach, Spaghetti Style

2 oz (56g)

Amount per serving	Amount per serving	Amount per serving
Calories 190	**Cholesterol** 0mg	**Total Carbohydrate** 42g
Total Fat 0.6g	**Sodium** 5mg	Dietary Fiber 3g
Saturated Fat 0g	**Protein** 4g	Sugars 3g

Pastariso Organic, Organic Brown Rice, Penne

2 oz (56g)

Amount per serving	Amount per serving	Amount per serving
Calories 190	**Cholesterol** 0mg	**Total Carbohydrate** 42g
Total Fat 0.6g	**Sodium** 5mg	Dietary Fiber 3g
Saturated Fat 0g	**Protein** 4g	Sugars 3g

Pastariso Organic, Organic Quick-Cooking Rice Mac & White Cheeze (Elephant)

2 oz (56g)

Amount per serving	Amount per serving	Amount per serving
Calories 194	**Cholesterol** 5mg	**Total Carbohydrate** 35g
Total Fat 2g	**Sodium** 206mg	Dietary Fiber 3g
Saturated Fat 0.5g	**Protein** 9g	Sugars 4g

Pastariso Organic, Organic Quick-Cooking White Rice Mac & Yellow Cheeze (Dolphin)

2 oz (56g)

Amount per serving	Amount per serving	Amount per serving
Calories 194	**Cholesterol** 5mg	**Total Carbohydrate** 35g
Total Fat 2g	**Sodium** 206mg	Dietary Fiber 3g
Saturated Fat 0.5g	**Protein** 9g	Sugars 4g

Pastariso Organic, Organic Quick-Cooking White Rice Mac & Yellow Cheeze (Orca)

2 oz (56g)

Amount per serving	Amount per serving	Amount per serving
Calories 194	**Cholesterol** 5mg	**Total Carbohydrate** 35g
Total Fat 2g	**Sodium** 206mg	Dietary Fiber 3g
Saturated Fat 0.5g	**Protein** 9g	Sugars 4g

Pastariso Organic, Organic Vegetable Rotini

2 oz (56g)

Amount per serving	Amount per serving	Amount per serving
Calories 190	**Cholesterol** 0mg	**Total Carbohydrate** 42g
Total Fat 0g	**Sodium** 5mg	Dietary Fiber 3g
Saturated Fat 0g	**Protein** 4g	Sugars 3g

Pastariso Organic, Organic Whole Grain Rice Elbows

2 oz (56g)

Amount per serving	Amount per serving	Amount per serving
Calories 190	**Cholesterol** 0mg	**Total Carbohydrate** 42g
Total Fat 0.6g	**Sodium** 5mg	Dietary Fiber 3g
Saturated Fat 0g	**Protein** 4g	Sugars 3g

Pastariso Organic, Organic Whole Grain Rice Vegetable Rotini

2 oz (56g)

Amount per serving	Amount per serving	Amount per serving
Calories 190	**Cholesterol** 0mg	**Total Carbohydrate** 42g
Total Fat 0g	**Sodium** 5mg	Dietary Fiber 3g
Saturated Fat 0g	**Protein** 4g	Sugars 3g

Tinkyada Organic, Gluten-Free Brown Rice Elbow Pasta, Dry

2 oz

Amount per serving	Amount per serving	Amount per serving
Calories 200	**Cholesterol** 0mg	**Total Carbohydrate** 44g
Total Fat 1.5g	**Sodium** 25mg	Dietary Fiber 1g
Saturated Fat 0g	**Protein** 4g	Sugars 0g

Tinkyada Organic, Gluten-Free Brown Rice Penne Pasta, Dry

2 oz

Amount per serving	Amount per serving	Amount per serving
Calories 210	**Cholesterol** 0mg	**Total Carbohydrate** 43g
Total Fat 2g	**Sodium** 15mg	Dietary Fiber 2g
Saturated Fat 1g	**Protein** 4g	Sugars 0g

Tinkyada Organic, Gluten-Free Brown Rice Spaghetti Style Pasta

2 oz

Amount per serving	Amount per serving	Amount per serving
Calories 200	**Cholesterol** 0mg	**Total Carbohydrate** 44g
Total Fat 1.5g	**Sodium** 25mg	Dietary Fiber 1g
Saturated Fat 0g	**Protein** 4g	Sugars 0g

Tolerant Foods, Organic Black Bean Mini Fettucine

3 oz (85g)

Amount per serving	Amount per serving	Amount per serving
Calories 320	**Cholesterol** 0mg	**Total Carbohydrate** 55g
Total Fat 1.5g	**Sodium** 10mg	Dietary Fiber 15g
Saturated Fat 0g	**Protein** 22g	Sugars 10g

Tolerant Foods, Organic Black Bean Penne

3 oz (85g)

Amount per serving	Amount per serving	Amount per serving
Calories 320	**Cholesterol** 0mg	**Total Carbohydrate** 55g
Total Fat 1.5g	**Sodium** 10mg	Dietary Fiber 15g
Saturated Fat 0g	**Protein** 22g	Sugars 10g

Tolerant Foods, Organic Black Bean Rotini

3 oz (85g)

Amount per serving	Amount per serving	Amount per serving
Calories 320	**Cholesterol** 0mg	**Total Carbohydrate** 55g
Total Fat 1.5g	**Sodium** 10mg	Dietary Fiber 15g
Saturated Fat 0g	**Protein** 22g	Sugars 10g

Tolerant Foods, Organic Mini Red Lentil Fettucine

3 oz (85g)

Amount per serving	Amount per serving	Amount per serving
Calories 310	**Cholesterol** 0mg	**Total Carbohydrate** 56g
Total Fat 1g	**Sodium** 10mg	Dietary Fiber 13g
Saturated Fat 0g	**Protein** 21g	Sugars 6g

Tolerant Foods, Organic Red Lentil Penne

3 oz (85g)

Amount per serving	Amount per serving	Amount per serving
Calories 310	**Cholesterol** 0mg	**Total Carbohydrate** 56g
Total Fat 1g	**Sodium** 10mg	Dietary Fiber 13g
Saturated Fat 0g	**Protein** 21g	Sugars 6g

Tolerant Foods, Organic Red Lentil Rotini

3 oz (85g)

Amount per serving	Amount per serving	Amount per serving
Calories 310	**Cholesterol** 0mg	**Total Carbohydrate** 56g
Total Fat 1g	**Sodium** 10mg	Dietary Fiber 13g
Saturated Fat 0g	**Protein** 21g	Sugars 6g

Westbrae Natural, Organic Spinach Spaghetti

2 oz dry (56g/about 1/8 of pkg)

Amount per serving	Amount per serving	Amount per serving
Calories 180	**Cholesterol** NA	**Total Carbohydrate** 38g
Total Fat 2g	**Sodium** 20mg	Dietary Fiber 8g
Saturated Fat NA	**Protein** 9g	Sugars 1g

Westbrae Natural, Organic Whole Wheat Lasagna

2 pieces dry (about 49g)

Amount per serving	Amount per serving	Amount per serving
Calories 180	**Cholesterol** NA	**Total Carbohydrate** 34g
Total Fat 1.5g	**Sodium** 5mg	Dietary Fiber 7g
Saturated Fat NA	**Protein** 8g	Sugars 1g

Westbrae Natural, Organic Whole Wheat Spaghetti

2 oz dry (56g/about 1/8 of pkg)

Amount per serving	Amount per serving	Amount per serving
Calories 200	**Cholesterol** NA	**Total Carbohydrate** 39g
Total Fat 1.5g	**Sodium** 10mg	Dietary Fiber 9g
Saturated Fat NA	**Protein** 9g	Sugars 1g

Wildwood Organic, Organic Pasta Slim, Low Calorie, Wheat Free Spaghetti

3.5 oz (100g)

Amount per serving	Amount per serving	Amount per serving
Calories 20	**Cholesterol** 0mg	**Total Carbohydrate** 4g
Total Fat 0.5g	**Sodium** 5mg	Dietary Fiber 3g
Saturated Fat 0g	**Protein** 1g	Sugars 0g

Wildwood Organic, Organic Pasta Slim, Low Calorie, Wheat Free Spinach Fettuccini

3.5 oz (100g)

Amount per serving	Amount per serving	Amount per serving
Calories 25	**Cholesterol** 0mg	**Total Carbohydrate** 5g
Total Fat 0g	**Sodium** 10mg	Dietary Fiber 3g
Saturated Fat 0g	**Protein** 1g	Sugars 0g

Wildwood Organic, Organic Pasta Slim, Wheat Free Tomato & Herb Angel Hair

3.5 oz (100g)

Amount per serving	Amount per serving	Amount per serving
Calories 20	**Cholesterol** 0mg	**Total Carbohydrate** 3g
Total Fat 0g	**Sodium** 5mg	Dietary Fiber 0g
Saturated Fat 0g	**Protein** 1g	Sugars 0g

Rice

Lotus Foods, Organic Brown Jasmine Rice

1/4 cup

Amount per serving	Amount per serving	Amount per serving
Calories 170	**Cholesterol** 0mg	**Total Carbohydrate** 36g
Total Fat 1.5g	**Sodium** 0mg	Dietary Fiber 2g
Saturated Fat 0.5g	**Protein** 4g	Sugars 0g

Lotus Foods, Organic Brown Jasmine Rice Heat & Eat Bowl

1 1/4 Cup (210g)

Amount per serving	Amount per serving	Amount per serving
Calories 350	**Cholesterol** 0mg	**Total Carbohydrate** 74g
Total Fat 3g	**Sodium** 13mg	Dietary Fiber 4g
Saturated Fat 1g	**Protein** 8g	Sugars 0.5g

Lotus Foods, Organic Brown Mekong Flower Rice™

1/3 cup (60g dry)

Amount per serving	Amount per serving	Amount per serving
Calories 210	**Cholesterol** 0mg	**Total Carbohydrate** 45g
Total Fat 1.5g	**Sodium** 0mg	Dietary Fiber 2g
Saturated Fat 0.5g	**Protein** 5g	Sugars 0g

Lotus Foods, Organic Carnaroli Rice

1/3 cup

Amount per serving	Amount per serving	Amount per serving
Calories 240	**Cholesterol** 0mg	**Total Carbohydrate** 53g
Total Fat 0g	**Sodium** 0mg	Dietary Fiber 2g
Saturated Fat 0g	**Protein** 5g	Sugars 0g

Lotus Foods, Organic Forbidden Rice®

1/3 cup (60g dry)

Amount per serving	Amount per serving	Amount per serving
Calories 200	**Cholesterol** 0mg	**Total Carbohydrate** 43g
Total Fat 2g	**Sodium** 0mg	Dietary Fiber 3g
Saturated Fat 0g	**Protein** 6g	Sugars 1g

Lotus Foods, Organic Forbidden Rice® Ramen

1/2 piece (35g)

Amount per serving	Amount per serving	Amount per serving
Calories 130	**Cholesterol** 0mg	**Total Carbohydrate** 27g
Total Fat 1.5g	**Sodium** 0mg	Dietary Fiber <1g
Saturated Fat 0g	**Protein** 3g	Sugars 0g

Lotus Foods, Organic Jade Pearl Rice™

1/3 cup

Amount per serving	Amount per serving	Amount per serving
Calories 210	**Cholesterol** 0mg	**Total Carbohydrate** 43g
Total Fat 0g	**Sodium** 0mg	Dietary Fiber 0g
Saturated Fat 0g	**Protein** 4g	Sugars 0g

Lotus Foods, Organic Jade Pearl Rice™ Ramen

1/2 piece (35g)

Amount per serving	Amount per serving	Amount per serving
Calories 120	**Cholesterol** 0mg	**Total Carbohydrate** 26g
Total Fat 1g	**Sodium** 0mg	Dietary Fiber <1g
Saturated Fat 0g	**Protein** 3g	Sugars 1g

Lotus Foods, Organic Jasmine Rice

1/3 cup (60g dry)

Amount per serving	Amount per serving	Amount per serving
Calories 210	**Cholesterol** 0mg	**Total Carbohydrate** 45g
Total Fat 1.5g	**Sodium** 0mg	Dietary Fiber 2g
Saturated Fat 0.5g	**Protein** 5g	Sugars 0g

Lotus Foods, Organic Millet & Brown Rice Ramen

1/2 piece (35g)

Amount per serving	Amount per serving	Amount per serving
Calories 130	**Cholesterol** 0mg	**Total Carbohydrate** 24g
Total Fat 1.5g	**Sodium** 0mg	Dietary Fiber 2g
Saturated Fat 0g	**Protein** 4g	Sugars 0g

Lotus Foods, Organic Volcano Rice™

1/3 cup (60g dry)

Amount per serving	Amount per serving	Amount per serving
Calories 200	**Cholesterol** 0mg	**Total Carbohydrate** 44g
Total Fat 0g	**Sodium** 0mg	Dietary Fiber 1g
Saturated Fat 0g	**Protein** 6g	Sugars 0g

Lotus Foods, Organic Volcano Rice™ Heat & Eat Bowl

1 1/4 cup (210g)

Amount per serving	Amount per serving	Amount per serving
Calories 340	**Cholesterol** 0mg	**Total Carbohydrate** 74g
Total Fat 1g	**Sodium** 0mg	Dietary Fiber 2g
Saturated Fat 0.5g	**Protein** 10g	Sugars 0g

Lundberg Family Farms, Heat & Eat, Organic Countrywild, Brown Rice Bowl

210g

Amount per serving	Amount per serving	Amount por serving
Calories 280	**Cholesterol** 0mg	**Total Carbohydrate** 65g
Total Fat 3g	**Sodium** 0mg	Dietary Fiber 6g
Saturated Fat 0g	**Protein** 6g	Sugars 0g

Lundberg Family Farms, Heat & Eat, Organic Long Grain Brown Rice Bowl

210g

Amount per serving	Amount per serving	Amount per serving
Calories 290	**Cholesterol** 0mg	**Total Carbohydrate** 65g
Total Fat 3g	**Sodium** 5mg	Dietary Fiber 6g
Saturated Fat 0.5g	**Protein** 6g	Sugars 1g

Lundberg Family Farms, Heat & Eat, Organic Short Grain Brown Rice Bowl

210g

Amount per serving	Amount per serving	Amount per serving
Calories 290	**Cholesterol** 0mg	**Total Carbohydrate** 65g
Total Fat 2.5g	**Sodium** 10mg	Dietary Fiber 5g
Saturated Fat 0.5g	**Protein** 5g	Sugars 1g

Lundberg Family Farms, Organic Brown Basmati and Wild Rice

1/4 cup (dry) (45g)

Amount per serving	Amount per serving	Amount per serving
Calories 150	**Cholesterol** 0mg	**Total Carbohydrate** 34g
Total Fat 1.5g	**Sodium** 0mg	Dietary Fiber 2g
Saturated Fat 0g	**Protein** 4g	Sugars 1g

Lundberg Family Farms, Organic Brown Long Grain Rice

1/4 cup (dry) (45g)

Amount per serving	Amount per serving	Amount per serving
Calories 150	**Cholesterol** 0mg	**Total Carbohydrate** 35g
Total Fat 1.5g	**Sodium** 0mg	Dietary Fiber 3g
Saturated Fat 0g	**Protein** 3g	Sugars 0g

Lundberg Family Farms, Organic California Brown Basmati Rice

1/4 cup (dry) (45g)

Amount per serving	Amount per serving	Amount per serving
Calories 150	**Cholesterol** 0mg	**Total Carbohydrate** 34g
Total Fat 1.5g	**Sodium** 0mg	Dietary Fiber 2g
Saturated Fat 0g	**Protein** 4g	Sugars 1g

Lundberg Family Farms, Organic California Brown Basmati Rice, Dry

1/4 cup

Amount per serving	Amount per serving	Amount per serving
Calories 150	**Cholesterol** 0mg	**Total Carbohydrate** 33g
Total Fat 1.5g	**Sodium** 0mg	Dietary Fiber 2g
Saturated Fat 0g	**Protein** 4g	Sugars 1g

Lundberg Family Farms, Organic California Brown Jasmine Rice, Dry

1/4 cup

Amount per serving	Amount per serving	Amount per serving
Calories 150	**Cholesterol** 0mg	**Total Carbohydrate** 33g
Total Fat 1.5g	**Sodium** 0mg	Dietary Fiber 2g
Saturated Fat 0g	**Protein** 4g	Sugars 1g

Lundberg Family Farms, Organic California White Basmati Rice

1/4 cup (dry) (45g)

Amount per serving	Amount per serving	Amount per serving
Calories 160	**Cholesterol** 0mg	**Total Carbohydrate** 34g
Total Fat 0.5g	**Sodium** 0mg	Dietary Fiber 1g
Saturated Fat 0g	**Protein** 3g	Sugars 0g

Lundberg Family Farms, Organic California White Jasmine Rice, Dry

1/4 cup

Amount per serving	Amount per serving	Amount per serving
Calories 160	**Cholesterol** 0mg	**Total Carbohydrate** 36g
Total Fat 0.5g	**Sodium** 0mg	Dietary Fiber 1g
Saturated Fat 0g	**Protein** 3g	Sugars 0g

Lundberg Family Farms, Organic California White Sushi Rice, Dry

1/4 cup

Amount per serving	Amount per serving	Amount per serving
Calories 150	**Cholesterol** 0mg	**Total Carbohydrate** 35g
Total Fat 0g	**Sodium** 5mg	Dietary Fiber 1g
Saturated Fat 0g	**Protein** 4g	Sugars 0g

Lundberg Family Farms, Organic Countrywild Brown Rice Bowl

1/4 cup (dry) (45g)

Amount per serving	Amount per serving	Amount per serving
Calories 280	**Cholesterol** 0mg	**Total Carbohydrate** 65g
Total Fat 3g	**Sodium** 0mg	Dietary Fiber 6g
Saturated Fat 0.5g	**Protein** 6g	Sugars 0g

Lundberg Family Farms, Organic Golden Rose Brown Rice, Dry

1/4 cup

Amount per serving	Amount per serving	Amount per serving
Calories 160	**Cholesterol** 0mg	**Total Carbohydrate** 34g
Total Fat 1g	**Sodium** 0mg	Dietary Fiber 1g
Saturated Fat 0g	**Protein** 3g	Sugars 0g

Lundberg Family Farms, Organic Long Grain Brown Rice, Dry

1/4 cup

Amount per serving	Amount per serving	Amount per serving
Calories 150	**Cholesterol** 0mg	**Total Carbohydrate** 35g
Total Fat 1.5g	**Sodium** 0mg	Dietary Fiber 3g
Saturated Fat 0g	**Protein** 3g	Sugars 0g

Lundberg Family Farms, Organic Lundberg Burgundy Red Rice

1/4 cup (dry) (45g)

Amount per serving	Amount per serving	Amount per serving
Calories 160	**Cholesterol** 0mg	**Total Carbohydrate** 32g
Total Fat 1g	**Sodium** 10mg	Dietary Fiber 2g
Saturated Fat 0g	**Protein** 4g	Sugars 0g

Lundberg Family Farms, Organic Quick Wild Rice, Dry

1/4 cup

Amount per serving	Amount per serving	Amount per serving
Calories 150	**Cholesterol** NA	**Total Carbohydrate** 33g
Total Fat 0.5g	**Sodium** 0mg	Dietary Fiber 2g
Saturated Fat 0g	**Protein** 6g	Sugars 1g

Lundberg Family Farms, Organic Short Grain Brown Rice, Dry

1/4 cup

Amount per serving	Amount per serving	Amount per serving
Calories 150	**Cholesterol** 0mg	**Total Carbohydrate** 35g
Total Fat 1.5g	**Sodium** 0mg	Dietary Fiber 3g
Saturated Fat 0g	**Protein** 3g	Sugars 1g

Lundberg Family Farms, Organic Sprouted Brown Basmati Rice

1/4 cup (dry) (45g)

Amount per serving	Amount per serving	Amount per serving
Calories 160	**Cholesterol** 0mg	**Total Carbohydrate** 33g
Total Fat 2g	**Sodium** 0mg	Dietary Fiber 2g
Saturated Fat 0g	**Protein** 4g	Sugars 1g

Lundberg Family Farms, Organic Sprouted Red Rice

1/4 cup (dry) (45g)

Amount per serving	Amount per serving	Amount per serving
Calories 160	**Cholesterol** 0mg	**Total Carbohydrate** 34g
Total Fat 1.5g	**Sodium** 0mg	Dietary Fiber 3g
Saturated Fat 0g	**Protein** 3g	Sugars 0g

Lundberg Family Farms, Organic Sprouted Short Brown Rice

1/4 cup (dry) (45g)

Amount per serving	Amount per serving	Amount per serving
Calories 160	**Cholesterol** 0mg	**Total Carbohydrate** 33g
Total Fat 1.5g	**Sodium** 0mg	Dietary Fiber 3g
Saturated Fat 0g	**Protein** 3g	Sugars 1g

Lundberg Family Farms, Organic Sprouted Tri-Colr Blend Rice

1/4 cup (dry) (45g)

Amount per serving	Amount per serving	Amount per serving
Calories 160	**Cholesterol** 0mg	**Total Carbohydrate** 33g
Total Fat 2g	**Sodium** 0mg	Dietary Fiber 3g
Saturated Fat 0g	**Protein** 3g	Sugars 0g

Lundberg Family Farms, Organic White Arborio Rice

1/4 cup

Amount per serving	Amount per serving	Amount per serving
Calories 160	**Cholesterol** 0mg	**Total Carbohydrate** 43g
Total Fat 1g	**Sodium** 0mg	Dietary Fiber 1g
Saturated Fat 0g	**Protein** 6g	Sugars 0g

Lundberg Family Farms, Organic White Long Grain Rice

1/4 cup (dry) (45g)

Amount per serving	Amount per serving	Amount per serving
Calories 160	**Cholesterol** 0mg	**Total Carbohydrate** 36g
Total Fat 0g	**Sodium** 0mg	Dietary Fiber 0g
Saturated Fat 0g	**Protein** 4g	Sugars 0g

Lundberg Family Farms, Organic Whole Grain & Wild Rice—Garlic & Basil

2 oz (56g—about 1/3 cup rice blend and 1 1/2 tsp seasoning mix) (1 cup prepared)

Amount per serving	Amount per serving	Amount per serving
Calories 210	**Cholesterol** 0mg	**Total Carbohydrate** 45g
Total Fat 1.5g	**Sodium** 470mg	Dietary Fiber 3g
Saturated Fat 0g	**Protein** 5g	Sugars 1g

Lundberg Family Farms, Organic Whole Grain & Wild Rice—Original

2 oz (56g—about 1/3 cup rice blend and 1 1/2 tsp seasoning mix) (1 cup prepared)

Amount per serving	Amount per serving	Amount per serving
Calories 210	**Cholesterol** 0mg	**Total Carbohydrate** 45g
Total Fat 1.5g	**Sodium** 470mg	Dietary Fiber 3g
Saturated Fat 0g	**Protein** 5g	Sugars 1g

Lundberg Family Farms, Organic Whole Grain & Wild Rice—Wild Porcini Mushroom

2 oz (56g—about 1/3 cup rice blend and 1 1/2 tsp seasoning mix) (1 cup prepared)

Amount per serving	Amount per serving	Amount per serving
Calories 210	**Cholesterol** 0mg	**Total Carbohydrate** 45g
Total Fat 1.5g	**Sodium** 470mg	Dietary Fiber 3g
Saturated Fat 0g	**Protein** 5g	Sugars 1g

Lundberg Family Farms, Organic Whole Grain Southwestern Rice

56g (about 1/4 cup rice and 2 tbsp seasoning mix) (1 cup prepared)

Amount per serving	Amount per serving	Amount per serving
Calories 220	**Cholesterol** 0mg	**Total Carbohydrate** 45g
Total Fat 2g	**Sodium** 410mg	Dietary Fiber 4g
Saturated Fat 0g	**Protein** 5g	Sugars 2g

Lundberg Family Farms, Organic Wild Blend

1/4 cup

Amount per serving	Amount per serving	Amount per serving
Calories 150	**Cholesterol** 0mg	**Total Carbohydrate** 35g
Total Fat 1.5g	**Sodium** 0mg	Dietary Fiber 3g
Saturated Fat 0g	**Protein** 4g	Sugars 0g

Lundberg Family Farms, Organic Wild Rice, Dry

1/4 cup

Amount per serving	Amount per serving	Amount per serving
Calories 150	**Cholesterol** 0mg	**Total Carbohydrate** 33g
Total Fat 1g	**Sodium** 0mg	Dietary Fiber 2g
Saturated Fat 0g	**Protein** 6g	Sugars 1g

Manna Organics, Organic Brown Rice

45g (1.6 oz)

Amount per serving	Amount per serving	Amount per serving
Calories 160	**Cholesterol** 0mg	**Total Carbohydrate** 34g
Total Fat 1g	**Sodium** 0mg	Dietary Fiber 2g
Saturated Fat 0g	**Protein** 3g	Sugars 0g

Vegetables

Eating a diet rich in vegetables and fruits may help reduce your risk for heart disease, obesity, and type 2 diabetes and may protect against certain types of cancers. Most vegetables are naturally low in fat, calories, and sodium. Vegetables do not have cholesterol, but adding sauces or seasonings can add cholesterol, in addition to calories, sodium, and fat.

Vegetables are important sources of key nutrients, including potassium, dietary fiber, folate (folic acid), vitamin A, and vitamin C. Potassium-rich vegetables include sweet potatoes, white potatoes, white beans, tomato products (paste, sauce, and juice), beet greens, soybeans, lima beans, spinach, lentils, and kidney beans. Diets rich in potassium may help to maintain healthy blood pressure, reduce the risk of developing kidney stones, and help to slow or decrease bone loss. Vitamin A keeps eyes and skin healthy and helps to protect against infections. Vitamin C aids in iron absorption, keeps teeth and gums healthy, and helps cuts and wounds heal.

Why Eat Organic Vegetables?

Choosing organic vegetables can substantially reduce the amount of synthetic pesticides in your diet. The Environmental Working Group (EWG) advises buying only USDA-certified organic bell peppers, carrots, celery, kale, lettuce, potatoes, and sweet peppers because theses vegetables generally have high concentrations of pesticide residue. It's not as critical to buy organic asparagus, avocados, cabbage, sweet corn, or onions since these vegetables tend to be very low in pesticide residues. While it may be ideal to go "all-organic," if you're on a budget, these guidelines can help you get the biggest bang for your organic buck.

Daily Goal

The USDA recommends filling half of your plate with fruits and vegetables, or about 2½ cups for an adult on a 2,000-calorie diet.

1 cup equivalents:
1 cup cooked vegetable	3" tomato
2 cups raw vegetables	1 cup cooked dry peas or beans
2 medium carrots	1 cup starchy vegetable

Lettuces

Earthbound Farm Organic, Deep Green Blends, Kale

3 oz (85g / about 2 cups)

Amount per serving	Amount per serving	Amount per serving
Calories 35	**Cholesterol** 0mg	**Total Carbohydrate** 5g
Total Fat 0.5g	**Sodium** 85mg	Dietary Fiber 2g
Saturated Fat 0g	**Protein** 2g	Sugars 1g

Earthbound Farm Organic, Deep Green Blends, Kale Italia

3 oz (85g / about 2 cups)

Amount per serving	Amount per serving	Amount per serving
Calories 30	**Cholesterol** 0mg	**Total Carbohydrate** 5g
Total Fat 0g	**Sodium** 70mg	Dietary Fiber 2g
Saturated Fat 0g	**Protein** 2g	Sugars 1g

Earthbound Farm Organic, Deep Green Blends, Power

3 oz (85g / about 2 cups)

Amount per serving	Amount per serving	Amount per serving
Calories 20	**Cholesterol** 0mg	**Total Carbohydrate** 3g
Total Fat 0g	**Sodium** 130mg	Dietary Fiber 2g
Saturated Fat 0g	**Protein** 2g	Sugars 0g

Earthbound Farm Organic, Deep Green Blends, Zen

3 oz (85g / about 2 cups)

Amount per serving	Amount per serving	Amount per serving
Calories 20	**Cholesterol** 0mg	**Total Carbohydrate** 4g
Total Fat 0g	**Sodium** 105mg	Dietary Fiber 1g
Saturated Fat 0g	**Protein** 2g	Sugars 0g

Earthbound Farm Organic, Easy Leaves, Butter Lettuce Leaves

3 oz (85g / about 2 cups)

Amount per serving	Amount per serving	Amount per serving
Calories 10	**Cholesterol** 0mg	**Total Carbohydrate** 2g
Total Fat 0g	**Sodium** 0mg	Dietary Fiber 1g
Saturated Fat 0g	**Protein** 1g	Sugars 1g

Earthbound Farm Organic, Easy Leaves, Petites

3 oz (85g / about 2 cups)

Amount per serving	Amount per serving	Amount per serving
Calories 15	**Cholesterol** 0mg	**Total Carbohydrate** 3g
Total Fat 0g	**Sodium** 50mg	Dietary Fiber 1g
Saturated Fat 0g	**Protein** 1g	Sugars 0g

Earthbound Farm Organic, Easy Leaves, Romaine

3 oz (85g / about 2 cups)

Amount per serving	Amount per serving	Amount per serving
Calories 10	**Cholesterol** 0mg	**Total Carbohydrate** 2g
Total Fat 0g	**Sodium** 5mg	Dietary Fiber 1g
Saturated Fat 0g	**Protein** 1g	Sugars 0g

Earthbound Farm Organic, Organic Romaine Hearts, 3 ct poly bag

3 oz (85g / about 2 cups)

Amount per serving	Amount per serving	Amount per serving
Calories 10	**Cholesterol** 0mg	**Total Carbohydrate** 2g
Total Fat 0g	**Sodium** 5mg	Dietary Fiber 1g
Saturated Fat 0g	**Protein** 1g	Sugars 0g

Organicgirl, 100% baby kale, 255g 100% recycled plastic clamshell - bilingual

2 cups (85g)

Amount per serving	Amount per serving	Amount per serving
Calories 45	**Cholesterol** 0mg	**Total Carbohydrate** 9g
Total Fat 0g	**Sodium** 35mg	Dietary Fiber 2g
Saturated Fat 0g	**Protein** 3g	Sugars 2g

Organicgirl, 100% baby kale, 9 oz 100% recycled plastic clamshell

2 cups (85g)

Amount per serving	Amount per serving	Amount per serving
Calories 45	**Cholesterol** 0mg	**Total Carbohydrate** 9g
Total Fat 0.5g	**Sodium** 35mg	Dietary Fiber 2g
Saturated Fat 0g	**Protein** 3g	Sugars 2g

Organicgirl, 50/50!, 10 oz 100% recycled plastic clamshell

2 cups (85g)

Amount per serving	Amount per serving	Amount per serving
Calories 20	**Cholesterol** 0mg	**Total Carbohydrate** 3g
Total Fat 0g	**Sodium** 70mg	Dietary Fiber 2g
Saturated Fat 0g	**Protein** 2g	Sugars <1g

Organicgirl, 50/50!, 142g 100% recycled plastic clamshell - bilingual

2 cups (85g)

Amount per serving	Amount per serving	Amount per serving
Calories 20	**Cholesterol** 0mg	**Total Carbohydrate** 3g
Total Fat 0g	**Sodium** 70mg	Dietary Fiber 2g
Saturated Fat 0g	**Protein** 2g	Sugars 1g

Organicgirl, 50/50!, 16 oz 100% recycled plastic clamshell

about 2 cups (85g)

Amount per serving	Amount per serving	Amount per serving
Calories 20	Cholesterol 0mg	Total Carbohydrate 3g
Total Fat 0g	Sodium 70mg	Dietary Fiber 2g
Saturated Fat 0g	Protein 2g	Sugars <1g

Organicgirl, 50/50!, 284g 100% recycled plastic clamshell - bilingual

2 cups (85g)

Amount per serving	Amount per serving	Amount per serving
Calories 20	Cholesterol 0mg	Total Carbohydrate 3g
Total Fat 0g	Sodium 70mg	Dietary Fiber 2g
Saturated Fat 0g	Protein 2g	Sugars 1g

Organicgirl, 50/50!, 454g 100% recycled plastic clamshell - bilingual

Per 2 cups (85g)

Amount per serving	Amount per serving	Amount per serving
Calories 20	Cholesterol 0mg	Total Carbohydrate 3g
Total Fat 0g	Sodium 70mg	Dietary Fiber 2g
Saturated Fat 0g	Protein 2g	Sugars 1g

Organicgirl, 50/50!, 5 oz 100% recycled plastic clamshell

2 cups (85g)

Amount per serving	Amount per serving	Amount per serving
Calories 20	Cholesterol 0mg	Total Carbohydrate 3g
Total Fat 0g	Sodium 70mg	Dietary Fiber 2g
Saturated Fat 0g	Protein 2g	Sugars <1g

Organicgirl, baby arugula, 10 oz 100% recycled plastic clamshell

about 2 cups (85g)

Amount per serving	Amount per serving	Amount per serving
Calories 25	Cholesterol 0mg	Total Carbohydrate 3g
Total Fat 0.5g	Sodium 25mg	Dietary Fiber 1g
Saturated Fat 0g	Protein 2g	Sugars 2g

Organicgirl, baby arugula, 142g 100% recycled plastic clamshell - bilingual

Per 2 cups (85g)

Amount per serving	Amount per serving	Amount per serving
Calories 25	Cholesterol 0mg	Total Carbohydrate 3g
Total Fat 0.5g	Sodium 25mg	Dietary Fiber 1g
Saturated Fat 0g	Protein 2g	Sugars 2g

Organicgirl, baby arugula, 284g 100% recycled plastic clamshell - bilingual

Per 2 cups (85g)

Amount per serving	Amount per serving	Amount per serving
Calories 25	**Cholesterol** 0mg	**Total Carbohydrate** 3g
Total Fat 0.5g	**Sodium** 25mg	Dietary Fiber 1g
Saturated Fat 0g	**Protein** 2g	Sugars 2g

Organicgirl, baby arugula, 5 oz 100% recycled plastic clamshell

about 2 cups (85g)

Amount per serving	Amount per serving	Amount per serving
Calories 25	**Cholesterol** 0mg	**Total Carbohydrate** 3g
Total Fat 0.5g	**Sodium** 25mg	Dietary Fiber 1g
Saturated Fat 0g	**Protein** 2g	Sugars 2g

Organicgirl, baby spinach & arugula, 14g clamshell - bilingual

Per 3 cups (85g)

Amount per serving	Amount per serving	Amount per serving
Calories 15	**Cholesterol** 0mg	**Total Carbohydrate** 3g
Total Fat 0g	**Sodium** 40mg	Dietary Fiber 2g
Saturated Fat 0g	**Protein** 2g	Sugars 1g

Organicgirl, baby spinach & arugula, 5 oz 100% recycled plastic clamshell

about 3 cups (85g)

Amount per serving	Amount per serving	Amount per serving
Calories 15	**Cholesterol** 0mg	**Total Carbohydrate** 3g
Total Fat 0g	**Sodium** 40mg	Dietary Fiber 2g
Saturated Fat 0g	**Protein** 2g	Sugars <1g

Organicgirl, baby spinach, 284g 100% recycled plastic clamshell - bilingual

Per 3 cups (85g)

Amount per serving	Amount per serving	Amount per serving
Calories 20	**Cholesterol** 0mg	**Total Carbohydrate** 3g
Total Fat 0g	**Sodium** 65mg	Dietary Fiber 2g
Saturated Fat 0g	**Protein** 2g	Sugars 0g

Organicgirl, baby spinach, 10 oz 100% recycled plastic clamshell

about 3 cups (85g)

Amount per serving	Amount per serving	Amount per serving
Calories 20	**Cholesterol** 0mg	**Total Carbohydrate** 3g
Total Fat 0g	**Sodium** 65mg	Dietary Fiber 2g
Saturated Fat 0g	**Protein** 2g	Sugars 0g

Organicgirl, baby spinach, 142g 100% recycled plastic clamshell - bilingual

Per 3 cups (85g)

Amount per serving	Amount per serving	Amount per serving
Calories 20	**Cholesterol** 0mg	**Total Carbohydrate** 3g
Total Fat 0g	**Sodium** 65mg	Dietary Fiber 2g
Saturated Fat 0g	**Protein** 2g	Sugars 0g

Organicgirl, baby spinach, 16 oz 100% recycled plastic clamshell

about 3 cups (85g)

Amount per serving	Amount per serving	Amount per serving
Calories 20	**Cholesterol** 0mg	**Total Carbohydrate** 3g
Total Fat 0g	**Sodium** 65mg	Dietary Fiber 2g
Saturated Fat 0g	**Protein** 2g	Sugars 0g

Organicgirl, baby spinach, 454g 100% recycled plastic clamshell - bilingual

Per 3 cups (85g)

Amount per serving	Amount per serving	Amount per serving
Calories 20	**Cholesterol** 0mg	**Total Carbohydrate** 3g
Total Fat 0g	**Sodium** 65mg	Dietary Fiber 2g
Saturated Fat 0g	**Protein** 2g	Sugars 0g

Organicgirl, baby spinach, 5 oz 100% recycled plastic clamshell

about 3 cups (85g)

Amount per serving	Amount per serving	Amount per serving
Calories 20	**Cholesterol** 0mg	**Total Carbohydrate** 3g
Total Fat 0g	**Sodium** 65mg	Dietary Fiber 2g
Saturated Fat 0g	**Protein** 2g	Sugars 0g

Organicgirl, baby spring mix, 10 oz 100% recycled plastic clamshell

about 3 cups (85g)

Amount per serving	Amount per serving	Amount per serving
Calories 15	**Cholesterol** 0mg	**Total Carbohydrate** 3g
Total Fat 0g	**Sodium** 70mg	Dietary Fiber 2g
Saturated Fat 0g	**Protein** 1g	Sugars <1g

Organicgirl, baby spring mix, 142g 100% recycled plastic clamshell - bilingual

Per 3 cups (85g)

Amount per serving	Amount per serving	Amount per serving
Calories 15	**Cholesterol** 0mg	**Total Carbohydrate** 3g
Total Fat 0g	**Sodium** 70mg	Dietary Fiber 2g
Saturated Fat 0g	**Protein** 1g	Sugars 1g

Organicgirl, baby spring mix, 16 oz 100% recycled plastic clamshell

about 3 cups (85g)

Amount per serving	Amount per serving	Amount per serving
Calories 15	**Cholesterol** 0mg	**Total Carbohydrate** 3g
Total Fat 0g	**Sodium** 70mg	Dietary Fiber 2g
Saturated Fat 0g	**Protein** 1g	Sugars <1g

Organicgirl, baby spring mix, 284g 100% recycled plastic clamshell - bilingual

Per 3 cups (85g)

Amount per serving	Amount per serving	Amount per serving
Calories 15	**Cholesterol** 0mg	**Total Carbohydrate** 3g
Total Fat 0g	**Sodium** 70mg	Dietary Fiber 2g
Saturated Fat 0g	**Protein** 1g	Sugars 1g

Organicgirl, baby spring mix, 454g 100% recycled plastic clamshell - bilingual

Per 3 cups (85g)

Amount per serving	Amount per serving	Amount per serving
Calories 15	**Cholesterol** 0mg	**Total Carbohydrate** 3g
Total Fat 0g	**Sodium** 70mg	Dietary Fiber 2g
Saturated Fat 0g	**Protein** 1g	Sugars 1g

Organicgirl, baby spring mix, 5 oz 100% recycled plastic clamshell

about 3 cups (85g)

Amount per serving	Amount per serving	Amount per serving
Calories 15	**Cholesterol** 0mg	**Total Carbohydrate** 3g
Total Fat 0g	**Sodium** 70mg	Dietary Fiber 2g
Saturated Fat 0g	**Protein** 1g	Sugars <1g

Organicgirl, fresh herbs & greens, 142g 5 oz clamshell - bilingual

2 cups (85g)

Amount per serving	Amount per serving	Amount per serving
Calories 15	**Cholesterol** 0mg	**Total Carbohydrate** 3g
Total Fat 0g	**Sodium** 80mg	Dietary Fiber 2g
Saturated Fat 0g	**Protein** 2g	Sugars <1g

Organicgirl, fresh herbs & greens, 5 oz 100% recycled plastic clamshell

2 cups (85g)

Amount per serving	Amount per serving	Amount per serving
Calories 0	**Cholesterol** 0mg	**Total Carbohydrate** 3g
Total Fat 0g	**Sodium** 80mg	Dietary Fiber 2g
Saturated Fat 0g	**Protein** 2g	Sugars <1g

Organicgirl, hearts of romaine, 12 oz protect pack!

2 cups (85g)

Amount per serving	Amount per serving	Amount per serving
Calories 10	**Cholesterol** 0mg	**Total Carbohydrate** 2g
Total Fat 0g	**Sodium** 5mg	Dietary Fiber 1g
Saturated Fat 0g	**Protein** 1g	Sugars 0g

Organicgirl, hearts of romaine, 340g protect pack! - bilingual

2 cups (85g)

Amount per serving	Amount per serving	Amount per serving
Calories 35	**Cholesterol** 0mg	**Total Carbohydrate** 2g
Total Fat 0g	**Sodium** 5mg	Dietary Fiber 1g
Saturated Fat 0g	**Protein** 1g	Sugars 0g

Organicgirl, I heart baby kale, 142g 100% recycled plastic clamshell - bilingual

Per 3 cups (85g)

Amount per serving	Amount per serving	Amount per serving
Calories 25	**Cholesterol** 0mg	**Total Carbohydrate** 5g
Total Fat 0g	**Sodium** 75mg	Dietary Fiber 2g
Saturated Fat 0g	**Protein** 2g	Sugars 1g

Organicgirl, I heart baby kale, 5 oz 100% recycled plastic clamshell

3 cups (85g)

Amount per serving	Amount per serving	Amount per serving
Calories 25	**Cholesterol** 0mg	**Total Carbohydrate** 5g
Total Fat 0g	**Sodium** 75mg	Dietary Fiber 2g
Saturated Fat 0g	**Protein** 2g	Sugars <1g

Organicgirl, mache rosettes, 99g 100% recycled plastic clamshell

Per cups (99g)

Amount per serving	Amount per serving	Amount per serving
Calories 35	**Cholesterol** 0mg	**Total Carbohydrate** 6g
Total Fat 0g	**Sodium** 25mg	Dietary Fiber 2g
Saturated Fat 0g	**Protein** 2g	Sugars 1g

Organicgirl, romaine heart leaves, 227g clamshell - bilingual

Per 2 cups (85g)

Amount per serving	Amount per serving	Amount per serving
Calories 10	**Cholesterol** 0mg	**Total Carbohydrate** 2g
Total Fat 0g	**Sodium** 5mg	Dietary Fiber 1g
Saturated Fat 0g	**Protein** 1g	Sugars 0g

Organicgirl, romaine heart leaves, 8 oz 100% recycled plastic clamshell

6 pieces (85g)

Amount per serving	Amount per serving	Amount per serving
Calories 15	**Cholesterol** 0mg	**Total Carbohydrate** 2g
Total Fat 0g	**Sodium** 5mg	Dietary Fiber 1g
Saturated Fat 0g	**Protein** 1g	Sugars 0g

Organicgirl, SUPER SPINACH!, 142g 100% recycled plastic clamshell - bilingual

Per 3 cups (85g)

Amount per serving	Amount per serving	Amount per serving
Calories 20	**Cholesterol** 0mg	**Total Carbohydrate** 3g
Total Fat 0g	**Sodium** 95mg	Dietary Fiber 2g
Saturated Fat 0g	**Protein** 2g	Sugars 1g

Organicgirl, SUPER SPINACH!, 5 oz 100% recycled plastic clamshell

about 3 cups (85g)

Amount per serving	Amount per serving	Amount per serving
Calories 20	**Cholesterol** 0mg	**Total Carbohydrate** 3g
Total Fat 0g	**Sodium** 95mg	Dietary Fiber 2g
Saturated Fat 0g	**Protein** 2g	Sugars <1g

Organicgirl, SUPERGREENS!, 10 oz 100% recycled plastic clamshell

about 3 cups (85g)

Amount per serving	Amount per serving	Amount per serving
Calories 20	**Cholesterol** 0mg	**Total Carbohydrate** 3g
Total Fat 0g	**Sodium** 95mg	Dietary Fiber 2g
Saturated Fat 0g	**Protein** 2g	Sugars <1g

Organicgirl, SUPERGREENS!, 142g 100% recycled plastic clamshell - bilingual

Per 3 cups (85g)

Amount per serving	Amount per serving	Amount per serving
Calories 20	**Cholesterol** 0mg	**Total Carbohydrate** 3g
Total Fat 0g	**Sodium** 95mg	Dietary Fiber 2g
Saturated Fat 0g	**Protein** 2g	Sugars 1g

Organicgirl, SUPERGREENS!, 16 oz 100% recycled plastic clamshell

about 3 cups (85g)

Amount per serving	Amount per serving	Amount per serving
Calories 20	**Cholesterol** 0mg	**Total Carbohydrate** 3g
Total Fat 0g	**Sodium** 95mg	Dietary Fiber 2g
Saturated Fat 0g	**Protein** 2g	Sugars <1g

Organicgirl, SUPERGREENS!, 284g 100% recycled plastic clamshell - bilingual

Per 3 cups (85g)

Amount per serving	Amount per serving	Amount per serving
Calories 20	**Cholesterol** 0mg	**Total Carbohydrate** 3g
Total Fat 0g	**Sodium** 95mg	Dietary Fiber 2g
Saturated Fat 0g	**Protein** 2g	Sugars 1g

Organicgirl, SUPERGREENS!, 454g 100% recycled plastic clamshell - bilingual

Per 3 cups (85g)

Amount per serving	Amount per serving	Amount per serving
Calories 20	**Cholesterol** 0mg	**Total Carbohydrate** 3g
Total Fat 0g	**Sodium** 95mg	Dietary Fiber 2g
Saturated Fat 0g	**Protein** 2g	Sugars 1g

Organicgirl, SUPERGREENS!, 5 oz 100% recycled plastic clamshell

about 3 cups (85g)

Amount per serving	Amount per serving	Amount per serving
Calories 20	**Cholesterol** 0mg	**Total Carbohydrate** 3g
Total Fat 0g	**Sodium** 95mg	Dietary Fiber 2g
Saturated Fat 0g	**Protein** 2g	Sugars <1g

Organicgirl, sweet mache blend, 3.5 oz 100% recycled plastic clamshell

3.5 oz (99g)

Amount per serving	Amount per serving	Amount per serving
Calories 25	**Cholesterol** 0mg	**Total Carbohydrate** 5g
Total Fat 0g	**Sodium** 105mg	Dietary Fiber 2g
Saturated Fat 0g	**Protein** 2g	Sugars <1g

Organicgirl, sweet mache blend, 99g 100% recycled plastic clamshell

Per 2 cups (99g)

Amount per serving	Amount per serving	Amount per serving
Calories 25	**Cholesterol** 0mg	**Total Carbohydrate** 5g
Total Fat 0g	**Sodium** 105mg	Dietary Fiber 2g
Saturated Fat 0g	**Protein** 2g	Sugars 1g

Vegetable Products

Native Forest, Organic Bamboo Shoots

1/2 cup

Amount per serving	Amount per serving	Amount per serving
Calories 15	**Cholesterol** 0mg	**Total Carbohydrate** 3g
Total Fat 0g	**Sodium** 5mg	Dietary Fiber 1g
Saturated Fat 0g	**Protein** 1g	Sugars 2g

Native Forest, Organic Cut Baby Corn
1/2 cup

Amount per serving	Amount per serving	Amount per serving
Calories 25	**Cholesterol** 0mg	**Total Carbohydrate** 4g
Total Fat 0g	**Sodium** 280mg	Dietary Fiber 2g
Saturated Fat 0g	**Protein** 2g	Sugars 1g

Native Forest, Organic Hearts of Palm
1 oz

Amount per serving	Amount per serving	Amount per serving
Calories 15	**Cholesterol** 0mg	**Total Carbohydrate** 2g
Total Fat 0g	**Sodium** 120mg	Dietary Fiber 1g
Saturated Fat 0g	**Protein** 1g	Sugars 0g

Native Forest, Organic Mushrooms Pieces & Stems
1/2 cup

Amount per serving	Amount per serving	Amount per serving
Calories 20	**Cholesterol** 0mg	**Total Carbohydrate** 3g
Total Fat 0g	**Sodium** 390mg	Dietary Fiber 1g
Saturated Fat 0g	**Protein** 2g	Sugars 1g

Vegetables

Earthbound Farm Organic, Farm Stand Favorites, Frozen Organic Collard Greens
1/3 cup (85g)

Amount per serving	Amount per serving	Amount per serving
Calories 30	**Cholesterol** 0mg	**Total Carbohydrate** 6g
Total Fat 0g	**Sodium** 45mg	Dietary Fiber 2g
Saturated Fat 0g	**Protein** 3g	Sugars 0g

Earthbound Farm Organic, Farm Stand Favorites, Frozen Organic Kale, 8 oz bag
1/3 cup (85g)

Amount per serving	Amount per serving	Amount per serving
Calories 25	**Cholesterol** 0mg	**Total Carbohydrate** 4g
Total Fat 0g	**Sodium** 15mg	Dietary Fiber 2g
Saturated Fat 0g	**Protein** 2g	Sugars 1g

Earthbound Farm Organic, Farm Stand Favorites, Frozen Organic Rainbow Chard Blend
1/3 cup (85g)

Amount per serving	Amount per serving	Amount per serving
Calories 15	**Cholesterol** 0mg	**Total Carbohydrate** 4g
Total Fat 0g	**Sodium** 150mg	Dietary Fiber 2g
Saturated Fat 0g	**Protein** 2g	Sugars 1g

Earthbound Farm Organic, Farm Stand Favorites, Frozen Organic Root Medley

2/3 cup (85g)

Amount per serving	Amount per serving	Amount per serving
Calories 40	**Cholesterol** 0mg	**Total Carbohydrate** 9g
Total Fat 0g	**Sodium** 35mg	Dietary Fiber 3g
Saturated Fat 0g	**Protein** 1g	Sugars 35g

Earthbound Farm Organic, Farm Stand Favorites, Frozen Organic Ruby Red Beets

2/3 cup (85g)

Amount per serving	Amount per serving	Amount per serving
Calories 45	**Cholesterol** 0mg	**Total Carbohydrate** 10g
Total Fat 0g	**Sodium** 35mg	Dietary Fiber 2g
Saturated Fat 0g	**Protein** 1g	Sugars 8g

Earthbound Farm Organic, Organic Avocados, Unpackaged, loose fruit

1/5 medium (30g)

Amount per serving	Amount per serving	Amount per serving
Calories 50	**Cholesterol** 0mg	**Total Carbohydrate** 3g
Total Fat 0.5g	**Sodium** 0mg	Dietary Fiber 2g
Saturated Fat 0g	**Protein** 1g	Sugars 0g

Earthbound Farm Organic, Organic Butternut Squash, Unpackaged, loose vegetables

1/2 cup (85g)

Amount per serving	Amount per serving	Amount per serving
Calories 35	**Cholesterol** 0mg	**Total Carbohydrate** 11g
Total Fat 0g	**Sodium** 0mg	Dietary Fiber 2g
Saturated Fat 0g	**Protein** 1g	Sugars 2g

Earthbound Farm Organic, Organic Celery Hearts, Sleeve

2 medium stalks (110g)

Amount per serving	Amount per serving	Amount per serving
Calories 15	**Cholesterol** 0mg	**Total Carbohydrate** 4g
Total Fat 0g	**Sodium** 115mg	Dietary Fiber 2g
Saturated Fat 0g	**Protein** 0g	Sugars 2g

Earthbound Farm Organic, Organic Celery, Sleeve, Bunch

2 medium stalks (110g)

Amount per serving	Amount per serving	Amount per serving
Calories 15	**Cholesterol** 0mg	**Total Carbohydrate** 4g
Total Fat 0g	**Sodium** 115mg	Dietary Fiber 2g
Saturated Fat 0g	**Protein** 0g	Sugars 2g

Earthbound Farm Organic, Organic Cucumber, Unpackaged, loose vegetables
1/3 medium (99g)

Amount per serving	Amount per serving	Amount per serving
Calories 10	**Cholesterol** 0mg	**Total Carbohydrate** 2g
Total Fat 0g	**Sodium** 0mg	Dietary Fiber 1g
Saturated Fat 0g	**Protein** 1g	Sugars 1g

Earthbound Farm Organic, Organic Garlic, 3 oz bag
1 clove (4g)

Amount per serving	Amount per serving	Amount per serving
Calories 5	**Cholesterol** 0mg	**Total Carbohydrate** 1g
Total Fat 0g	**Sodium** 0mg	Dietary Fiber 0g
Saturated Fat 0g	**Protein** 0g	Sugars 0g

Earthbound Farm Organic, Organic Garnet Yams, 3 lb bag, Unpackaged, loose yams
3/4 cup (85g)

Amount per serving	Amount per serving	Amount per serving
Calories 80	**Cholesterol** 0mg	**Total Carbohydrate** 22g
Total Fat 0g	**Sodium** 15mg	Dietary Fiber 2g
Saturated Fat 0g	**Protein** 1g	Sugars 2g

Earthbound Farm Organic, Organic Grape Tomatoes, 10 oz clamshell
1/2 cup (85g)

Amount per serving	Amount per serving	Amount per serving
Calories 15	**Cholesterol** 0mg	**Total Carbohydrate** 7g
Total Fat 0g	**Sodium** 15mg	Dietary Fiber 1g
Saturated Fat 0g	**Protein** 1g	Sugars 1g

Earthbound Farm Organic, Organic Green Onions
1/4 cup chopped (25g)

Amount per serving	Amount per serving	Amount per serving
Calories 10	**Cholesterol** 0mg	**Total Carbohydrate** 2g
Total Fat 0g	**Sodium** 10mg	Dietary Fiber 1g
Saturated Fat 0g	**Protein** 0g	Sugars 1g

Earthbound Farm Organic, Organic Heirloom Potatoes French Fingerling, 1.5 lb bag
2 potatoes (110g)

Amount per serving	Amount per serving	Amount per serving
Calories 90	**Cholesterol** 0mg	**Total Carbohydrate** 19g
Total Fat 0g	**Sodium** 5mg	Dietary Fiber 1g
Saturated Fat 0g	**Protein** 3g	Sugars 0g

Earthbound Farm Organic, Organic Heirloom Potatoes Ruby Crescent, 1.5 lb bag

2 potatoes (110g)

Amount per serving	Amount per serving	Amount per serving
Calories 70	**Cholesterol** 0mg	**Total Carbohydrate** 19g
Total Fat 0g	**Sodium** 0mg	Dietary Fiber 2g
Saturated Fat 0g	**Protein** 3g	Sugars 0g

Earthbound Farm Organic, Organic Heirloom Potatoes Russian Banana, 1.5 lb bag

2 potatoes (110g)

Amount per serving	Amount per serving	Amount per serving
Calories 70	**Cholesterol** 0mg	**Total Carbohydrate** 19g
Total Fat 0g	**Sodium** 0mg	Dietary Fiber 2g
Saturated Fat 0g	**Protein** 3g	Sugars 0g

Earthbound Farm Organic, Organic Jewel Yams, 3 lb bag, Unpackaged, loose yams

3/4 cup (85g)

Amount per serving	Amount per serving	Amount per serving
Calories 70	**Cholesterol** 0mg	**Total Carbohydrate** 23g
Total Fat 0g	**Sodium** 15mg	Dietary Fiber 2g
Saturated Fat 0g	**Protein** 1g	Sugars 2g

Earthbound Farm Organic, Organic Red Cherry Tomatoes, 10 oz clamshell

1/2 cup (85g)

Amount per serving	Amount per serving	Amount per serving
Calories 15	**Cholesterol** 0mg	**Total Carbohydrate** 7g
Total Fat 0g	**Sodium** 15mg	Dietary Fiber 1g
Saturated Fat 0g	**Protein** 1g	Sugars 1g

Earthbound Farm Organic, Organic Red Onions, 3 lb bag

1/2 cup (85g)

Amount per serving	Amount per serving	Amount per serving
Calories 25	**Cholesterol** 0mg	**Total Carbohydrate** 6g
Total Fat 0g	**Sodium** 5mg	Dietary Fiber 1g
Saturated Fat 0g	**Protein** 1g	Sugars 4g

Earthbound Farm Organic, Organic Red Potatoes, 3 lb bag

1 potato (85g)

Amount per serving	Amount per serving	Amount per serving
Calories 70	**Cholesterol** 0mg	**Total Carbohydrate** 14g
Total Fat 0g	**Sodium** 5mg	Dietary Fiber 1g
Saturated Fat 0g	**Protein** 2g	Sugars 2g

Earthbound Farm Organic, Organic Round Slicer Tomatoes
1/2 cup (85g)

Amount per serving	Amount per serving	Amount per serving
Calories 15	**Cholesterol** 0mg	**Total Carbohydrate** 7g
Total Fat 0g	**Sodium** 15mg	Dietary Fiber 1g
Saturated Fat 0g	**Protein** 1g	Sugars 1g

Earthbound Farm Organic, Organic Russet Potatoes, 5 lb bag
1 potato (200g)

Amount per serving	Amount per serving	Amount per serving
Calories 190	**Cholesterol** 0mg	**Total Carbohydrate** 43g
Total Fat 0g	**Sodium** 20mg	Dietary Fiber 5g
Saturated Fat 0g	**Protein** 5g	Sugars 2g

Earthbound Farm Organic, Organic Yellow Onions, 3 lb bag
1/2 cup (85g)

Amount per serving	Amount per serving	Amount per serving
Calories 25	**Cholesterol** 0mg	**Total Carbohydrate** 6g
Total Fat 0g	**Sodium** 5mg	Dietary Fiber 1g
Saturated Fat 0g	**Protein** 1g	Sugars 4g

Earthbound Farm Organic, Organic Yellow Potatoes, 3 lb bag
1 potato (110g)

Amount per serving	Amount per serving	Amount per serving
Calories 100	**Cholesterol** 0mg	**Total Carbohydrate** 25g
Total Fat 0g	**Sodium** 5mg	Dietary Fiber 1g
Saturated Fat 0g	**Protein** 2g	Sugars 1g

Earthbound Farm Organic, Organic Zucchini, Bulk (individual vegetable)
1/2 cup (85g)

Amount per serving	Amount per serving	Amount per serving
Calories 35	**Cholesterol** 0mg	**Total Carbohydrate** 11g
Total Fat 0g	**Sodium** 0mg	Dietary Fiber 2g
Saturated Fat 0g	**Protein** 1g	Sugars 2g

Frieda's, Organic Amarosa Fingerling Potatoes
4 potatoes (148g)

Amount per serving	Amount per serving	Amount per serving
Calories 100	**Cholesterol** 0mg	**Total Carbohydrate** 25g
Total Fat 0g	**Sodium** 0mg	Dietary Fiber 3g
Saturated Fat 0g	**Protein** 4g	Sugars 3g

Frieda's, Organic Cucumber

4 oz (113g)

Amount per serving	Amount per serving	Amount per serving
Calories 15	**Cholesterol** 0mg	**Total Carbohydrate** 4g
Total Fat 0g	**Sodium** 0mg	Dietary Fiber 1g
Saturated Fat 0g	**Protein** 1g	Sugars 2g

Frieda's, Organic Finger Lime

2 oz (55g)

Amount per serving	Amount per serving	Amount per serving
Calories 15	**Cholesterol** 0mg	**Total Carbohydrate** 6g
Total Fat 0g	**Sodium** 0mg	Dietary Fiber 2g
Saturated Fat 0g	**Protein** 0g	Sugars 1g

Frieda's, Organic Garlic

1 tsp (3g)

Amount per serving	Amount per serving	Amount per serving
Calories 5	**Cholesterol** 0mg	**Total Carbohydrate** 1g
Total Fat 0g	**Sodium** 0mg	Dietary Fiber 1g
Saturated Fat 0g	**Protein** 0g	Sugars 0g

Frieda's, Organic Heirloom Apples

1 medium (140g)

Amount per serving	Amount per serving	Amount per serving
Calories 70	**Cholesterol** 0mg	**Total Carbohydrate** 19g
Total Fat 0g	**Sodium** 0mg	Dietary Fiber 3g
Saturated Fat 0g	**Protein** 0g	Sugars 15g

Frieda's, Organic Klamath Pearl Potatoes

1/2 cup (85g)

Amount per serving	Amount per serving	Amount per serving
Calories 70	**Cholesterol** 0mg	**Total Carbohydrate** 15g
Total Fat 0g	**Sodium** 5mg	Dietary Fiber 1g
Saturated Fat 0g	**Protein** 2g	Sugars 0g

Frieda's, Organic Purple Fiesta Fingerling Potatoes

4 potatoes (148g)

Amount per serving	Amount per serving	Amount per serving
Calories 100	**Cholesterol** 0mg	**Total Carbohydrate** 25g
Total Fat 0g	**Sodium** 0mg	Dietary Fiber 3g
Saturated Fat 0g	**Protein** 4g	Sugars 3g

Westbrae Natural, Organic Cut Green Beans

1/2 cup (120g)

Amount per serving	Amount per serving	Amount per serving
Calories 20	**Cholesterol** 0mg	**Total Carbohydrate** 4g
Total Fat 0g	**Sodium** 370mg	Dietary Fiber 1g
Saturated Fat 0g	**Protein** 1g	Sugars 2g

Westbrae Natural, Organic French Cut Green Beans

1/2 cup (120g)

Amount per serving	Amount per serving	Amount per serving
Calories 20	**Cholesterol** 0mg	**Total Carbohydrate** 4g
Total Fat 0g	**Sodium** 370mg	Dietary Fiber 1g
Saturated Fat 0g	**Protein** 1g	Sugars 2g

Westbrae Natural, Organic Golden Corn

1/2 cup (125g)

Amount per serving	Amount per serving	Amount per serving
Calories 90	**Cholesterol** 0mg	**Total Carbohydrate** 14g
Total Fat 1g	**Sodium** 340mg	Dietary Fiber 2g
Saturated Fat 0g	**Protein** 2g	Sugars 5g

Westbrae Natural, Organic Sweet Peas

1/2 cup (125g)

Amount per serving	Amount per serving	Amount per serving
Calories 60	**Cholesterol** 0mg	**Total Carbohydrate** 10g
Total Fat 0g	**Sodium** 360mg	Dietary Fiber 3g
Saturated Fat 0g	**Protein** 4g	Sugars 4g

Westbrae Natural, Organic White Corn

1/2 cup (125g)

Amount per serving	Amount per serving	Amount per serving
Calories 100	**Cholesterol** 0mg	**Total Carbohydrate** 20g
Total Fat 1g	**Sodium** 340mg	Dietary Fiber 1g
Saturated Fat 0g	**Protein** 2g	Sugars 5g

Fruits

Why Eat Organic Fruit?

Naturally low in fat, sodium, and calories, fruits are a healthy choice to satisfy a craving for something sweet. They contain many essential nutrients including vitamins and minerals—potassium, vitamin C, folate (folic acid), and dietary fiber. Diets rich in potassium may help to maintain healthy blood pressure. Dietary fiber from fruits, as part of an overall healthy diet, helps reduce blood cholesterol levels and may lower the risk of heart disease. Vitamin C is important for growth and repair of all body tissues, helps heal cuts and wounds, and keeps teeth and gums healthy. Fruits also contain a variety of phytonutrients that often act as antioxidants, protecting the cells of the body from the damaging effects of free radicals.

Organic fruits are grown in accordance with organic agriculture standards, which means they have not been exposed to synthetic chemical fertilizers, herbicides, or pesticides. Unlike conventionally grown, non-organic fruit, they contain no pesticide residues. According to the Environmental Working Group (EWG), it's most important to buy organic apples, cherries, grapes, imported nectarines, peaches, and strawberries because when these are grown conventionally, they have high levels of pesticides and may harbor residue from several different pesticides. The EWG identifies cantaloupe, grapefruit, kiwi, mangos, papayas, and pineapples as fruits with the least pesticide residue.

Daily Goal

Two cups for an adult on a 2,000-calorie diet.

1 cup equivalents:
    2.5" whole fruit   8 oz. fruit juice (100%)
    1 cup chopped or sliced fruit   32 seedless grapes
    ½ cup dried fruit   8 large strawberries

Fruit Juices

Earthbound Farm Organic, Organic Smoothie Kickstart, Kale Berry

1/2 package (113g)

Amount per serving	Amount per serving	Amount per serving
Calories 40	**Cholesterol** 0mg	**Total Carbohydrate** 9g
Total Fat 0g	**Sodium** 10mg	Dietary Fiber 3g
Saturated Fat 0g	**Protein** 1g	Sugars 5g

Earthbound Farm Organic, Organic Smoothie Kickstart, Mango Peach Carrot

1/2 package (113g)

Amount per serving	Amount per serving	Amount per serving
Calories 50	**Cholesterol** 0mg	**Total Carbohydrate** 14g
Total Fat 0g	**Sodium** 20mg	Dietary Fiber 3g
Saturated Fat 0g	**Protein** 1g	Sugars 10g

Eden Foods, Apple Juice, Organic

8 oz

Amount per serving	Amount per serving	Amount per serving
Calories 90	**Cholesterol** 24mg	**Total Carbohydrate** 0g
Total Fat 0g	**Sodium** 0mg	Dietary Fiber 12g
Saturated Fat 0g	**Protein** 0g	Sugars 0g

Eden Foods, Cherry Juice Concentrate, Organic

2 tbsp

Amount per serving	Amount per serving	Amount per serving
Calories 110	**Cholesterol** 26mg	**Total Carbohydrate** 0g
Total Fat 0g	**Sodium** 0mg	Dietary Fiber 21g
Saturated Fat 0g	**Protein** 20g	Sugars 1g

Eden Foods, Concord Grape Juice, Organic

8 oz

Amount per serving	Amount per serving	Amount per serving
Calories 150	**Cholesterol** 37mg	**Total Carbohydrate** <1g
Total Fat 0g	**Sodium** 0mg	Dietary Fiber 32g
Saturated Fat NA	**Protein** 35g	Sugars <1g

Eden Foods, Montmorency Tart Cherry Juice, Organic

8 oz

Amount per serving	Amount per serving	Amount per serving
Calories 140	**Cholesterol** 33mg	**Total Carbohydrate** 0g
Total Fat 0g	**Sodium** 4mg	Dietary Fiber 25g
Saturated Fat 0g	**Protein** 30g	Sugars 1g

Hansen's Natural, Hansen's Organic Junior Juice, Apple

1 package / 125 ml

Amount per serving	Amount per serving	Amount per serving
Calories 60	**Cholesterol** 15mg	**Total Carbohydrate** NA
Total Fat 0g	**Sodium** 0mg	Dietary Fiber 15g
Saturated Fat NA	**Protein** 10g	Sugars NA

Hansen's Natural, Hansen's Organic Junior Juice, Berry Medley

1 package / 125 ml

Amount per serving	Amount per serving	Amount per serving
Calories 60	**Cholesterol** 15mg	**Total Carbohydrate** NA
Total Fat 0g	**Sodium** 0mg	Dietary Fiber 15g
Saturated Fat NA	**Protein** 10g	Sugars NA

Nature Factor, Organic Coconut Water

1 can

Amount per serving	Amount per serving	Amount per serving
Calories 80	**Cholesterol** 16mg	**Total Carbohydrate** NA
Total Fat 0g	**Sodium** 0mg	Dietary Fiber 9g
Saturated Fat NA	**Protein** 50g	Sugars 0g

Fruit Products

Eden Foods, Apple Butter, Organic

1 tbsp

Amount per serving	Amount per serving	Amount per serving
Calories 20	**Cholesterol** NA	**Total Carbohydrate** 4g
Total Fat 0g	**Sodium** 0mg	Dietary Fiber 1g
Saturated Fat 0g	**Protein** 0g	Sugars 4g

Eden Foods, Apple Cherry Butter, Organic

1 tbsp

Amount per serving	Amount per serving	Amount per serving
Calories 25	**Cholesterol** NA	**Total Carbohydrate** 6g
Total Fat 0g	**Sodium** 0mg	Dietary Fiber <1g
Saturated Fat 0g	**Protein** 0g	Sugars 5g

Eden Foods, Apple Cherry Sauce, Organic

1/2 cup

Amount per serving	Amount per serving	Amount per serving
Calories 70	**Cholesterol** 0mg	**Total Carbohydrate** 17g
Total Fat 0g	**Sodium** 10mg	Dietary Fiber 3g
Saturated Fat 0g	**Protein** 0g	Sugars 12g

Eden Foods, Apple Cinnamon Sauce, Organic

1/2 cup

Amount per serving	Amount per serving	Amount per serving
Calories 60	**Cholesterol** 0mg	**Total Carbohydrate** 14g
Total Fat 0g	**Sodium** 10mg	Dietary Fiber 2g
Saturated Fat 0g	**Protein** 0g	Sugars 12g

Eden Foods, Apple Sauce, Organic

1/2 cup

Amount per serving	Amount per serving	Amount per serving
Calories 60	**Cholesterol** NA	**Total Carbohydrate** 13g
Total Fat 0g	**Sodium** 10mg	Dietary Fiber 2g
Saturated Fat 0g	**Protein** 0g	Sugars 10g

Eden Foods, Apple Strawberry Sauce, Organic

1/2 cup

Amount per serving	Amount per serving	Amount per serving
Calories 60	**Cholesterol** NA	**Total Carbohydrate** 13g
Total Fat 0g	**Sodium** 10mg	Dietary Fiber 2g
Saturated Fat 0g	**Protein** 0g	Sugars 10g

Eden Foods, Cherry Butter, Montmorency Tart, Organic

1 tbsp

Amount per serving	Amount per serving	Amount per serving
Calories 35	**Cholesterol** NA	**Total Carbohydrate** 9g
Total Fat 0g	**Sodium** 0mg	Dietary Fiber 1g
Saturated Fat NA	**Protein** 0g	Sugars 8g

Eden Foods, Thompson Raisins, Organic

1/4 cup

Amount per serving	Amount per serving	Amount per serving
Calories 130	**Cholesterol** 0mg	**Total Carbohydrate** 32g
Total Fat 0g	**Sodium** 0mg	Dietary Fiber 1.5g
Saturated Fat 0g	**Protein** 1g	Sugars 24g

Eden Foods, Wild Berry Mix, Organic

3 tbsp

Amount per serving	Amount per serving	Amount per serving
Calories 150	**Cholesterol** 0mg	**Total Carbohydrate** 13g
Total Fat 8g	**Sodium** 10mg	Dietary Fiber 4g
Saturated Fat 1g	**Protein** 5g	Sugars 1g

Let's Do...Organic, Organic Coconut Flakes

3 tbsp

Amount per serving	Amount per serving	Amount per serving
Calories 110	**Cholesterol** 0mg	**Total Carbohydrate** 4g
Total Fat 10g	**Sodium** 5mg	Dietary Fiber 2g
Saturated Fat 9g	**Protein** 1g	Sugars <1g

Let's Do...Organic, Organic Creamed Coconut

1 tbsp

Amount per serving	Amount per serving	Amount per serving
Calories 190	**Cholesterol** 0mg	**Total Carbohydrate** 7g
Total Fat 18g	**Sodium** 10mg	Dietary Fiber 5g
Saturated Fat 16g	**Protein** 2g	Sugars 2g

Let's Do...Organic, Organic Reduced Fat Shredded Coconut

4 tbsp

Amount per serving	Amount per serving	Amount per serving
Calories 70	**Cholesterol** 0mg	**Total Carbohydrate** 4g
Total Fat 6g	**Sodium** 0mg	Dietary Fiber 2g
Saturated Fat 5g	**Protein** 1g	Sugars 0g

Let's Do...Organic, Organic Shredded Coconut

3 tbsp

Amount per serving	Amount per serving	Amount per serving
Calories 110	**Cholesterol** 0mg	**Total Carbohydrate** 4g
Total Fat 10g	**Sodium** 5mg	Dietary Fiber 2g
Saturated Fat 9g	**Protein** 1g	Sugars <1g

Manna Organics, Organic Dates (Extruded)

1 oz (28g/1 oz)

Amount per serving	Amount per serving	Amount per serving
Calories 90	**Cholesterol** 0mg	**Total Carbohydrate** 24g
Total Fat 0g	**Sodium** 10mg	Dietary Fiber 3g
Saturated Fat 0g	**Protein** 1g	Sugars 19g

Manna Organics, Organic Raisins

1 oz (28g)

Amount per serving	Amount per serving	Amount per serving
Calories 90	**Cholesterol** 0mg	**Total Carbohydrate** 22g
Total Fat 0g	**Sodium** 5mg	Dietary Fiber 2g
Saturated Fat 0g	**Protein** 1g	Sugars 20g

Native Forest, Organic Mango Chunks

1/2 cup

Amount per serving	Amount per serving	Amount per serving
Calories 70	**Cholesterol** 0mg	**Total Carbohydrate** 19g
Total Fat 0g	**Sodium** 0mg	Dietary Fiber 2g
Saturated Fat 0g	**Protein** 0g	Sugars 17g

Native Forest, Organic Papaya Chunks

1/2 cup

Amount per serving	Amount per serving	Amount per serving
Calories 60	**Cholesterol** 0mg	**Total Carbohydrate** 14g
Total Fat 0g	**Sodium** 0mg	Dietary Fiber 1g
Saturated Fat 0g	**Protein** <1g	Sugars 11g

Native Forest, Organic Pineapple Chunks

1/2 cup

Amount per serving	Amount per serving	Amount per serving
Calories 60	**Cholesterol** 0mg	**Total Carbohydrate** 15g
Total Fat 0g	**Sodium** 10mg	Dietary Fiber 1g
Saturated Fat 0g	**Protein** 0g	Sugars 13g

Native Forest, Organic Pineapple Crushed

1/2 cup

Amount per serving	Amount per serving	Amount per serving
Calories 60	**Cholesterol** 0mg	**Total Carbohydrate** 15g
Total Fat 0g	**Sodium** 10mg	Dietary Fiber 1g
Saturated Fat 0g	**Protein** 0g	Sugars 13g

Native Forest, Organic Pineapple Slices

1/2 cup

Amount per serving	Amount per serving	Amount per serving
Calories 60	**Cholesterol** 0mg	**Total Carbohydrate** 15g
Total Fat 0g	**Sodium** 10mg	Dietary Fiber 1g
Saturated Fat 0g	**Protein** 0g	Sugars 13g

Native Forest, Organic Sliced Peaches

1/2 cup

Amount per serving	Amount per serving	Amount per serving
Calories 60	**Cholesterol** 0mg	**Total Carbohydrate** 14g
Total Fat 0g	**Sodium** 5mg	Dietary Fiber 2g
Saturated Fat 0g	**Protein** <1g	Sugars 12g

Native Forest, Organic Tropical Fruit Salad

1/2 cup

Amount per serving	Amount per serving	Amount per serving
Calories 70	**Cholesterol** 0mg	**Total Carbohydrate** 16g
Total Fat 0g	**Sodium** 0mg	Dietary Fiber 1g
Saturated Fat 0g	**Protein** <1g	Sugars 14g

Newman's Own Organics, Organic Dried Fruit, Apples

1/4 cup (40g)

Amount per serving	Amount per serving	Amount per serving
Calories 120	**Cholesterol** 0mg	**Total Carbohydrate** 29g
Total Fat 0g	**Sodium** 0mg	Dietary Fiber 2g
Saturated Fat 0g	**Protein** 0g	Sugars 22g

Newman's Own Organics, Organic Dried Fruit, Apricots

1/4 cup (40g)

Amount per serving	Amount per serving	Amount per serving
Calories 110	**Cholesterol** 0mg	**Total Carbohydrate** 25g
Total Fat 0g	**Sodium** 0mg	Dietary Fiber 2g
Saturated Fat 0g	**Protein** 1g	Sugars 15g

Newman's Own Organics, Organic Dried Fruit, Berry Blend

1/4 cup (40g)

Amount per serving	Amount per serving	Amount per serving
Calories 120	**Cholesterol** 0mg	**Total Carbohydrate** 31g
Total Fat 0g	**Sodium** 5mg	Dietary Fiber 2g
Saturated Fat 0g	**Protein** 1g	Sugars 25g

Newman's Own Organics, Organic Dried Fruit, Cranberries

1/4 cup (40g)

Amount per serving	Amount per serving	Amount per serving
Calories 130	**Cholesterol** 0mg	**Total Carbohydrate** 34g
Total Fat 0g	**Sodium** 0mg	Dietary Fiber 2g
Saturated Fat 0g	**Protein** 0g	Sugars 31g

Newman's Own Organics, Organic Dried Fruit, Prunes

1/4 cup (40g)

Amount per serving	Amount per serving	Amount per serving
Calories 110	**Cholesterol** 0mg	**Total Carbohydrate** 26g
Total Fat 0g	**Sodium** 5mg	Dietary Fiber 2g
Saturated Fat 0g	**Protein** 1g	Sugars 13g

Newman's Own Organics, Organic Dried Fruit, Raisins

1/4 cup (40g)

Amount per serving	Amount per serving	Amount per serving
Calories 130	Cholesterol 0mg	Total Carbohydrate 31g
Total Fat 0g	Sodium 10mg	Dietary Fiber 2g
Saturated Fat 0g	Protein 1g	Sugars 29g

Santa Cruz Organic, Apple Apricot Sauce

1/2 cup (126g)

Amount per serving	Amount per serving	Amount per serving
Calories 70	Cholesterol NA	Total Carbohydrate 19g
Total Fat 0g	Sodium 0mg	Dietary Fiber 2g
Saturated Fat NA	Protein <1g	Sugars 15g

Santa Cruz Organic, Apple Apricot Sauce Cups

1 unit (113g)

Amount per serving	Amount per serving	Amount per serving
Calories 70	Cholesterol NA	Total Carbohydrate 17g
Total Fat 0g	Sodium 10mg	Dietary Fiber 2g
Saturated Fat NA	Protein <1g	Sugars 14g

Santa Cruz Organic, Apple Peach Sauce

1/2 cup (127g)

Amount per serving	Amount per serving	Amount per serving
Calories 60	Cholesterol NA	Total Carbohydrate 15g
Total Fat 0g	Sodium 0mg	Dietary Fiber 2g
Saturated Fat NA	Protein <1g	Sugars 12g

Santa Cruz Organic, Apple Peach Sauce Cups

1 unit

Amount per serving	Amount per serving	Amount per serving
Calories 70	Cholesterol 0mg	Total Carbohydrate 17g
Total Fat 0g	Sodium 10mg	Dietary Fiber 2g
Saturated Fat 0g	Protein <1g	Sugars 14g

Santa Cruz Organic, Apple Sauce

1/2 cup (125g)

Amount per serving	Amount per serving	Amount per serving
Calories 60	Cholesterol NA	Total Carbohydrate 15g
Total Fat 0g	Sodium 0mg	Dietary Fiber 2g
Saturated Fat NA	Protein 0g	Sugars 12g

Santa Cruz Organic, Apple Sauce Cups

1 unit (113g)

Amount per serving	Amount per serving	Amount per serving
Calories 50	**Cholesterol** NA	**Total Carbohydrate** 14g
Total Fat 0g	**Sodium** 10mg	Dietary Fiber 1g
Saturated Fat NA	**Protein** 0g	Sugars 11g

Santa Cruz Organic, Apple Sauce Pouch

1 pouch

Amount per serving	Amount per serving	Amount per serving
Calories 45	**Cholesterol** NA	**Total Carbohydrate** 13g
Total Fat 0g	**Sodium** 0mg	Dietary Fiber 2g
Saturated Fat NA	**Protein** 0g	Sugars 11g

Santa Cruz Organic, Apple Strawberry Sauce

1/2 cup (126g)

Amount per serving	Amount per serving	Amount per serving
Calories 60	**Cholesterol** NA	**Total Carbohydrate** 16g
Total Fat 0g	**Sodium** 0mg	Dietary Fiber 2g
Saturated Fat NA	**Protein** 0g	Sugars 13g

Santa Cruz Organic, Apple Strawberry Sauce Pouch

1 pouch

Amount per serving	Amount per serving	Amount per serving
Calories 45	**Cholesterol** NA	**Total Carbohydrate** 13g
Total Fat 0g	**Sodium** 0mg	Dietary Fiber 2g
Saturated Fat NA	**Protein** NA	Sugars 10g

Santa Cruz Organic, Apricot Fruit Spread

1 tbsp

Amount per serving	Amount per serving	Amount per serving
Calories 40	**Cholesterol** NA	**Total Carbohydrate** 10g
Total Fat 0g	**Sodium** 5mg	Dietary Fiber NA
Saturated Fat NA	**Protein** 0g	Sugars 10g

Santa Cruz Organic, Blackberry Pomegranate Fruit Spread

1 tbsp (19g)

Amount per serving	Amount per serving	Amount per serving
Calories 45	**Cholesterol** NA	**Total Carbohydrate** 11g
Total Fat 0g	**Sodium** 5mg	Dietary Fiber NA
Saturated Fat NA	**Protein** 0g	Sugars 10g

Santa Cruz Organic, Cinnamon Apple Sauce

1/2 cup (127g)

Amount per serving	Amount per serving	Amount per serving
Calories 70	Cholesterol NA	Total Carbohydrate 19g
Total Fat 0g	Sodium 0mg	Dietary Fiber 2g
Saturated Fat NA	Protein 0g	Sugars 16g

Santa Cruz Organic, Cinnamon Apple Sauce Cups

1 unit (113g)

Amount per serving	Amount per serving	Amount per serving
Calories 60	Cholesterol NA	Total Carbohydrate 17g
Total Fat 0g	Sodium 10mg	Dietary Fiber 1g
Saturated Fat NA	Protein 0g	Sugars 14g

Santa Cruz Organic, Cinnamon Apple Sauce Pouch

1 pouch

Amount per serving	Amount per serving	Amount per serving
Calories 60	Cholesterol NA	Total Carbohydrate 15g
Total Fat 0g	Sodium 0mg	Dietary Fiber 2g
Saturated Fat NA	Protein 0g	Sugars 12g

Santa Cruz Organic, Concord Grape Fruit Spread

1 tbsp (19g)

Amount per serving	Amount per serving	Amount per serving
Calories 40	Cholesterol NA	Total Carbohydrate 10g
Total Fat 0g	Sodium 10mg	Dietary Fiber NA
Saturated Fat NA	Protein 0g	Sugars 10g

Santa Cruz Organic, Mango Fruit Spread

1 tbsp (19g)

Amount per serving	Amount per serving	Amount per serving
Calories 45	Cholesterol NA	Total Carbohydrate 11g
Total Fat 0g	Sodium 5mg	Dietary Fiber NA
Saturated Fat NA	Protein 0g	Sugars 10g

Santa Cruz Organic, Seedless Red Raspberry Fruit Spread

1 tbsp (19g)

Amount per serving	Amount per serving	Amount per serving
Calories 40	Cholesterol NA	Total Carbohydrate 10g
Total Fat 0g	Sodium 5mg	Dietary Fiber NA
Saturated Fat NA	Protein 0g	Sugars 10g

Santa Cruz Organic, Strawberry Fruit Spread

1 tbsp (19g)

Amount per serving	Amount per serving	Amount per serving
Calories 40	**Cholesterol** NA	**Total Carbohydrate** 10g
Total Fat 0g	**Sodium** 5mg	Dietary Fiber NA
Saturated Fat NA	**Protein** 0g	Sugars 10g

Fruits

Driscoll's, Organic Blackberries

1 cup (144g)

Amount per serving	Amount per serving	Amount per serving
Calories 43	**Cholesterol** 0mg	**Total Carbohydrate** 10g
Total Fat 0.5g	**Sodium** 1mg	Dietary Fiber 5g
Saturated Fat 0g	**Protein** 1g	Sugars 5g

Driscoll's, Organic Blueberries

1 cup (148g)

Amount per serving	Amount per serving	Amount per serving
Calories 84	**Cholesterol** 0mg	**Total Carbohydrate** 14g
Total Fat 0.3g	**Sodium** 1mg	Dietary Fiber 2g
Saturated Fat 0g	**Protein** 1g	Sugars 10g

Driscoll's, Organic Raspberries

1 cup (123g)

Amount per serving	Amount per serving	Amount per serving
Calories 52	**Cholesterol** 0mg	**Total Carbohydrate** 12g
Total Fat 0.7g	**Sodium** 1mg	Dietary Fiber 7g
Saturated Fat 0g	**Protein** 1g	Sugars 4g

Driscoll's, Organic Strawberries

1 cup (144g)

Amount per serving	Amount per serving	Amount per serving
Calories 50	**Cholesterol** 0mg	**Total Carbohydrate** 11g
Total Fat 0g	**Sodium** 0mg	Dietary Fiber 2g
Saturated Fat 0g	**Protein** 1g	Sugars 8g

Earthbound Farm Organic, Frozen Organic Blueberries, 10 oz bag, 2 lb bag

1 cup (140g)

Amount per serving	Amount per serving	Amount per serving
Calories 70	**Cholesterol** 0mg	**Total Carbohydrate** 17g
Total Fat 1g	**Sodium** 0mg	Dietary Fiber 4g
Saturated Fat 0g	**Protein** 1g	Sugars 12g

Earthbound Farm Organic, Organic Apples, 3 lb bag

1 medium (155g)

Amount per serving	Amount per serving	Amount per serving
Calories 80	**Cholesterol** 0mg	**Total Carbohydrate** 20g
Total Fat 0g	**Sodium** 0mg	Dietary Fiber 3g
Saturated Fat 0g	**Protein** 0g	Sugars 19g

Earthbound Farm Organic, Organic Berry Basket Blend, 10 oz bag

1 cup (140g)

Amount per serving	Amount per serving	Amount per serving
Calories 70	**Cholesterol** 0mg	**Total Carbohydrate** 16g
Total Fat 0g	**Sodium** 0mg	Dietary Fiber 4g
Saturated Fat 0g	**Protein** 1g	Sugars 10g

Earthbound Farm Organic, Organic Blueberries

1 cup (140g)

Amount per serving	Amount per serving	Amount per serving
Calories 80	**Cholesterol** 0mg	**Total Carbohydrate** 19g
Total Fat 0g	**Sodium** 10mg	Dietary Fiber 4g
Saturated Fat 0g	**Protein** 1g	Sugars 16g

Earthbound Farm Organic, Organic Grapefruit, 4 lb bag

1/2 medium (154g)

Amount per serving	Amount per serving	Amount per serving
Calories 60	**Cholesterol** 0mg	**Total Carbohydrate** 15g
Total Fat 0g	**Sodium** 0mg	Dietary Fiber 2g
Saturated Fat 0g	**Protein** 1g	Sugars 11g

Earthbound Farm Organic, Organic Green Seedless Grapes

3/4 cup (140g)

Amount per serving	Amount per serving	Amount per serving
Calories 90	**Cholesterol** 0mg	**Total Carbohydrate** 20g
Total Fat 0g	**Sodium** 0mg	Dietary Fiber 1g
Saturated Fat 0g	**Protein** 1g	Sugars 22g

Earthbound Farm Organic, Organic Kiwifruit, 1 lb bag

2 medium (148g)

Amount per serving	Amount per serving	Amount per serving
Calories 90	**Cholesterol** 0mg	**Total Carbohydrate** 20g
Total Fat 1g	**Sodium** 0mg	Dietary Fiber 4g
Saturated Fat 0g	**Protein** 1g	Sugars 13g

Earthbound Farm Organic, Organic Lemons, 2 lb bag

1 medium (58g)

Amount per serving	Amount per serving	Amount per serving
Calories 15	**Cholesterol** 0mg	**Total Carbohydrate** 5g
Total Fat 0g	**Sodium** 0mg	Dietary Fiber 2g
Saturated Fat 0g	**Protein** 0g	Sugars 2g

Earthbound Farm Organic, Organic Navel Oranges, 4 lb bag

1 large (184g)

Amount per serving	Amount per serving	Amount per serving
Calories 90	**Cholesterol** 0mg	**Total Carbohydrate** 22g
Total Fat 0g	**Sodium** 0mg	Dietary Fiber 4g
Saturated Fat 0g	**Protein** 2g	Sugars 12g

Earthbound Farm Organic, Organic Pears, 3 lb bag

1 medium (166g)

Amount per serving	Amount per serving	Amount per serving
Calories 100	**Cholesterol** 0mg	**Total Carbohydrate** 26g
Total Fat 0g	**Sodium** 0mg	Dietary Fiber 6g
Saturated Fat 0g	**Protein** 1g	Sugars 16g

Earthbound Farm Organic, Organic Red Mangos, Unpackaged, loose fruit

1 medium (207g)

Amount per serving	Amount per serving	Amount per serving
Calories 140	**Cholesterol** 0mg	**Total Carbohydrate** 35g
Total Fat 0.5g	**Sodium** 0mg	Dietary Fiber 4g
Saturated Fat 0g	**Protein** 1g	Sugars 30g

Earthbound Farm Organic, Organic Red Seedless Grapes

3/4 cup (140g)

Amount per serving	Amount per serving	Amount per serving
Calories 100	**Cholesterol** 0mg	**Total Carbohydrate** 22g
Total Fat 0g	**Sodium** 0mg	Dietary Fiber 1g
Saturated Fat 0g	**Protein** 1g	Sugars 18g

Earthbound Farm Organic, Organic Strawberries, 8.8 oz clamshell, 1 lb clamshell

8 medium (147g)

Amount per serving	Amount per serving	Amount per serving
Calories 50	**Cholesterol** 0mg	**Total Carbohydrate** 11g
Total Fat 0g	**Sodium** 0mg	Dietary Fiber 2g
Saturated Fat 0g	**Protein** 1g	Sugars 8g

Earthbound Farm Organic, Organic Valencia Oranges, 4 lb bag

1 large (184g)

Amount per serving	Amount per serving	Amount per serving
Calories 90	**Cholesterol** 0mg	**Total Carbohydrate** 22g
Total Fat 0g	**Sodium** 0mg	Dietary Fiber 4g
Saturated Fat 0g	**Protein** 2g	Sugars 12g

Earthbound Farm Organic, Organic Yellow Mangos, Unpackaged, loose fruit

1 medium (207g)

Amount per serving	Amount per serving	Amount per serving
Calories 140	**Cholesterol** 0mg	**Total Carbohydrate** 35g
Total Fat 0.5g	**Sodium** 0mg	Dietary Fiber 4g
Saturated Fat 0g	**Protein** 1g	Sugars 30g

Dairy Foods

Dairy foods are excellent sources of key nutrients—calcium, potassium, vitamin D, and protein—that are essential for health, especially for nurturing strong bones and teeth. Dairy is vitally important for children and teens to ensure bone growth and development, and it may even reduce the risk of osteoporosis in older adults. People who consume dairy products may reduce their risk of developing high blood pressure, cardiovascular disease, and type 2 diabetes.

The USDA recommends substituting low-fat or fat-free dairy foods for full-fat versions, such as cheeses made from whole milk that are high in saturated fat. Saturated fats raise LDL (low-density lipoprotein) cholesterol, and elevated levels of LDL cholesterol are associated with increased risk of heart disease.

Why Choose Organic Dairy Products?

There are many reasons to choose organic dairy products. USDA organic standards require that the cows are raised in safe, clean, uncrowded environments with opportunities for exercise and ample grazing time. The animals must be fed organic feed and cannot be treated with antibiotics or given growth hormones. Buying organic dairy products also helps to ensure humane treatment of cows and encourage agricultural practices that support human and environmental health.

Daily Goal

Three cups for an adult on a 2,000-calorie diet.

1 cup equivalents:

1 cup milk	2 oz. processed cheese
6 oz. yogurt	2 cups cottage cheese
1.5 oz. hard cheese	2 egg whites
1/3 cup shredded cheese	

Butter

Horizon®, Organic Salted Butter

1 tbsp (14g)

Amount per serving	Amount per serving	Amount per serving
Calories 100	**Cholesterol** 30mg	**Total Carbohydrate** 0g
Total Fat 11g	**Sodium** 115mg	Dietary Fiber NA
Saturated Fat 7g	**Protein** 0g	Sugars NA

Horizon®, Organic Unsalted Butter

1 tbsp (14g)

Amount per serving	Amount per serving	Amount per serving
Calories 100	**Cholesterol** 30mg	**Total Carbohydrate** 0g
Total Fat 11g	**Sodium** 0mg	Dietary Fiber NA
Saturated Fat 7g	**Protein** 0g	Sugars NA

Organic Valley, Cultured Butter, Unsalted

1 tbsp (14g)

Amount per serving	Amount per serving	Amount per serving
Calories 100	**Cholesterol** 30mg	**Total Carbohydrate** 0g
Total Fat 11g	**Sodium** 0mg	Dietary Fiber 0g
Saturated Fat 7g	**Protein** 0g	Sugars 0g

Organic Valley, European Style Butter

1 tbsp (14g)

Amount per serving	Amount per serving	Amount per serving
Calories 110	**Cholesterol** 35mg	**Total Carbohydrate** 0g
Total Fat 12g	**Sodium** 0mg	Dietary Fiber 0g
Saturated Fat 8g	**Protein** 0g	Sugars 0g

Stonyfield Organic, Organic Salted Butter

1 tbsp

Amount per serving	Amount per serving	Amount per serving
Calories 100	**Cholesterol** 30mg	**Total Carbohydrate** 0g
Total Fat 11g	**Sodium** 75mg	Dietary Fiber 0g
Saturated Fat 7g	**Protein** 0g	Sugars 0g

Stonyfield Organic, Organic Unsalted Butter

1 tbsp

Amount per serving	Amount per serving	Amount per serving
Calories 100	**Cholesterol** 30mg	**Total Carbohydrate** 0g
Total Fat 11g	**Sodium** 0mg	Dietary Fiber 0g
Saturated Fat 7g	**Protein** 0g	Sugars 0g

Straus Family Creamery, European-Style Organic Salted Butter

1 tbsp (14g)

Amount per serving	Amount per serving	Amount per serving
Calories 110	**Cholesterol** 30mg	**Total Carbohydrate** 0g
Total Fat 12g	**Sodium** 45mg	Dietary Fiber 0g
Saturated Fat 8g	**Protein** 0g	Sugars 0g

Straus Family Creamery, European-Style Organic Unsalted Butter

1 tbsp (14g)

Amount per serving	Amount per serving	Amount per serving
Calories 110	**Cholesterol** 30mg	**Total Carbohydrate** 0g
Total Fat 12g	**Sodium** 0mg	Dietary Fiber 0g
Saturated Fat 8g	**Protein** 0g	Sugars 0g

Cheese

Applegate Farms, Organic American Cheese

1 slice

Amount per serving	Amount per serving	Amount per serving
Calories 80	**Cholesterol** 25mg	**Total Carbohydrate** 1g
Total Fat 7g	**Sodium** 270mg	Dietary Fiber 0g
Saturated Fat 5g	**Protein** 5g	Sugars 0g

Applegate Farms, Organic Mild Cheddar Cheese

1 slice

Amount per serving	Amount per serving	Amount per serving
Calories 80	**Cholesterol** 20mg	**Total Carbohydrate** 0g
Total Fat 6g	**Sodium** 130mg	Dietary Fiber 0g
Saturated Fat 4g	**Protein** 5g	Sugars 0g

Applegate Farms, Organic Monterey Jack Cheese

1 slice

Amount per serving	Amount per serving	Amount per serving
Calories 80	**Cholesterol** 20mg	**Total Carbohydrate** 0g
Total Fat 6g	**Sodium** 130mg	Dietary Fiber 0g
Saturated Fat 4g	**Protein** 5g	Sugars 0g

Applegate Farms, Organic Muenster Cheese

1 slice

Amount per serving	Amount per serving	Amount per serving
Calories 85	**Cholesterol** 20mg	**Total Carbohydrate** 0g
Total Fat 6g	**Sodium** 130mg	Dietary Fiber 0g
Saturated Fat 4g	**Protein** 5g	Sugars 0g

Applegate Farms, Organic Provolone Cheese

1 slice

Amount per serving	Amount per serving	Amount per serving
Calories 70	**Cholesterol** 15mg	**Total Carbohydrate** 0g
Total Fat 5g	**Sodium** 160mg	Dietary Fiber 0g
Saturated Fat 3g	**Protein** 5g	Sugars 0g

Green Valley Organics, Cream Cheese

2 tbsp

Amount per serving	Amount per serving	Amount per serving
Calories 90	**Cholesterol** 25mg	**Total Carbohydrate** 2g
Total Fat 9g	**Sodium** 35mg	Dietary Fiber 0g
Saturated Fat 6g	**Protein** 1g	Sugars 0g

Horizon®, Mexican, Organic Shredded Mexican Cheese

1/4 cup (28g)

Amount per serving	Amount per serving	Amount per serving
Calories 110	**Cholesterol** 25mg	**Total Carbohydrate** 1g
Total Fat 9g	**Sodium** 170mg	Dietary Fiber 0g
Saturated Fat 5g	**Protein** 7g	Sugars 0g

Horizon®, Organic Lowfat Cottage Cheese

1/2 cup (113g)

Amount per serving	Amount per serving	Amount per serving
Calories 100	**Cholesterol** 10mg	**Total Carbohydrate** 4g
Total Fat 2.5g	**Sodium** 390mg	Dietary Fiber 0g
Saturated Fat 1.5g	**Protein** 14g	Sugars 4g

Horizon®, Organic Regular Cottage Cheese

1/2 cup (113g)

Amount per serving	Amount per serving	Amount per serving
Calories 120	**Cholesterol** 20mg	**Total Carbohydrate** 4g
Total Fat 5g	**Sodium** 400mg	Dietary Fiber 0g
Saturated Fat 3g	**Protein** 14g	Sugars 4g

Horizon®, Original Cream Cheese

2 tbsp (30g)

Amount per serving	Amount per serving	Amount per serving
Calories 100	**Cholesterol** 30mg	**Total Carbohydrate** 1g
Total Fat 10g	**Sodium** 90mg	Dietary Fiber 0g
Saturated Fat 6g	**Protein** 2g	Sugars 0g

Horizon®, Reduced Fat Cream Cheese

2 tbsp (30g)

Amount per serving	Amount per serving	Amount per serving
Calories 80	**Cholesterol** 25mg	**Total Carbohydrate** 2g
Total Fat 7g	**Sodium** 100mg	Dietary Fiber 0g
Saturated Fat 4g	**Protein** 2g	Sugars 1g

Horizon®, Shreds, Organic Shredded Cheddar Cheese

1/4 cup (28g)

Amount per serving	Amount per serving	Amount per serving
Calories 110	**Cholesterol** 25mg	**Total Carbohydrate** 1g
Total Fat 9g	**Sodium** 180mg	Dietary Fiber 0g
Saturated Fat 5g	**Protein** 7g	Sugars 0g

Horizon®, Shreds, Organic Shredded Monterey Jack Cheese

1/4 cup (28g)

Amount per serving	Amount per serving	Amount per serving
Calories 100	**Cholesterol** 25mg	**Total Carbohydrate** 0g
Total Fat 8g	**Sodium** 170mg	Dietary Fiber 0g
Saturated Fat 4.5g	**Protein** 6g	Sugars 0g

Horizon®, Shreds, Organic Shredded Mozzarella Cheese

1/4 cup (28g)

Amount per serving	Amount per serving	Amount per serving
Calories 80	**Cholesterol** 15mg	**Total Carbohydrate** 1g
Total Fat 5g	**Sodium** 170mg	Dietary Fiber 0g
Saturated Fat 3g	**Protein** 8g	Sugars 0g

Horizon®, Singles, Organic American Cheese Slices

1 slice (19g)

Amount per serving	Amount per serving	Amount per serving
Calories 60	**Cholesterol** 15mg	**Total Carbohydrate** 2g
Total Fat 5g	**Sodium** 230mg	Dietary Fiber 0g
Saturated Fat 3g	**Protein** 3g	Sugars 1g

Horizon®, Slices, Organic Cheddar Cheese Slices

1 slice (21g)

Amount per serving	Amount per serving	Amount per serving
Calories 80	**Cholesterol** 20mg	**Total Carbohydrate** 0g
Total Fat 7g	**Sodium** 135mg	Dietary Fiber 0g
Saturated Fat 4g	**Protein** 5g	Sugars 0g

Horizon®, Slices, Organic Provolone Cheese Slices

1 slice (21g)

Amount per serving	Amount per serving	Amount per serving
Calories 70	**Cholesterol** 15mg	**Total Carbohydrate** 0g
Total Fat 6g	**Sodium** 180mg	Dietary Fiber 0g
Saturated Fat 3.5g	**Protein** 5g	Sugars 0g

Horizon®, Sticks, Mozzarella Cheese Sticks

1 stick (28g)

Amount per serving	Amount per serving	Amount per serving
Calories 80	**Cholesterol** 15mg	**Total Carbohydrate** <1g
Total Fat 6g	**Sodium** 200mg	Dietary Fiber 0g
Saturated Fat 3.5g	**Protein** 8g	Sugars 0g

Horizon®, Sticks, Organic Colby Cheese Sticks

1 stick (28g)

Amount per serving	Amount per serving	Amount per serving
Calories 110	**Cholesterol** 1mg	**Total Carbohydrate** 1g
Total Fat 9g	**Sodium** 170mg	Dietary Fiber 0g
Saturated Fat 5g	**Protein** 7g	Sugars 0g

Lifeway Foods, Organic Farmer Cheese

2 tbsp

Amount per serving	Amount per serving	Amount per serving
Calories 40	**Cholesterol** 6mg	**Total Carbohydrate** 4g
Total Fat 1.5g	**Sodium** 10mg	Dietary Fiber 0g
Saturated Fat 1g	**Protein** 3g	Sugars 4g

Organic Valley, American Singles

1.5 slice (28g)

Amount per serving	Amount per serving	Amount per serving
Calories 110	**Cholesterol** 25mg	**Total Carbohydrate** <1g
Total Fat 9g	**Sodium** 170mg	Dietary Fiber 0g
Saturated Fat 6g	**Protein** 7g	Sugars <1g

Organic Valley, Baby Swiss Cheese

1 oz (28g)

Amount per serving	Amount per serving	Amount per serving
Calories 110	**Cholesterol** 25mg	**Total Carbohydrate** 0g
Total Fat 9g	**Sodium** 125mg	Dietary Fiber 0g
Saturated Fat 6g	**Protein** 7g	Sugars 0g

Organic Valley, Baby Swiss Slices

1 slice (21g)

Amount per serving	Amount per serving	Amount per serving
Calories 80	**Cholesterol** 20mg	**Total Carbohydrate** 0g
Total Fat 7g	**Sodium** 95mg	Dietary Fiber 0g
Saturated Fat 3.5g	**Protein** 5g	Sugars 0g

Organic Valley, Colby Cheese

1 oz (28g)

Amount per serving	Amount per serving	Amount per serving
Calories 110	**Cholesterol** 25mg	**Total Carbohydrate** <1g
Total Fat 9g	**Sodium** 170mg	Dietary Fiber 0g
Saturated Fat 6g	**Protein** 7g	Sugars <1g

Organic Valley, Cream Cheese Spread, Tub

2 tbsp (30g)

Amount per serving	Amount per serving	Amount per serving
Calories 90	**Cholesterol** 25mg	**Total Carbohydrate** 3g
Total Fat 9g	**Sodium** 150mg	Dietary Fiber 0g
Saturated Fat 6g	**Protein** 1g	Sugars 3g

Organic Valley, Cream Cheese, Bar

2 tbsp (30g)

Amount per serving	Amount per serving	Amount per serving
Calories 100	**Cholesterol** 30mg	**Total Carbohydrate** 2g
Total Fat 10g	**Sodium** 100mg	Dietary Fiber 0g
Saturated Fat 6g	**Protein** 2g	Sugars <1g

Organic Valley, Feta Cheese

1 oz (28g)

Amount per serving	Amount per serving	Amount per serving
Calories 60	**Cholesterol** 10mg	**Total Carbohydrate** <1g
Total Fat 4g	**Sodium** 430mg	Dietary Fiber 0g
Saturated Fat 2.5g	**Protein** 5g	Sugars 0g

Organic Valley, Feta Cheese Crumbles

1 oz (28g)

Amount per serving	Amount per serving	Amount per serving
Calories 70	**Cholesterol** 15mg	**Total Carbohydrate** 2g
Total Fat 4g	**Sodium** 430mg	Dietary Fiber 0g
Saturated Fat 2.5g	**Protein** 6g	Sugars 0g

Organic Valley, Grassmilk Raw Cheddar Cheese

1 oz (28g)

Amount per serving	Amount per serving	Amount per serving
Calories 110	**Cholesterol** 30mg	**Total Carbohydrate** 0g
Total Fat 9g	**Sodium** 170mg	Dietary Fiber 0g
Saturated Fat 6g	**Protein** 7g	Sugars 0g

Organic Valley, Grassmilk, Raw Sharp Cheddar Cheese

1 oz (28g)

Amount per serving	Amount per serving	Amount per serving
Calories 110	**Cholesterol** 30mg	**Total Carbohydrate** 0g
Total Fat 9g	**Sodium** 170mg	Dietary Fiber 0g
Saturated Fat 6g	**Protein** 7g	Sugars 0g

Organic Valley, Grated Parmesan

1/4 cup (28g)

Amount per serving	Amount per serving	Amount per serving
Calories 110	**Cholesterol** 20mg	**Total Carbohydrate** 2g
Total Fat 7g	**Sodium** 350mg	Dietary Fiber 0g
Saturated Fat 4g	**Protein** 10g	Sugars 0g

Organic Valley, Italian Blend, Shredded

1/4 cup (28g)

Amount per serving	Amount per serving	Amount per serving
Calories 90	**Cholesterol** 20mg	**Total Carbohydrate** 1g
Total Fat 7g	**Sodium** 220mg	Dietary Fiber 0g
Saturated Fat 4g	**Protein** 7g	Sugars 0g

Organic Valley, Mexican Blend, Shredded

1/4 cup (28g)

Amount per serving	Amount per serving	Amount per serving
Calories 110	**Cholesterol** 30mg	**Total Carbohydrate** 1g
Total Fat 9g	**Sodium** 170mg	Dietary Fiber 0g
Saturated Fat 6g	**Protein** 7g	Sugars 0g

Organic Valley, Mild Cheddar Slices

1 slice (21g)

Amount per serving	Amount per serving	Amount per serving
Calories 80	**Cholesterol** 20mg	**Total Carbohydrate** 0g
Total Fat 7g	**Sodium** 130mg	Dietary Fiber 0g
Saturated Fat 4.5g	**Protein** 5g	Sugars 0g

Organic Valley, Mild Cheddar, Shredded

1/4 cup (28g)

Amount per serving	Amount per serving	Amount per serving
Calories 110	**Cholesterol** 30mg	**Total Carbohydrate** 1g
Total Fat 9g	**Sodium** 180mg	Dietary Fiber 0g
Saturated Fat 6g	**Protein** 7g	Sugars 0g

Organic Valley, Monterey Jack, Reduced Fat, Shredded

1/4 cup (28g)

Amount per serving	Amount per serving	Amount per serving
Calories 80	**Cholesterol** 15mg	**Total Carbohydrate** 1g
Total Fat 5g	**Sodium** 180mg	Dietary Fiber 0g
Saturated Fat 3.5g	**Protein** 8g	Sugars 0g

Organic Valley, Montery Jack Cheese

1 oz (28g)

Amount per serving	Amount per serving	Amount per serving
Calories 100	**Cholesterol** 30mg	**Total Carbohydrate** 0g
Total Fat 9g	**Sodium** 170mg	Dietary Fiber 0g
Saturated Ful 4.5g	**Protein** 7g	Sugars 0g

Organic Valley, Mozzarella Cheese

1 oz (28g)

Amount per serving	Amount per serving	Amount per serving
Calories 80	**Cholesterol** 20mg	**Total Carbohydrate** <1g
Total Fat 6g	**Sodium** 190mg	Dietary Fiber 0g
Saturated Fat 3.5g	**Protein** 7g	Sugars 0g

Organic Valley, Mozzarella, Low Moisture, Part Skim, Shredded

1/4 cup (28g)

Amount per serving	Amount por serving	Amount per serving
Calories 90	**Cholesterol** 20mg	**Total Carbohydrate** 1g
Total Fat 6g	**Sodium** 190mg	Dietary Fiber 0g
Saturated Fat 4g	**Protein** 7g	Sugars 0g

Organic Valley, Muenster Cheese

1 oz (28g)

Amount per serving	Amount per serving	Amount per serving
Calories 100	**Cholesterol** 25mg	**Total Carbohydrate** 0g
Total Fat 8g	**Sodium** 180mg	Dietary Fiber 0g
Saturated Fat 5g	**Protein** 7g	Sugars 0g

Organic Valley, Muenster Slices

1 slice (21g)

Amount per serving	Amount per serving	Amount per serving
Calories 80	**Cholesterol** 20mg	**Total Carbohydrate** 0g
Total Fat 6g	**Sodium** 160mg	Dietary Fiber 0g
Saturated Fat 4g	**Protein** 5g	Sugars 0g

Organic Valley, Organic Lowfat Sour Cream

2 tbsp (30g)

Amount per serving	Amount per serving	Amount per serving
Calories 30	**Cholesterol** 10mg	**Total Carbohydrate** 3g
Total Fat 2g	**Sodium** 20mg	Dietary Fiber 0g
Saturated Fat 1g	**Protein** 1g	Sugars 2g

Organic Valley, Organic Neufchatel Cheese Spread, Tub

2 tbsp (30g)

Amount per serving	Amount per serving	Amount per serving
Calories 70	**Cholesterol** 20mg	**Total Carbohydrate** 2g
Total Fat 6g	**Sodium** 160mg	Dietary Fiber 0g
Saturated Fat 4g	**Protein** 2g	Sugars 2g

Organic Valley, Organic Neufchatel Cheese, Bar

2 tbsp (30g)

Amount per serving	Amount per serving	Amount per serving
Calories 80	**Cholesterol** 20mg	**Total Carbohydrate** 1g
Total Fat 6g	**Sodium** 115mg	Dietary Fiber 0g
Saturated Fat 4g	**Protein** 2g	Sugars 1g

Organic Valley, Organic Small Curd Cottage Cheese

1/2 cup (110g)

Amount per serving	Amount per serving	Amount per serving
Calories 110	**Cholesterol** 15mg	**Total Carbohydrate** 5g
Total Fat 5g	**Sodium** 450mg	Dietary Fiber 0g
Saturated Fat 3g	**Protein** 14g	Sugars 4g

Organic Valley, Organic Small Curd Lowfat Cottage Cheese

1/2 cup (110g)

Amount per serving	Amount per serving	Amount per serving
Calories 100	**Cholesterol** 10mg	**Total Carbohydrate** 4g
Total Fat 2g	**Sodium** 450mg	Dietary Fiber 0g
Saturated Fat 1.5g	**Protein** 15g	Sugars 3g

Organic Valley, Organic Sour Cream

2 tbsp (30g)

Amount per serving	Amount per serving	Amount per serving
Calories 60	**Cholesterol** 25mg	**Total Carbohydrate** 2g
Total Fat 5g	**Sodium** 20mg	Dietary Fiber 0g
Saturated Fat 3.5g	**Protein** 1g	Sugars 1g

Organic Valley, Parmesan Cheese, Shredded

1/4 cup (28g)

Amount per serving	Amount per serving	Amount per serving
Calories 110	**Cholesterol** 20mg	**Total Carbohydrate** 0g
Total Fat 7g	**Sodium** 350mg	Dietary Fiber 0g
Saturated Fat 4g	**Protein** 10g	Sugars 0g

Organic Valley, Pepper Jack Cheese

1 oz (28g)

Amount por serving	Amount per serving	Amount per serving
Calories 100	**Cholesterol** 25mg	**Total Carbohydrate** 0g
Total Fat 8g	**Sodium** 220mg	Dietary Fiber 0g
Saturated Fat 5g	**Protein** 6g	Sugars 0g

Organic Valley, Provolone Cheese

1 oz (28g)

Amount per serving	Amount per serving	Amount per serving
Calories 100	**Cholesterol** 20mg	**Total Carbohydrate** 1g
Total Fat 8g	**Sodium** 250mg	Dietary Fiber 0g
Saturated Fat 5g	**Protein** 7g	Sugars 0g

Organic Valley, Provolone Slices

1 slice (21g)

Amount per serving	Amount per serving	Amount per serving
Calories 70	**Cholesterol** 15mg	**Total Carbohydrate** 0g
Total Fat 6g	**Sodium** 190mg	Dietary Fiber 0g
Saturated Fat 4g	**Protein** 5g	Sugars 0g

Organic Valley, Reduced Fat Monterey Jack Slices

1 slice (21g)

Amount per serving	Amount per serving	Amount per serving
Calories 60	**Cholesterol** 15mg	**Total Carbohydrate** 0g
Total Fat 4g	**Sodium** 140mg	Dietary Fiber 0g
Saturated Fat 3g	**Protein** 5g	Sugars 0g

Organic Valley, Stringles, Cheddar, 6 pack

1 unit (28g)

Amount per serving	Amount per serving	Amount per serving
Calories 110	**Cholesterol** 30mg	**Total Carbohydrate** 0g
Total Fat 9g	**Sodium** 170mg	Dietary Fiber 0g
Saturated Fat 6g	**Protein** 7g	Sugars 0g

Organic Valley, Stringles, Colby Jack, 6 pack

1 unit (28g)

Amount per serving	Amount per serving	Amount per serving
Calories 110	**Cholesterol** 30mg	**Total Carbohydrate** 0g
Total Fat 9g	**Sodium** 200mg	Dietary Fiber 0g
Saturated Fat 6g	**Protein** 7g	Sugars 0g

Organic Valley, Stringles, Mozzarella, Low Moisture, Part Skim, 6 pack

1 unit (28g)

Amount per serving	Amount per serving	Amount per serving
Calories 80	**Cholesterol** 20mg	**Total Carbohydrate** 0g
Total Fat 6g	**Sodium** 210mg	Dietary Fiber 0g
Saturated Fat 3.5g	**Protein** 7g	Sugars 0g

Organic Valley, Vermont Extra Sharp Cheddar Cheese

1 oz (28g)

Amount per serving	Amount per serving	Amount per serving
Calories 110	**Cholesterol** 30mg	**Total Carbohydrate** 0g
Total Fat 9g	**Sodium** 170mg	Dietary Fiber 0g
Saturated Fat 6g	**Protein** 7g	Sugars 0g

Organic Valley, Whole Milk Ricotta Cheese

1/4 cup (55g)

Amount per serving	Amount per serving	Amount per serving
Calories 100	**Cholesterol** 20mg	**Total Carbohydrate** 3g
Total Fat 7g	**Sodium** 100mg	Dietary Fiber 0g
Saturated Fat 4g	**Protein** 6g	Sugars 3g

Organic Valley, Wisconsin Kickapoo Blue Cheese Wedge

1 oz (28g)

Amount per serving	Amount per serving	Amount per serving
Calories 100	**Cholesterol** 25mg	**Total Carbohydrate** 1g
Total Fat 8g	**Sodium** 310mg	Dietary Fiber 0g
Saturated Fat 5g	**Protein** 6g	Sugars 0g

Organic Valley, Wisconsin Raw Jack Style Cheese

1 oz (28g)

Amount per serving	Amount per serving	Amount per serving
Calories 100	**Cholesterol** 25mg	**Total Carbohydrate** 0g
Total Fat 8g	**Sodium** 170mg	Dietary Fiber 0g
Saturated Fat 5g	**Protein** 7g	Sugars 0g

Dairy Alternative Desserts

SOY DREAM®, Rice Dream Cocoa Marble Fudge Frozen Dessert

1/2 cup (90g)

Amount per serving	Amount per serving	Amount per serving
Calories 170	**Cholesterol** 0mg	**Total Carbohydrate** 31g
Total Fat 6g	**Sodium** 90mg	Dietary Fiber 1g
Saturated Fat 0.5g	**Protein** <1g	Sugars 17g

SOY DREAM®, Rice Dream Neapolitan Frozen Dessert

1/2 cup (90g)

Amount per serving	Amount per serving	Amount per serving
Calories 160	**Cholesterol** 0mg	**Total Carbohydrate** 26g
Total Fat 6g	**Sodium** 80mg	Dietary Fiber >1g
Saturated Fat 0.5g	**Protein** 0g	Sugars 13g

SOY DREAM®, Rice Dream Strawberry Frozen Dessert

1/2 cup (80g)

Amount per serving	Amount per serving	Amount per serving
Calories 170	**Cholesterol** 0mg	**Total Carbohydrate** 30g
Total Fat 6g	**Sodium** 85mg	Dietary Fiber 0g
Saturated Fat 0.5g	**Protein** 0g	Sugars 16g

SOY DREAM®, Rice Dream Vanilla Frozen Dessert

1/2 cup (90g)

Amount por serving	Amount per serving	Amount per serving
Calories 160	**Cholesterol** 0mg	**Total Carbohydrate** 26g
Total Fat 6g	**Sodium** 85mg	Dietary Fiber 0g
Saturated Fat 0.5g	**Protein** 0g	Sugars 14g

ZenSoy, Chocolate Pudding (Made with Soymilk)

108g

Amount per serving	Amount per serving	Amount per serving
Calories 110	**Cholesterol** 0mg	**Total Carbohydrate** 23g
Total Fat 1g	**Sodium** 75mg	Dietary Fiber 1g
Saturated Fat 0g	**Protein** 3g	Sugars 18g

ZenSoy, Chocolate/Vanilla Swirl Pudding (Made with Soymilk)

108g

Amount per serving	Amount per serving	Amount per serving
Calories 110	**Cholesterol** 0mg	**Total Carbohydrate** 22g
Total Fat 1g	**Sodium** 70mg	Dietary Fiber 1g
Saturated Fat 0g	**Protein** 3g	Sugars 17g

ZenSoy, Vanilla Pudding (Made with Soymilk)

108g

Amount per serving	Amount per serving	Amount per serving
Calories 100	**Cholesterol** 0mg	**Total Carbohydrate** 20g
Total Fat 1g	**Sodium** 60mg	Dietary Fiber <1g
Saturated Fat 0g	**Protein** 2g	Sugars 14g

Dairy Alternatives

Eden Foods, EdenBlend, Organic Rice and Soymilk

8 fl oz

Amount per serving	Amount per serving	Amount per serving
Calories 120	**Cholesterol** 0mg	**Total Carbohydrate** 18g
Total Fat 3g	**Sodium** 90mg	Dietary Fiber <1g
Saturated Fat 0.5g	**Protein** 7g	Sugars 8g

Eden Foods, Unsweetened Edensoy, Organic Soymilk

8 fl oz

Amount per serving	Amount per serving	Amount per serving
Calories 120	**Cholesterol** 0mg	**Total Carbohydrate** 5g
Total Fat 6g	**Sodium** 5mg	Dietary Fiber <1g
Saturated Fat 1g	**Protein** 12g	Sugars 2g

Good Karma, Organic, Chocolate Whole Grain Ricemilk

1 cup / 8 fl oz

Amount per serving	Amount per serving	Amount per serving
Calories 120	**Cholesterol** 0mg	**Total Carbohydrate** 25g
Total Fat 2.5g	**Sodium** 180mg	Dietary Fiber 3g
Saturated Fat 0g	**Protein** 1g	Sugars 18g

Good Karma, Organic, Original Whole Grain Ricemilk

1 cup / 8 fl oz

Amount per serving	Amount per serving	Amount per serving
Calories 100	**Cholesterol** 0mg	**Total Carbohydrate** 19g
Total Fat 3g	**Sodium** 150mg	Dietary Fiber 3g
Saturated Fat 0g	**Protein** 1g	Sugars 9g

Good Karma, Organic, Vanilla Whole Grain Ricemilk

1 cup / 8 fl oz

Amount per serving	Amount per serving	Amount per serving
Calories 120	**Cholesterol** 0mg	**Total Carbohydrate** 26g
Total Fat 3g	**Sodium** 150mg	Dietary Fiber 3g
Saturated Fat 0g	**Protein** 1g	Sugars 13g

Horizon®, Fat-Free Lactose-Free Milk

1 cup (240 ml)

Amount per serving	Amount per serving	Amount per serving
Calories 90	**Cholesterol** 5mg	**Total Carbohydrate** 13g
Total Fat 0g	**Sodium** 135mg	Dietary Fiber 0g
Saturated Fat 0g	**Protein** 8g	Sugars 12g

Horizon®, Reduced Fat Lactose-Free Milk

1 cup (240 ml)

Amount per serving	Amount per serving	Amount per serving
Calories 130	**Cholesterol** 20mg	**Total Carbohydrate** 12g
Total Fat 5g	**Sodium** 130mg	Dietary Fiber 0g
Saturated Fat 3g	**Protein** 8g	Sugars 12g

Native Forest, Organic Coconut Milk

1/4 cup

Amount per serving	Amount per serving	Amount per serving
Calories 100	**Cholesterol** 0mg	**Total Carbohydrate** 3g
Total Fat 10g	**Sodium** 25mg	Dietary Fiber 0g
Saturated Fat 9g	**Protein** <1g	Sugars 1g

Native Forest, Organic Light Coconut Milk

1/4 cup

Amount per serving	Amount per serving	Amount per serving
Calories 45	**Cholesterol** 0mg	**Total Carbohydrate** 2g
Total Fat 4g	**Sodium** 15mg	Dietary Fiber 0g
Saturated Fat 3.5g	**Protein** <1g	Sugars <1g

Organic Valley, Chocolate Soy Milk

1 cup (240 ml)

Amount per serving	Amount per serving	Amount per serving
Calories 130	**Cholesterol** 0mg	**Total Carbohydrate** 20g
Total Fat 3g	**Sodium** 160mg	Dietary Fiber 3g
Saturated Fat 0.5g	**Protein** 5g	Sugars 16g

Organic Valley, Original Soy Milk

1 cup (240 ml)

Amount per serving	Amount per serving	Amount per serving
Calories 110	**Cholesterol** 0mg	**Total Carbohydrate** 11g
Total Fat 4g	**Sodium** 100mg	Dietary Fiber 3g
Saturated Fat 0.5g	**Protein** 7g	Sugars 6g

Organic Valley, Pasture Butter, Salted

1 tbsp (14g)

Amount per serving	Amount per serving	Amount per serving
Calories 110	**Cholesterol** 30mg	**Total Carbohydrate** 0g
Total Fat 12g	**Sodium** 40mg	Dietary Fiber 0g
Saturated Fat 7g	**Protein** 0g	Sugars 0g

Organic Valley, Salted Butter

1 tbsp (14g)

Amount per serving	Amount per serving	Amount per serving
Calories 100	**Cholesterol** 30mg	**Total Carbohydrate** 0g
Total Fat 11g	**Sodium** 75mg	Dietary Fiber 0g
Saturated Fat 7g	**Protein** 0g	Sugars 0g

Organic Valley, Soy Creamer, French Vanilla

1 tbsp (15 ml)

Amount per serving	Amount per serving	Amount per serving
Calories 25	**Cholesterol** 0mg	**Total Carbohydrate** 4g
Total Fat 1g	**Sodium** 30mg	Dietary Fiber 0g
Saturated Fat 0g	**Protein** 0g	Sugars 3g

Organic Valley, Soy Creamer, Original

1 tbsp (15 ml)

Amount per serving	Amount per serving	Amount per serving
Calories 15	**Cholesterol** 0mg	**Total Carbohydrate** 1g
Total Fat 1g	**Sodium** 30mg	Dietary Fiber 0g
Saturated Fat 0g	**Protein** 0g	Sugars 1g

Organic Valley, Unsweetened Soy Milk

1 cup (240 ml)

Amount per serving	Amount per serving	Amount per serving
Calories 80	**Cholesterol** 0mg	**Total Carbohydrate** 3g
Total Fat 4g	**Sodium** 110mg	Dietary Fiber 1g
Saturated Fat 0g	**Protein** 7g	Sugars 1g

Organic Valley, Vanilla Soy Milk

1 cup (240 ml)

Amount per serving	Amount per serving	Amount per serving
Calories 110	**Cholesterol** 0mg	**Total Carbohydrate** 14g
Total Fat 3.5g	**Sodium** 100mg	Dietary Fiber 2g
Saturated Fat 0g	**Protein** 6g	Sugars 10g

Organic Valley, Whipped Butter

1 tbsp (7g)

Amount per serving	Amount per serving	Amount per serving
Calories 50	**Cholesterol** 15mg	**Total Carbohydrate** 0g
Total Fat 6g	**Sodium** 40mg	Dietary Fiber 0g
Saturated Fat 3.5g	**Protein** 0g	Sugars 0g

Pacific, Organic 7 Grain Original Non-Dairy Beverage

1 cup (8 fl oz) 240 ml

Amount per serving	Amount per serving	Amount per serving
Calories 140	**Cholesterol** 0mg	**Total Carbohydrate** 27g
Total Fat 2g	**Sodium** 75mg	Dietary Fiber 1g
Saturated Fat 0g	**Protein** 3g	Sugars 16g

Pacific, Organic 7 Grain Vanilla Non-Dairy Beverage

1 cup (8 fl oz) 240 ml

Amount per serving	Amount per serving	Amount per serving
Calories 140	**Cholesterol** 0mg	**Total Carbohydrate** 28g
Total Fat 2g	**Sodium** 75mg	Dietary Fiber 1g
Saturated Fat 0g	**Protein** 3g	Sugars 16g

Pacific, Organic Almond Chocolate Single Serve 4 Pack Non-Dairy Beverage

1 cup (8 fl oz) 240 ml

Amount per serving	Amount per serving	Amount per serving
Calories 100	**Cholesterol** 0mg	**Total Carbohydrate** 19g
Total Fat 3g	**Sodium** 150mg	Dietary Fiber 1g
Saturated Fat 0g	**Protein** 1g	Sugars 17g

Pacific, Organic Almond Original Non-Dairy Beverage

1 cup (8 fl oz) 240 ml

Amount per serving	Amount per serving	Amount per serving
Calories 60	**Cholesterol** 0mg	**Total Carbohydrate** 8g
Total Fat 3g	**Sodium** 150mg	Dietary Fiber 0g
Saturated Fat 0g	**Protein** 1g	Sugars 7g

Pacific, Organic Almond Vanilla Non-Dairy Beverage

1 cup (8 fl oz) 240 ml

Amount per serving	Amount per serving	Amount per serving
Calories 70	**Cholesterol** 0mg	**Total Carbohydrate** 11g
Total Fat 3g	**Sodium** 150mg	Dietary Fiber 0g
Saturated Fat 0g	**Protein** 1g	Sugars 10g

Pacific, Organic Almond Vanilla Single Serve 4 Pack Non-Dairy Beverage

1 cup (8 fl oz) 240 ml

Amount per serving	Amount per serving	Amount per serving
Calories 70	**Cholesterol** 0mg	**Total Carbohydrate** 11g
Total Fat 3g	**Sodium** 150mg	Dietary Fiber 0g
Saturated Fat 0g	**Protein** 1g	Sugars 10g

Pacific, Organic Oat Original Non-Dairy Beverage

1 cup (8 fl oz) 240 ml

Amount per serving	Amount per serving	Amount per serving
Calories 130	**Cholesterol** 0mg	**Total Carbohydrate** 24g
Total Fat 2.5g	**Sodium** 115mg	Dietary Fiber 2g
Saturated Fat 0g	**Protein** 4g	Sugars 19g

Pacific, Organic Oat Vanilla Non-Dairy Beverage

1 cup (8 fl oz) 240 ml

Amount per serving	Amount per serving	Amount per serving
Calories 130	**Cholesterol** 0mg	**Total Carbohydrate** 25g
Total Fat 2.5g	**Sodium** 110mg	Dietary Fiber 2g
Saturated Fat 0g	**Protein** 4g	Sugars 20g

Pacific, Organic Unsweetened Almond Original Non-Dairy Beverage

1 cup (8 fl oz) 240 ml

Amount per serving	Amount per serving	Amount per serving
Calories 35	**Cholesterol** 0mg	**Total Carbohydrate** 2g
Total Fat 2.5g	**Sodium** 190mg	Dietary Fiber 0g
Saturated Fat 0g	**Protein** 1g	Sugars 0g

Pacific, Organic Unsweetened Almond Vanilla Non-Dairy Beverage

1 cup (8 fl oz) 240 ml

Amount per serving	Amount per serving	Amount per serving
Calories 35	**Cholesterol** 0mg	**Total Carbohydrate** 3g
Total Fat 2.5g	**Sodium** 190mg	Dietary Fiber 0g
Saturated Fat 0g	**Protein** 1g	Sugars 0g

Pacific, Organic Unsweetened Soy Original Non-Dairy Beverage

1 cup (8 fl oz) 240 ml

Amount per serving	Amount per serving	Amount per serving
Calories 90	**Cholesterol** 0mg	**Total Carbohydrate** 4g
Total Fat 4.5g	**Sodium** 85mg	Dietary Fiber 2g
Saturated Fat 0.5g	**Protein** 9g	Sugars 2g

So Delicious® Dairy Free, Cashew Milk Beverages, Cashew Milk Unsweetened

1 cup (240 ml)

Amount per serving	Amount per serving	Amount per serving
Calories 35	**Cholesterol** 0mg	**Total Carbohydrate** 1g
Total Fat 3.5g	**Sodium** 85mg	Dietary Fiber 0g
Saturated Fat 0g	**Protein** 0g	Sugars 0g

So Delicious® Dairy Free, Cashew Milk Beverages, Vanilla Cashew Milk Unsweetened

1 cup (240 ml)

Amount per serving	Amount per serving	Amount per serving
Calories 35	**Cholesterol** 0mg	**Total Carbohydrate** 1g
Total Fat 3.5g	**Sodium** 85mg	Dietary Fiber 0g
Saturated Fat 0g	**Protein** 0g	Sugars 0g

So Delicious® Dairy Free, Coconut Milk Beverages, Chocolate Coconut Milk

1 cup (240 ml)

Amount per serving	Amount per serving	Amount per serving
Calories 100	**Cholesterol** 0mg	**Total Carbohydrate** 12g
Total Fat 5g	**Sodium** 160mg	Dietary Fiber 1g
Saturated Fat 4g	**Protein** 1g	Sugars 10g

So Delicious® Dairy Free, Coconut Milk Beverages, Cococcino Latte

8 oz

Amount per serving	Amount per serving	Amount per serving
Calories 100	**Cholesterol** 0mg	**Total Carbohydrate** 19g
Total Fat 2.5g	**Sodium** 105mg	Dietary Fiber 1g
Saturated Fat 2.5g	**Protein** 1g	Sugars 16g

So Delicious® Dairy Free, Coconut Milk Beverages, Cococcino Latte Single-Serve

1 container

Amount per serving	Amount per serving	Amount per serving
Calories 130	**Cholesterol** 0mg	**Total Carbohydrate** 26g
Total Fat 4g	**Sodium** 150mg	Dietary Fiber 2g
Saturated Fat 3.5g	**Protein** 1g	Sugars 22g

So Delicious® Dairy Free, Coconut Milk Beverages, Cococcino Mocha

8 oz

Amount per serving	Amount per serving	Amount per serving
Calories 110	**Cholesterol** 0mg	**Total Carbohydrate** 21g
Total Fat 3g	**Sodium** 105mg	Dietary Fiber 2g
Saturated Fat 2.5g	**Protein** 1g	Sugars 18g

So Delicious® Dairy Free, Coconut Milk Beverages, Cococcino Mocha Single-Serve

1 container

Amount per serving	Amount per serving	Amount per serving
Calories 130	**Cholesterol** 0mg	**Total Carbohydrate** 30g
Total Fat 4g	**Sodium** 150mg	Dietary Fiber 2g
Saturated Fat 3.5g	**Protein** 2g	Sugars 25g

So Delicious® Dairy Free, Coconut Milk Beverages, Mint Chocolate Coconut Beverage

1/2 cup (120 ml)

Amount per serving	Amount per serving	Amount per serving
Calories 50	**Cholesterol** 0mg	**Total Carbohydrate** 7g
Total Fat 2.5g	**Sodium** 80mg	Dietary Fiber 1g
Saturated Fat 2g	**Protein** 0g	Sugars 6g

So Delicious® Dairy Free, Coconut Milk Beverages, Nog Coconut Beverage

1/2 cup (120 ml)

Amount per serving	Amount per serving	Amount per serving
Calories 90	**Cholesterol** 0mg	**Total Carbohydrate** 15g
Total Fat 3g	**Sodium** 115mg	Dietary Fiber 1g
Saturated Fat 3g	**Protein** 0g	Sugars 14g

So Delicious® Dairy Free, Coconut Milk Beverages, Pumpkin Spice Coconut Beverage

1/2 cup (120 ml)

Amount per serving	Amount per serving	Amount per serving
Calories 70	**Cholesterol** 0mg	**Total Carbohydrate** 15g
Total Fat 1g	**Sodium** 100mg	Dietary Fiber 1g
Saturated Fat 1g	**Protein** 0g	Sugars 14g

So Delicious® Dairy Free, Coconut Milk Beverages, Sugar Free Vanilla Coconut Milk

1 cup (240 ml)

Amount per serving	Amount per serving	Amount per serving
Calories 50	**Cholesterol** 0mg	**Total Carbohydrate** 2g
Total Fat 4.5g	**Sodium** 65mg	Dietary Fiber 1g
Saturated Fat 4g	**Protein** 0g	Sugars 0g

So Delicious® Dairy Free, Coconut Milk Beverages, Unsweetened Coconut Milk

1 cup (240 ml)

Amount per serving	Amount per serving	Amount per serving
Calories 45	**Cholesterol** 0mg	**Total Carbohydrate** 2g
Total Fat 4.5g	**Sodium** 15mg	Dietary Fiber 1g
Saturated Fat 4g	**Protein** 0g	Sugars 1g

So Delicious® Dairy Free, Coconut Milk Beverages, Vanilla Coconut Milk

1 cup (240 ml)

Amount per serving	Amount per serving	Amount per serving
Calories 80	**Cholesterol** 0mg	**Total Carbohydrate** 10g
Total Fat 4.5g	**Sodium** 15mg	Dietary Fiber 1g
Saturated Fat 4g	**Protein** 0g	Sugars 8g

So Delicious® Dairy Free, Coconut Milk, Chocolate Coconut Milk Single-Serve

1 carton (240 ml)

Amount per serving	Amount per serving	Amount per serving
Calories 90	**Cholesterol** 0mg	**Total Carbohydrate** 12g
Total Fat 5g	**Sodium** 160mg	Dietary Fiber 1g
Saturated Fat 4g	**Protein** 1g	Sugars 9g

So Delicious® Dairy Free, Coconut Milk, Sugar Free Original Coconut Milk

1 cup (240 ml)

Amount per serving	Amount per serving	Amount per serving
Calories 45	**Cholesterol** 0mg	**Total Carbohydrate** 2g
Total Fat 4.5g	**Sodium** 65mg	Dietary Fiber 1g
Saturated Fat 4g	**Protein** 0g	Sugars 0g

So Delicious® Dairy Free, Coconut Milk, Unsweetened Vanilla Coconut Milk

1 cup (240 ml)

Amount per serving	Amount per serving	Amount per serving
Calories 45	**Cholesterol** 0mg	**Total Carbohydrate** 2g
Total Fat 4.5g	**Sodium** 15mg	Dietary Fiber 1g
Saturated Fat 4g	**Protein** 0g	Sugars 0g

So Delicious® Dairy Free, Dairy Free Beverages, Original Almond Plus™ 5X

1 cup (240 ml)

Amount per serving	Amount per serving	Amount per serving
Calories 70	**Cholesterol** 0mg	**Total Carbohydrate** 8g
Total Fat 2g	**Sodium** 95mg	Dietary Fiber 0g
Saturated Fat 0g	**Protein** 5g	Sugars 8g

So Delicious® Dairy Free, Dairy Free Beverages, Original Coconut Milk Beverage

1 cup (240 ml)

Amount per serving	Amount per serving	Amount per serving
Calories 70	Cholesterol 0mg	Total Carbohydrate 8g
Total Fat 4.5g	Sodium 15mg	Dietary Fiber 1g
Saturated Fat 4g	Protein 0g	Sugars 7g

So Delicious® Dairy Free, Dairy Free Beverages, Unsweetened Almond Plus™ 5X

1 cup (240 ml)

Amount per serving	Amount per serving	Amount per serving
Calories 40	Cholesterol 0mg	Total Carbohydrate 0g
Total Fat 2g	Sodium 95mg	Dietary Fiber 0g
Saturated Fat 0g	Protein 5g	Sugars 0g

So Delicious® Dairy Free, Dairy Free Beverages, Vanilla Almond Plus™ 5X

1 cup (240 ml)

Amount per serving	Amount per serving	Amount per serving
Calories 70	Cholesterol 0mg	Total Carbohydrate 8g
Total Fat 2g	Sodium 95mg	Dietary Fiber 0g
Saturated Fat 0g	Protein 5g	Sugars 8g

So Delicious® Dairy Free, Vanilla Single-Serve Almond Plus™ 5X

1 cup (240 ml)

Amount per serving	Amount per serving	Amount per serving
Calories 70	Cholesterol 0mg	Total Carbohydrate 8g
Total Fat 2g	Sodium 95mg	Dietary Fiber 0g
Saturated Fat 0g	Protein 5g	Sugars 8g

So Delicious®, French Vanilla Almond Milk "Creamer"

1 tbsp (15 ml)

Amount per serving	Amount per serving	Amount per serving
Calories 15	Cholesterol 0mg	Total Carbohydrate 3g
Total Fat 0g	Sodium 0mg	Dietary Fiber 0g
Saturated Fat 0g	Protein 0g	Sugars 3g

So Delicious®, Original Almond Milk "Creamer"

1 tbsp (15 ml)

Amount per serving	Amount per serving	Amount per serving
Calories 5	Cholesterol 0mg	Total Carbohydrate 1g
Total Fat 0g	Sodium 0mg	Dietary Fiber 0g
Saturated Fat 0g	Protein 0g	Sugars 0g

SOY DREAM®, Dream Blends, Enriched Rice & Quinoa Original Drink

1 cup, 8 fl oz (240 ml)

Amount per serving	Amount per serving	Amount per serving
Calories 90	**Cholesterol** 0mg	**Total Carbohydrate** 16g
Total Fat 3g	**Sodium** 140mg	Dietary Fiber 0g
Saturated Fat 0g	**Protein** <1g	Sugars 7g

SOY DREAM®, Dream Blends, Enriched Rice & Quinoa Original Drink, Unsweetened

1 cup, 8 fl oz (240 ml)

Amount per serving	Amount per serving	Amount per serving
Calories 60	**Cholesterol** 0mg	**Total Carbohydrate** 9g
Total Fat 2.5g	**Sodium** 105mg	Dietary Fiber 0g
Saturated Fat 0g	**Protein** <1g	Sugars <1g

SOY DREAM®, Dream Blends, Sprouted Rice Dream Original Rice Drink

1 cup, 8 fl oz (240 ml)

Amount per serving	Amount per serving	Amount per serving
Calories 120	**Cholesterol** 0mg	**Total Carbohydrate** 23g
Total Fat 2.5g	**Sodium** 100mg	Dietary Fiber 0g
Saturated Fat 0g	**Protein** 1g	Sugars 10g

SOY DREAM®, Dream Blends, Sprouted Rice Dream Rice Drink, Unsweetened

1 cup, 8 fl oz (240 ml)

Amount per serving	Amount per serving	Amount per serving
Calories 70	**Cholesterol** 0mg	**Total Carbohydrate** 11g
Total Fat 2.5g	**Sodium** 110mg	Dietary Fiber 0g
Saturated Fat 0g	**Protein** 0g	Sugars >1g

SOY DREAM®, Refrigerated, Enriched Original Soymilk

1 cup, 8 fl oz (240 ml)

Amount per serving	Amount per serving	Amount per serving
Calories 100	**Cholesterol** 0mg	**Total Carbohydrate** 9g
Total Fat 3.5g	**Sodium** 140mg	Dietary Fiber 2g
Saturated Fat 0.5g	**Protein** 8g	Sugars 5g

SOY DREAM®, Refrigerated, Enriched Vanilla Soymilk

1 cup, 8 fl oz (240 ml)

Amount per serving	Amount per serving	Amount per serving
Calories 120	**Cholesterol** 0mg	**Total Carbohydrate** 14g
Total Fat 3.5g	**Sodium** 130mg	Dietary Fiber 2g
Saturated Fat 0.5g	**Protein** 8g	Sugars 10g

SOY DREAM®, Shelf Stable, Enriched Original Soymilk

1 cup, 8 fl oz (240 ml)

Amount per serving	Amount per serving	Amount per serving
Calories 100	**Cholesterol** 0mg	**Total Carbohydrate** 8g
Total Fat 4g	**Sodium** 135mg	Dietary Fiber 2g
Saturated Fat 0.5g	**Protein** 7g	Sugars 4g

SOY DREAM®, Shelf Stable, Enriched Vanilla Soymilk

1 cup, 8 fl oz (240 ml)

Amount per serving	Amount per serving	Amount per serving
Calories 120	**Cholesterol** 0mg	**Total Carbohydrate** 14g
Total Fat 4g	**Sodium** 135mg	Dietary Fiber 2g
Saturated Fat 0.5g	**Protein** 7g	Sugars 10g

SOY DREAM®, Shelf Stable, Original Classic Soymilk

8 fl oz (240 ml)

Amount per serving	Amount per serving	Amount per serving
Calories 130	**Cholesterol** 0mg	**Total Carbohydrate** 16g
Total Fat 4g	**Sodium** 135mg	Dietary Fiber 2g
Saturated Fat 0.5g	**Protein** 7g	Sugars 10g

SOY DREAM®, Shelf Stable, Rice Dream Original Classic Rice Drink

1 cup, 8 fl oz (240 ml)

Amount per serving	Amount per serving	Amount per serving
Calories 120	**Cholesterol** 0mg	**Total Carbohydrate** 24g
Total Fat 2.5g	**Sodium** 100mg	Dietary Fiber 0g
Saturated Fat 0g	**Protein** 1g	Sugars 11g

SOY DREAM®, Shelf Stable, Rice Dream Original Enriched Rice Drink

1 cup, 8 fl oz (240 ml)

Amount per serving	Amount per serving	Amount per serving
Calories 120	**Cholesterol** 0mg	**Total Carbohydrate** 23g
Total Fat 2.5g	**Sodium** 100mg	Dietary Fiber 0g
Saturated Fat 0g	**Protein** 1g	Sugars 10g

SOY DREAM®, Shelf Stable, Rice Dream Original Enriched Unsweetened Rice Drink

1 cup, 8 fl oz (240 ml)

Amount per serving	Amount per serving	Amount per serving
Calories 70	**Cholesterol** 0mg	**Total Carbohydrate** 11g
Total Fat 2.5g	**Sodium** 110mg	Dietary Fiber 0g
Saturated Fat 0g	**Protein** 0g	Sugars <1g

SOY DREAM®, Shelf Stable, Vanilla Classic Soymilk

1 cup, 8 fl oz (240 ml)

Amount per serving	Amount per serving	Amount per serving
Calories 140	**Cholesterol** 0mg	**Total Carbohydrate** 18g
Total Fat 4g	**Sodium** 135mg	Dietary Fiber 2g
Saturated Fat 0.5g	**Protein** 7g	Sugars 10g

Thai Kitchen, Organic Lite Coconut Milk

1/3 cup

Amount per serving	Amount per serving	Amount per serving
Calories 50	**Cholesterol** 0mg	**Total Carbohydrate** 1g
Total Fat 5g	**Sodium** 5mg	Dietary Fiber 0g
Saturated Fat 4g	**Protein** 0g	Sugars 0g

WESTSOY®, Organic Original Soymilk

1 cup / 8 fl oz

Amount per serving	Amount per serving	Amount per serving
Calories 130	**Cholesterol** 0mg	**Total Carbohydrate** 18g
Total Fat 3.5g	**Sodium** 125mg	Dietary Fiber 3g
Saturated Fat 0.5g	**Protein** 8g	Sugars 12g

WESTSOY®, Organic Soymilk Plus Plain

1 cup / 8 fl oz

Amount per serving	Amount per serving	Amount per serving
Calories 110	**Cholesterol** 0mg	**Total Carbohydrate** 11g
Total Fat 4.5g	**Sodium** 125mg	Dietary Fiber 1g
Saturated Fat 0.5g	**Protein** 8g	Sugars 10g

WESTSOY®, Organic Soymilk Plus Vanilla

1 cup / 8 fl oz

Amount per serving	Amount per serving	Amount per serving
Calories 110	**Cholesterol** 0mg	**Total Carbohydrate** 11g
Total Fat 4.5g	**Sodium** 125mg	Dietary Fiber 1g
Saturated Fat 0.5g	**Protein** 8g	Sugars 10g

WESTSOY®, Organic Unsweetened Soymilk

1 cup / 8 fl oz

Amount per serving	Amount per serving	Amount per serving
Calories 90	**Cholesterol** 0mg	**Total Carbohydrate** 5g
Total Fat 4.5g	**Sodium** 30mg	Dietary Fiber 4g
Saturated Fat 0.5g	**Protein** 9g	Sugars 1g

WESTSOY®, Organic Unsweetened Vanilla Soymilk

1 cup / 8 fl oz

Amount per serving	Amount per serving	Amount per serving
Calories 100	**Cholesterol** 0mg	**Total Carbohydrate** 5g
Total Fat 4.5g	**Sodium** 30mg	Dietary Fiber 4g
Saturated Fat 0.5g	**Protein** 9g	Sugars 1g

Wildwood Organic, Organic Original Soy Creamer

1 tbsp (15 ml)

Amount per serving	Amount per serving	Amount per serving
Calories 15	**Cholesterol** 0mg	**Total Carbohydrate** 1g
Total Fat 1.5g	**Sodium** 0mg	Dietary Fiber 0g
Saturated Fat 0g	**Protein** 0g	Sugars 1g

Wildwood Organic, Organic Original Soymilk

8 fl oz (240 ml)

Amount per serving	Amount per serving	Amount per serving
Calories 90	**Cholesterol** 0mg	**Total Carbohydrate** 7g
Total Fat 3.5g	**Sodium** 70mg	Dietary Fiber 1g
Saturated Fat 0.5g	**Protein** 7g	Sugars 6g

Wildwood Organic, Organic Vanilla Soymilk

8 fl oz (240 ml)

Amount per serving	Amount per serving	Amount per serving
Calories 90	**Cholesterol** 0mg	**Total Carbohydrate** 8g
Total Fat 3.5g	**Sodium** 70mg	Dietary Fiber 1g
Saturated Fat 0.5g	**Protein** 7g	Sugars 7g

Wildwood Organic, Unsweetened Soymilk

8 fl oz (240 ml)

Amount per serving	Amount per serving	Amount per serving
Calories 70	**Cholesterol** 0mg	**Total Carbohydrate** 3g
Total Fat 3.5g	**Sodium** 70mg	Dietary Fiber 1g
Saturated Fat 0.5g	**Protein** 7g	Sugars 2g

ZenSoy, Half Gallon, Cappuccino Soymilk

1 cup (240 ml)

Amount per serving	Amount per serving	Amount per serving
Calories 150	**Cholesterol** 0mg	**Total Carbohydrate** 22g
Total Fat 3.5g	**Sodium** 160mg	Dietary Fiber 1g
Saturated Fat 1g	**Protein** 7g	Sugars 17g

ZenSoy, Half Gallon, Chocolate Soymilk

1 cup (240 ml)

Amount per serving	Amount per serving	Amount per serving
Calories 170	**Cholesterol** 0mg	**Total Carbohydrate** 27g
Total Fat 4g	**Sodium** 160mg	Dietary Fiber 2g
Saturated Fat 1g	**Protein** 7g	Sugars 160g

ZenSoy, Half Gallon, Plain Soymilk

1 cup (240 ml)

Amount per serving	Amount per serving	Amount per serving
Calories 110	**Cholesterol** 0mg	**Total Carbohydrate** 14g
Total Fat 3.5g	**Sodium** 80mg	Dietary Fiber 1g
Saturated Fat 1g	**Protein** 7g	Sugars 12g

ZenSoy, Half Gallon, Vanilla Soymilk

1 cup (240 ml)

Amount per serving	Amount per serving	Amount per serving
Calories 110	**Cholesterol** 0mg	**Total Carbohydrate** 14g
Total Fat 3.5g	**Sodium** 80mg	Dietary Fiber 1g
Saturated Fat 1g	**Protein** 7g	Sugars 12g

ZenSoy, Soy on the Go (8.25 oz), Cappuccino Soymilk

8.25 fl oz (244 ml)

Amount per serving	Amount per serving	Amount per serving
Calories 150	**Cholesterol** 0mg	**Total Carbohydrate** 22g
Total Fat 3.5g	**Sodium** 160mg	Dietary Fiber 1g
Saturated Fat 1g	**Protein** 7g	Sugars 17g

ZenSoy, Soy on the Go (8.25 oz), Chocolate Soymilk

8.25 fl oz (244 ml)

Amount per serving	Amount per serving	Amount per serving
Calories 170	**Cholesterol** 0mg	**Total Carbohydrate** 27g
Total Fat 4g	**Sodium** 160mg	Dietary Fiber 2g
Saturated Fat 1g	**Protein** 7g	Sugars 23g

ZenSoy, Soy on the Go (8.25 oz), Vanilla Soymilk

8.25 fl oz (244 ml)

Amount per serving	Amount per serving	Amount per serving
Calories 110	**Cholesterol** 0mg	**Total Carbohydrate** 14g
Total Fat 3.5g	**Sodium** 80mg	Dietary Fiber 1g
Saturated Fat 1g	**Protein** 7g	Sugars 12g

Dairy-based Desserts

Let's Do...Organic, Organic Tapioca Granules

1 tbsp (6g)

Amount per serving	Amount per serving	Amount per serving
Calories 20	**Cholesterol** 0mg	**Total Carbohydrate** 6g
Total Fat 0g	**Sodium** 0mg	Dietary Fiber 0g
Saturated Fat 0g	**Protein** 0g	Sugars 0g

Let's Do...Organic, Organic Tapioca Pearls

1 tbsp (13g)

Amount per serving	Amount per serving	Amount per serving
Calories 35	**Cholesterol** 0mg	**Total Carbohydrate** 9g
Total Fat 0g	**Sodium** 0mg	Dietary Fiber 0g
Saturated Fat 0g	**Protein** 0g	Sugars 0g

Let's Do...Organic, Organic Tapioca Starch

1 tbsp (8g)

Amount per serving	Amount per serving	Amount per serving
Calories 30	**Cholesterol** 0mg	**Total Carbohydrate** 7g
Total Fat 0g	**Sodium** 0mg	Dietary Fiber 0g
Saturated Fat 0g	**Protein** 0g	Sugars 0g

Eggs

Horizon®, Organic Egg Whites

3 tbsp (46g)

Amount per serving	Amount per serving	Amount per serving
Calories 25	**Cholesterol** 0mg	**Total Carbohydrate** 0g
Total Fat 0g	**Sodium** 75mg	Dietary Fiber 0g
Saturated Fat 0g	**Protein** 5g	Sugars 0g

Horizon®, Organic Extra Large Eggs

1 egg (56g)

Amount per serving	Amount per serving	Amount per serving
Calories 80	**Cholesterol** 240mg	**Total Carbohydrate** <1g
Total Fat 5g	**Sodium** 70mg	Dietary Fiber NA
Saturated Fat 1.5g	**Protein** 7g	Sugars NA

Horizon®, Organic Large Eggs

1 egg (50g)

Amount per serving	Amount per serving	Amount per serving
Calories 70	**Cholesterol** 215mg	**Total Carbohydrate** <1g
Total Fat 4.5g	**Sodium** 65mg	Dietary Fiber NA
Saturated Fat 1.5g	**Protein** 6g	Sugars NA

Horizon®, Organic Omega-3 Eggs

1 egg (50g)

Amount per serving	Amount per serving	Amount per serving
Calories 70	**Cholesterol** 215mg	**Total Carbohydrate** <1g
Total Fat 4.5g	**Sodium** 65mg	Dietary Fiber NA
Saturated Fat 1.5g	**Protein** 6g	Sugars NA

Land O'Lakes, Organic All-Natural Eggs

1 large egg (50g)

Amount per serving	Amount per serving	Amount per serving
Calories 70	**Cholesterol** 185mg	**Total Carbohydrate** 0g
Total Fat 5g	**Sodium** 70mg	Dietary Fiber 0g
Saturated Fat 1.5g	**Protein** 6g	Sugars 0g

Organic Valley, California Organic Large Brown Eggs

1 egg (50g)

Amount per serving	Amount per serving	Amount per serving
Calories 60	**Cholesterol** 210mg	**Total Carbohydrate** <1g
Total Fat 4g	**Sodium** 70mg	Dietary Fiber 0g
Saturated Fat 1.5g	**Protein** 6g	Sugars 0g

Organic Valley, Omega-3 Organic Large Brown Eggs

1 egg (50g)

Amount per serving	Amount per serving	Amount per serving
Calories 60	**Cholesterol** 210mg	**Total Carbohydrate** <1g
Total Fat 4g	**Sodium** 70mg	Dietary Fiber 0g
Saturated Fat 1.5g	**Protein** 6g	Sugars 0g

Organic Valley, Organic California Extra-Large Brown Eggs

1 egg (58g)

Amount per serving	Amount per serving	Amount per serving
Calories 70	**Cholesterol** 245mg	**Total Carbohydrate** <1g
Total Fat 4.5g	**Sodium** 80mg	Dietary Fiber 0g
Saturated Fat 1.5g	**Protein** 7g	Sugars 0g

Organic Valley, Organic California Extra-Large, Omega-3 Eggs

1 egg (58g)

Amount per serving	Amount per serving	Amount per serving
Calories 70	**Cholesterol** 245mg	**Total Carbohydrate** <1g
Total Fat 4.5g	**Sodium** 80mg	Dietary Fiber 0g
Saturated Fat 1.5g	**Protein** 7g	Sugars 0g

Organic Valley, Organic California Large Brown Eggs

1 egg (50g)

Amount per serving	Amount per serving	Amount per serving
Calories 60	**Cholesterol** 210mg	**Total Carbohydrate** <1g
Total Fat 4g	**Sodium** 70mg	Dietary Fiber 0g
Saturated Fat 1.5g	**Protein** 6g	Sugars 0g

Organic Valley, Organic Egg Whites, Pasteurized

1/4 cup (60g)

Amount per serving	Amount per serving	Amount per serving
Calories 25	**Cholesterol** 0mg	**Total Carbohydrate** 1g
Total Fat 0g	**Sodium** 95mg	Dietary Fiber 0g
Saturated Fat 0g	**Protein** 6g	Sugars 0g

Organic Valley, Organic Extra-Large Brown Eggs

1 egg (58g)

Amount per serving	Amount per serving	Amount per serving
Calories 70	**Cholesterol** 245mg	**Total Carbohydrate** <1g
Total Fat 4.5g	**Sodium** 80mg	Dietary Fiber 0g
Saturated Fat 1.5g	**Protein** 7g	Sugars 0g

Organic Valley, Organic Large Brown Eggs

1 egg (50g)

Amount per serving	Amount per serving	Amount per serving
Calories 60	**Cholesterol** 210mg	**Total Carbohydrate** <1g
Total Fat 4g	**Sodium** 70mg	Dietary Fiber 0g
Saturated Fat 1.5g	**Protein** 6g	Sugars 0g

Organic Valley, Organic Medium Brown Eggs

1 egg (44g)

Amount per serving	Amount per serving	Amount per serving
Calories 50	**Cholesterol** 185mg	**Total Carbohydrate** <1g
Total Fat 3.5g	**Sodium** 60mg	Dietary Fiber 0g
Saturated Fat 1g	**Protein** 6g	Sugars 0g

Organic Valley, Organic Omega-3 Extra Large Eggs

1 egg (58g)

Amount per serving	Amount per serving	Amount per serving
Calories 70	**Cholesterol** 245mg	**Total Carbohydrate** <1g
Total Fat 4.5g	**Sodium** 80mg	Dietary Fiber 0g
Saturated Fat 1.5g	**Protein** 7g	Sugars 0g

Frozen Desserts

Good Karma, Organic, Rice Divine, Banana Fudge Non-Dairy Frozen Dessert

1/2 cup

Amount per serving	Amount per serving	Amount per serving
Calories 150	**Cholesterol** 0mg	**Total Carbohydrate** 25g
Total Fat 6g	**Sodium** 85mg	Dietary Fiber 1g
Saturated Fat 0g	**Protein** 0g	Sugars 16g

Good Karma, Organic, Rice Divine, Carrot Cake Non-Dairy Frozen Dessert

1/2 cup

Amount per serving	Amount per serving	Amount per serving
Calories 160	**Cholesterol** 0mg	**Total Carbohydrate** 25g
Total Fat 7g	**Sodium** 105mg	Dietary Fiber 1g
Saturated Fat 1g	**Protein** 0g	Sugars 15g

Good Karma, Organic, Rioc Divine, Chocolate Chip Non-Dairy Frozen Dessert

1/2 cup

Amount per serving	Amount per serving	Amount per serving
Calories 170	**Cholesterol** 0mg	**Total Carbohydrate** 23g
Total Fat 9g	**Sodium** 60mg	Dietary Fiber 2g
Saturated Fat 3g	**Protein** 0g	Sugars 13g

Good Karma, Organic, Rice Divine, Coconut Mango Non-Dairy Frozen Dessert

1/2 cup

Amount per serving	Amount per serving	Amount per serving
Calories 150	**Cholesterol** 0mg	**Total Carbohydrate** 23g
Total Fat 6g	**Sodium** 75mg	Dietary Fiber 1g
Saturated Fat 1g	**Protein** 0g	Sugars 14g

Good Karma, Organic, Rice Divine, Key Lime Pie Non-Dairy Frozen Dessert

1/2 cup

Amount per serving	Amount per serving	Amount per serving
Calories 140	**Cholesterol** 0mg	**Total Carbohydrate** 23g
Total Fat 6g	**Sodium** 55mg	Dietary Fiber 1g
Saturated Fat 0g	**Protein** 0g	Sugars 13g

Good Karma, Organic, Rice Divine, Mint Chocolate Swirl Non-Dairy Frozen Dessert

1/2 cup

Amount per serving	Amount per serving	Amount per serving
Calories 150	**Cholesterol** 0mg	**Total Carbohydrate** 24g
Total Fat 6g	**Sodium** 80mg	Dietary Fiber 1g
Saturated Fat 0.5g	**Protein** 0g	Sugars 15g

Good Karma, Organic, Rice Divine, Mudd Pie Non-Dairy Frozen Dessert

1/2 cup

Amount per serving	Amount per serving	Amount per serving
Calories 170	**Cholesterol** 0mg	**Total Carbohydrate** 26g
Total Fat 8g	**Sodium** 85mg	Dietary Fiber 2g
Saturated Fat 1g	**Protein** 1g	Sugars 15g

Good Karma, Organic, Rice Divine, Non-Dairy Chocolate Chocolate Bars

1 bar

Amount per serving	Amount per serving	Amount per serving
Calories 200	**Cholesterol** 0mg	**Total Carbohydrate** 22g
Total Fat 13g	**Sodium** 55mg	Dietary Fiber 1g
Saturated Fat 7g	**Protein** 0g	Sugars 12g

Good Karma, Organic, Rice Divine, Non-Dairy Chocolate Peanut Butter Fudge

1/2 cup

Amount per serving	Amount per serving	Amount per serving
Calories 200	**Cholesterol** 0mg	**Total Carbohydrate** 27g
Total Fat 10g	**Sodium** 120mg	Dietary Fiber 2g
Saturated Fat 1g	**Protein** 1g	Sugars 16g

Good Karma, Organic, Rice Divine, Very Cherry Non-Dairy Frozen Dessert

1/2 cup

Amount per serving	Amount per serving	Amount per serving
Calories 160	**Cholesterol** 0mg	**Total Carbohydrate** 26g
Total Fat 6g	**Sodium** 55mg	Dietary Fiber 1g
Saturated Fat 0g	**Protein** 0g	Sugars 17g

Good Karma, Organic, Rice Divine, Very Vanilla Bars Non-Dairy Frozen Dessert

1 bar

Amount per serving	Amount per serving	Amount per serving
Calories 200	**Cholesterol** 0mg	**Total Carbohydrate** 21g
Total Fat 13g	**Sodium** 55mg	Dietary Fiber 1g
Saturated Fat 7g	**Protein** 0g	Sugars 13g

Good Karma, Organic, Rice Divine, Very Vanilla Non-Dairy Frozen Dessert

1/2 cup

Amount per serving	Amount per serving	Amount per serving
Calories 150	**Cholesterol** 0mg	**Total Carbohydrate** 22g
Total Fat 7g	**Sodium** 75mg	Dietary Fiber 1g
Saturated Fat 0.5g	**Protein** 0g	Sugars 12g

Julie's, Organic Blackberry Frozen Yogurt, Pint

1/2 cup (90g)

Amount per serving	Amount per serving	Amount per serving
Calories 140	**Cholesterol** 10mg	**Total Carbohydrate** 27g
Total Fat 2.5g	**Sodium** 50mg	Dietary Fiber 2g
Saturated Fat 1.5g	**Protein** 3g	Sugars 20g

Julie's, Organic Blackberry Ice Cream & Dark Chocolate Single Bar (12/Pack)

1 bar (81g)

Amount per serving	Amount per serving	Amount per serving
Calories 250	**Cholesterol** 45mg	**Total Carbohydrate** 22g
Total Fat 17g	**Sodium** 30mg	Dietary Fiber 0g
Saturated Fat 10g	**Protein** 3g	Sugars 15g

Julie's, Organic Blackberry Ice Cream, Pint

1/2 cup (96g)

Amount per serving	Amount per serving	Amount per serving
Calories 210	**Cholesterol** 70mg	**Total Carbohydrate** 23g
Total Fat 13g	**Sodium** 45mg	Dietary Fiber <1g
Saturated Fat 8g	**Protein** 3g	Sugars 21g

Julie's, Organic Blackberry Sorbet Bars (4/Pack)

1 bar (54g)

Amount per serving	Amount per serving	Amount per serving
Calories 60	**Cholesterol** 0mg	**Total Carbohydrate** 16g
Total Fat 0g	**Sodium** 20mg	Dietary Fiber <1g
Saturated Fat 0g	**Protein** 0g	Sugars 14g

Julie's, Organic Blackberry Sorbet Single Bar (12/Pack)

1 bar (54g)

Amount per serving	Amount per serving	Amount per serving
Calories 60	**Cholesterol** 0mg	**Total Carbohydrate** 16g
Total Fat 0g	**Sodium** 20mg	Dietary Fiber <1g
Saturated Fat 0g	**Protein** 0g	Sugars 14g

Julie's, Organic Blackberry Sorbet, Pint

1/2 cup (96g)

Amount per serving	Amount per serving	Amount per serving
Calories 110	**Cholesterol** 0mg	**Total Carbohydrate** 28g
Total Fat 0g	**Sodium** 35mg	Dietary Fiber 1g
Saturated Fat 0g	**Protein** 0g	Sugars 26g

Julie's, Organic Blueberry Frozen Yogurt, Pint

1/2 cup (90g)

Amount per serving	Amount per serving	Amount per serving
Calories 140	**Cholesterol** 10mg	**Total Carbohydrate** 27g
Total Fat 2.5g	**Sodium** 50mg	Dietary Fiber 2g
Saturated Fat 1.5g	**Protein** 3g	Sugars 19g

Julie's, Organic Caramel Sorbet, Pint

1/2 cup (96g)

Amount per serving	Amount per serving	Amount per serving
Calories 230	**Cholesterol** 75mg	**Total Carbohydrate** 24g
Total Fat 14g	**Sodium** 85mg	Dietary Fiber 0g
Saturated Fat 8g	**Protein** 4g	Sugars 23g

Julie's, Organic Chocolate Frozen Yogurt, Pint

1/2 cup (90g)

Amount per serving	Amount per serving	Amount per serving
Calories 130	**Cholesterol** 10mg	**Total Carbohydrate** 25g
Total Fat 3g	**Sodium** 75mg	Dietary Fiber 3g
Saturated Fat 2g	**Protein** 4g	Sugars 17g

Julie's, Organic Chocolate Ice Cream & Dark Chocolate Single Bar (12/Pack)

1 bar (81g)

Amount per serving	Amount per serving	Amount per serving
Calories 270	**Cholesterol** 55mg	**Total Carbohydrate** 24g
Total Fat 18g	**Sodium** 35mg	Dietary Fiber 0g
Saturated Fat 11g	**Protein** 4g	Sugars 17g

Julie's, Organic Chocolate Ice Cream Sandwiches (6/Pack)

1 sandwich (60g)

Amount per serving	Amount per serving	Amount per serving
Calories 140	**Cholesterol** 30mg	**Total Carbohydrate** 20g
Total Fat 7g	**Sodium** 115mg	Dietary Fiber 1g
Saturated Fat 4.5g	**Protein** 3g	Sugars 10g

Julie's, Organic Chocolate Ice Cream, Pint

1/2 cup (96g)

Amount per serving	Amount per serving	Amount per serving
Calories 220	**Cholesterol** 70mg	**Total Carbohydrate** 23g
Total Fat 13g	**Sodium** 75mg	Dietary Fiber 2g
Saturated Fat 8g	**Protein** 4g	Sugars 20g

Julie's, Organic Chocolate Ice Cream, Quart

1/2 cup (92g)

Amount per serving	Amount per serving	Amount per serving
Calories 210	**Cholesterol** 65mg	**Total Carbohydrate** 22g
Total Fat 12g	**Sodium** 70mg	Dietary Fiber 1g
Saturated Fat 8g	**Protein** 4g	Sugars 19g

Julie's, Organic Cinnamon Apple Frozen Yogurt, Pint

1/2 cup (90g)

Amount per serving	Amount per serving	Amount per serving
Calories 140	**Cholesterol** 10mg	**Total Carbohydrate** 27g
Total Fat 2.5g	**Sodium** 50mg	Dietary Fiber 2g
Saturated Fat 1.5g	**Protein** 3g	Sugars 19g

Julie's, Organic Coconut Pineapple Frozen Yogurt, Pint

1/2 cup (90g)

Amount per serving	Amount per serving	Amount per serving
Calories 130	**Cholesterol** 10mg	**Total Carbohydrate** 26g
Total Fat 3g	**Sodium** 55mg	Dietary Fiber 2g
Saturated Fat 1.5g	**Protein** 3g	Sugars 18g

Julie's, Organic Coffee Ice Cream & Dark Chocolate Single Bar (12/Pack)

1 bar (81g)

Amount per serving	Amount per serving	Amount per serving
Calories 260	**Cholesterol** 55mg	**Total Carbohydrate** 22g
Total Fat 18g	**Sodium** 35mg	Dietary Fiber 0g
Saturated Fat 11g	**Protein** 3g	Sugars 15g

Julie's, Organic Cookies & Cream Ice Cream, Pint

1/2 cup (96g)

Amount per serving	Amount per serving	Amount per serving
Calories 240	**Cholesterol** 75mg	**Total Carbohydrate** 24g
Total Fat 15g	**Sodium** 100mg	Dietary Fiber 0g
Saturated Fat 8g	**Protein** 1g	Sugars 20g

Julie's, Organic Lemon Frozen Yogurt, Pint

1/2 cup (90g)

Amount per serving	Amount per serving	Amount per serving
Calories 130	**Cholesterol** 10mg	**Total Carbohydrate** 24g
Total Fat 3g	**Sodium** 55mg	Dietary Fiber 2g
Saturated Fat 2g	**Protein** 4g	Sugars 17g

Julie's, Organic Lemon Sorbet Bars (4/Pack)

1 bar (55g)

Amount per serving	Amount per serving	Amount per serving
Calories 60	**Cholesterol** 0mg	**Total Carbohydrate** 16g
Total Fat 0g	**Sodium** 30mg	Dietary Fiber 0g
Saturated Fat 0g	**Protein** 0g	Sugars 15g

Julie's, Organic Mandarin Sorbet & Cream, Pint

1/2 cup (96g)

Amount per serving	Amount per serving	Amount per serving
Calories 160	**Cholesterol** 35mg	**Total Carbohydrate** 25g
Total Fat 6g	**Sodium** 45mg	Dietary Fiber 0g
Saturated Fat 3.5g	**Protein** 4g	Sugars 24g

Julie's, Organic Mandarin Sorbet Bars (4/Pack)

1 Bar (54g)

Amount per serving	Amount per serving	Amount per serving
Calories 60	**Cholesterol** 0mg	**Total Carbohydrate** 19g
Total Fat 0g	**Sodium** 30mg	Dietary Fiber 0g
Saturated Fat 0g	**Protein** 0g	Sugars 15g

Julie's, Organic Mango Passion Sorbet Bars (4/Pack)

1 bar (55g)

Amount per serving	Amount per serving	Amount per serving
Calories 60	**Cholesterol** 0mg	**Total Carbohydrate** 15g
Total Fat 0g	**Sodium** 25mg	Dietary Fiber 0g
Saturated Fat 0g	**Protein** 0g	Sugars 13g

Julie's, Organic Mango Passion Sorbet Single Bar (12/Pack)

1 bar (55g)

Amount per serving	Amount per serving	Amount per serving
Calories 60	**Cholesterol** 0mg	**Total Carbohydrate** 15g
Total Fat 0g	**Sodium** 25mg	Dietary Fiber 0g
Saturated Fat 0g	**Protein** 0g	Sugars 13g

Julie's, Organic Mango Passion Sorbet, Pint

1/2 cup (96g)

Amount per serving	Amount per serving	Amount per serving
Calories 100	**Cholesterol** 0mg	**Total Carbohydrate** 27g
Total Fat 0g	**Sodium** 35mg	Dietary Fiber <1g
Saturated Fat 0g	**Protein** 0g	Sugars 24g

Julie's, Organic Mint Fudge Ice Cream, Pint

1/2 cup (96g)

Amount per serving	Amount per serving	Amount per serving
Calories 220	**Cholesterol** 75mg	**Total Carbohydrate** 24g
Total Fat 13g	**Sodium** 60mg	Dietary Fiber 0g
Saturated Fat 8g	**Protein** 3g	Sugars 22g

Julie's, Organic Mocha Java Ice Cream, Pint

1/2 cup (96g)

Amount per serving	Amount per serving	Amount per serving
Calories 220	**Cholesterol** 75mg	**Total Carbohydrate** 24g
Total Fat 13g	**Sodium** 60mg	Dietary Fiber 0g
Saturated Fat 8g	**Protein** 4g	Sugars 22g

Julie's, Organic Peanut Butter Fudge Ice Cream, Pint

1/2 cup (90g)

Amount per serving	Amount per serving	Amount per serving
Calories 260	**Cholesterol** 70mg	**Total Carbohydrate** 24g
Total Fat 17g	**Sodium** 125mg	Dietary Fiber <1g
Saturated Fat 8g	**Protein** 4g	Sugars 22g

Julie's, Organic Petite Juliette (Vanilla) Sandwiches (8/Pack)

1 sandwich (40g)

Amount per serving	Amount per serving	Amount per serving
Calories 100	**Cholesterol** 25mg	**Total Carbohydrate** 12g
Total Fat 5g	**Sodium** 70mg	Dietary Fiber 0g
Saturated Fat 3g	**Protein** 2g	Sugars 6g

Julie's, Organic Raspberry Truffle Sorbet, Pint

1/2 cup (96g)

Amount per serving	Amount per serving	Amount per serving
Calories 250	**Cholesterol** 70mg	**Total Carbohydrate** 24g
Total Fat 16g	**Sodium** 45mg	Dietary Fiber <1g
Saturated Fat 9g	**Protein** 3g	Sugars 22g

Julie's, Organic Strawberry Lowfat Frozen Yogurt Single Bar (12/Pack)

1 bar (63g)

Amount per serving	Amount per serving	Amount per serving
Calories 100	**Cholesterol** 10mg	**Total Carbohydrate** 20g
Total Fat 2g	**Sodium** 35mg	Dietary Fiber 3g
Saturated Fat 1g	**Protein** 2g	Sugars 14g

Julie's, Organic Strawberry Sorbet & Cream, Pint

1/2 cup (96g)

Amount per serving	Amount per serving	Amount per serving
Calories 160	**Cholesterol** 35mg	**Total Carbohydrate** 26g
Total Fat 6g	**Sodium** 45mg	Dietary Fiber 0g
Saturated Fat 3.5g	**Protein** 2g	Sugars 24g

Julie's, Organic Strawberry Sorbet, Pint

1/2 cup (96g)

Amount per serving	Amount per serving	Amount per serving
Calories 210	**Cholesterol** 75mg	**Total Carbohydrate** 22g
Total Fat 13g	**Sodium** 50mg	Dietary Fiber 0g
Saturated Fat 8g	**Protein** 3g	Sugars 21g

Julie's, Organic Vanilla Bean Frozen Yogurt, Pint

1/2 cup (90g)

Amount per serving	Amount per serving	Amount per serving
Calories 140	**Cholesterol** 10mg	**Total Carbohydrate** 25g
Total Fat 3g	**Sodium** 60mg	Dietary Fiber 2g
Saturated Fat 2g	**Protein** 4g	Sugars 17g

Julie's, Organic Vanilla Ice Cream & Dark Chocolate Single Bar (12/Pack)

1 bar (81g)

Amount per serving	Amount per serving	Amount per serving
Calories 260	**Cholesterol** 55mg	**Total Carbohydrate** 22g
Total Fat 18g	**Sodium** 35mg	Dietary Fiber 0g
Saturated Fat 11g	**Protein** 3g	Sugars 17g

Julie's, Organic Vanilla Ice Cream Sandwich (Single) (24/Pack)

1 sandwich (80g)

Amount per serving	Amount per serving	Amount per serving
Calories 200	**Cholesterol** 55mg	**Total Carbohydrate** 23g
Total Fat 11g	**Sodium** 115mg	Dietary Fiber 0g
Saturated Fat 7g	**Protein** 4g	Sugars 13g

Julie's, Organic Vanilla Ice Cream Sandwich Single (12/Pack)

1 sandwich (80g)

Amount per serving	Amount per serving	Amount per serving
Calories 200	**Cholesterol** 55mg	**Total Carbohydrate** 23g
Total Fat 11g	**Sodium** 115mg	Dietary Fiber 0g
Saturated Fat 7g	**Protein** 4g	Sugars 13g

Julie's, Organic Vanilla Ice Cream, Pint

1/2 cup (96g)

Amount per serving	Amount per serving	Amount per serving
Calories 220	**Cholesterol** 85mg	**Total Carbohydrate** 20g
Total Fat 15g	**Sodium** 55mg	Dietary Fiber 0g
Saturated Fat 9g	**Protein** 4g	Sugars 18g

Julie's, Organic Vanilla Ice Cream, Quart

1/2 cup (92g)

Amount per serving	Amount per serving	Amount per serving
Calories 210	**Cholesterol** 80mg	**Total Carbohydrate** 19g
Total Fat 14g	**Sodium** 50mg	Dietary Fiber 0g
Saturated Fat 8g	**Protein** 4g	Sugars 18g

SOY DREAM®, Butter Pecan Frozen Dessert

1/2 cup (70g)

Amount per serving	Amount per serving	Amount per serving
Calories 190	**Cholesterol** 0mg	**Total Carbohydrate** 23g
Total Fat 11g	**Sodium** 140mg	Dietary Fiber 1g
Saturated Fat 2g	**Protein** 1g	Sugars 14g

SOY DREAM®, French Vanilla Frozen Dessert

1/2 cup (70g)

Amount per serving	Amount per serving	Amount per serving
Calories 170	**Cholesterol** 0mg	**Total Carbohydrate** 21g
Total Fat 9g	**Sodium** 150mg	Dietary Fiber <1g
Saturated Fat 1.5g	**Protein** 1g	Sugars 13g

SOY DREAM®, Vanilla Fudge Frozen Dessert

1/2 cup (70g)

Amount per serving	Amount per serving	Amount per serving
Calories 170	**Cholesterol** 0mg	**Total Carbohydrate** 23g
Total Fat 9g	**Sodium** 150mg	Dietary Fiber 1g
Saturated Fat 1.5g	**Protein** <1g	Sugars 16g

Stonyfield Organic, After Dark, Chocolate Frozen Nonfat Yogurt

1/2 cup (85g)

Amount per serving	Amount per serving	Amount per serving
Calories 100	**Cholesterol** <5mg	**Total Carbohydrate** 21g
Total Fat 0g	**Sodium** 55mg	Dietary Fiber 1g
Saturated Fat 0g	**Protein** 4g	Sugars 18g

Stonyfield Organic, After Dark, Chocolate Frozen Nonfat Yogurt Bar

1 bar (70g)

Amount per serving	Amount per serving	Amount per serving
Calories 170	**Cholesterol** 0mg	**Total Carbohydrate** 21g
Total Fat 8g	**Sodium** 35mg	Dietary Fiber 1g
Saturated Fat 7g	**Protein** 3g	Sugars 18g

Stonyfield Organic, Crème Caramel Frozen Nonfat Yogurt

1/2 cup (85g)

Amount per serving	Amount per serving	Amount per serving
Calories 130	**Cholesterol** 5mg	**Total Carbohydrate** 26g
Total Fat 1.5g	**Sodium** 95mg	Dietary Fiber 0g
Saturated Fat 1g	**Protein** 4g	Sugars 25g

Stonyfield Organic, Frozen Yogurt Pearls Cocount-Chocolate

2 pearls (46g)

Amount per serving	Amount per serving	Amount per serving
Calories 60	**Cholesterol** 0mg	**Total Carbohydrate** 9g
Total Fat 2.5g	**Sodium** 15mg	Dietary Fiber 1g
Saturated Fat 2g	**Protein** 1g	Sugars 7g

Stonyfield Organic, Frozen Yogurt Pearls Peach-Vanilla

2 pearls (46g)

Amount per serving	Amount per serving	Amount per serving
Calories 50	**Cholesterol** 0mg	**Total Carbohydrate** 11g
Total Fat 0g	**Sodium** 75mg	Dietary Fiber 1g
Saturated Fat 0g	**Protein** 1g	Sugars 9g

Stonyfield Organic, Frozen Yogurt Pearls Strawberry-Chocolate

2 pearls (46g)

Amount per serving	Amount per serving	Amount per serving
Calories 40	**Cholesterol** 0mg	**Total Carbohydrate** 10g
Total Fat 0g	**Sodium** 75mg	Dietary Fiber 0g
Saturated Fat 0g	**Protein** 1g	Sugars 8g

Stonyfield Organic, Frozen Yogurt Pearls Strawberry-Vanilla

2 pearls (46g)

Amount per serving	Amount per serving	Amount per serving
Calories 40	**Cholesterol** 0mg	**Total Carbohydrate** 10g
Total Fat 0g	**Sodium** 75mg	Dietary Fiber 0g
Saturated Fat 0g	**Protein** 1g	Sugars 8g

Stonyfield Organic, Gotta Have Java Frozen Nonfat Yogurt

1/2 cup (85g)

Amount per serving	Amount per serving	Amount per serving
Calories 100	**Cholesterol** <5mg	**Total Carbohydrate** 21g
Total Fat 0g	**Sodium** 65mg	Dietary Fiber 0g
Saturated Fat 0g	**Protein** 5g	Sugars 18g

Stonyfield Organic, Gotta Have Vanilla Frozen Nonfat Yogurt

1/2 cup (85g)

Amount per serving	Amount per serving	Amount per serving
Calories 100	**Cholesterol** <5mg	**Total Carbohydrate** 20g
Total Fat 0g	**Sodium** 65mg	Dietary Fiber 0g
Saturated Fat 0g	**Protein** 4g	Sugars 19g

Stonyfield Organic, Gotta Have Vanilla Frozen Nonfat Yogurt Bar

1 bar (70g)

Amount per serving	Amount per serving	Amount per serving
Calories 170	**Cholesterol** 0mg	**Total Carbohydrate** 21g
Total Fat 8g	**Sodium** 40mg	Dietary Fiber 1g
Saturated Fat 7g	**Protein** 3g	Sugars 18g

Stonyfield Organic, Greek Frozen Nonfat Yogurt Blueberry

1 bar (70g)

Amount per serving	Amount per serving	Amount per serving
Calories 170	**Cholesterol** 0mg	**Total Carbohydrate** 21g
Total Fat 8g	**Sodium** 40mg	Dietary Fiber 1g
Saturated Fat 7g	**Protein** 3g	Sugars 18g

Stonyfield Organic, Greek Frozen Nonfat Yogurt Chocolate

1/2 cup (85g)

Amount per serving	Amount per serving	Amount per serving
Calories 100	**Cholesterol** <5mg	**Total Carbohydrate** 19g
Total Fat 0g	**Sodium** 55mg	Dietary Fiber 1g
Saturated Fat 0g	**Protein** 6g	Sugars 16g

Stonyfield Organic, Greek Frozen Nonfat Yogurt Honey

1/2 cup (85g)

Amount per serving	Amount per serving	Amount per serving
Calories 110	**Cholesterol** <5mg	**Total Carbohydrate** 22g
Total Fat 0g	**Sodium** 60mg	Dietary Fiber 0g
Saturated Fat 0g	**Protein** 6g	Sugars 20g

Stonyfield Organic, Greek Frozen Nonfat Yogurt Super Fruits

1/2 cup (85g)

Amount per serving	Amount per serving	Amount per serving
Calories 110	**Cholesterol** <5mg	**Total Carbohydrate** 21g
Total Fat 0g	**Sodium** 60mg	Dietary Fiber 0g
Saturated Fat 0g	**Protein** 6g	Sugars 20g

Stonyfield Organic, Greek Frozen Nonfat Yogurt Vanilla

1/2 cup (85g)

Amount per serving	Amount per serving	Amount per serving
Calories 100	**Cholesterol** <5mg	**Total Carbohydrate** 19g
Total Fat 0g	**Sodium** 65mg	Dietary Fiber 0g
Saturated Fat 0g	**Protein** 6g	Sugars 17g

Stonyfield Organic, Minty Chocolate Chip Frozen Nonfat Yogurt

1/2 cup (85g)

Amount per serving	Amount per serving	Amount per serving
Calories 140	**Cholesterol** <5mg	**Total Carbohydrate** 25g
Total Fat 2.5g	**Sodium** 50mg	Dietary Fiber 1g
Saturated Fat 1.5g	**Protein** 4g	Sugars 21g

Stonyfield Organic, Vanilla Fudge Swirl Frozen Nonfat Yogurt

1/2 cup (85g)

Amount per serving	Amount per serving	Amount per serving
Calories 120	**Cholesterol** <5mg	**Total Carbohydrate** 25g
Total Fat 0g	**Sodium** 65mg	Dietary Fiber 0g
Saturated Fat 0g	**Protein** 4g	Sugars 23g

Straus Family Creamery, NuScoop Organic Chocolate Dessert

4 fl oz (96g)

Amount per serving	Amount per serving	Amount per serving
Calories 170	**Cholesterol** 10mg	**Total Carbohydrate** 22g
Total Fat 6g	**Sodium** 65mg	Dietary Fiber 3g
Saturated Fat 3g	**Protein** 6g	Sugars 17g

Straus Family Creamery, NuScoop Organic Coffee Dessert

4 fl oz (96g)

Amount per serving	Amount per serving	Amount per serving
Calories 180	**Cholesterol** 14mg	**Total Carbohydrate** 23g
Total Fat 7g	**Sodium** 60mg	Dietary Fiber 2g
Saturated Fat 3.5g	**Protein** 6g	Sugars 17g

Straus Family Creamery, NuScoop Organic Strawberry Dessert

4 fl oz (96g)

Amount per serving	Amount per serving	Amount per serving
Calories 180	**Cholesterol** 12mg	**Total Carbohydrate** 24g
Total Fat 6g	**Sodium** 65mg	Dietary Fiber 2g
Saturated Fat 3g	**Protein** 6g	Sugars 19g

Straus Family Creamery, Organic Brown Sugar Banana Ice Cream

1/2 cup (91g)

Amount per serving	Amount per serving	Amount per serving
Calories 250	**Cholesterol** 55mg	**Total Carbohydrate** 32g
Total Fat 11g	**Sodium** 45mg	Dietary Fiber 0g
Saturated Fat 7g	**Protein** 3g	Sugars 31g

Straus Family Creamery, Organic Caramel Toffee Crunch Ice Cream

1/2 cup (91g)

Amount per serving	Amount per serving	Amount per serving
Calories 240	**Cholesterol** 70mg	**Total Carbohydrate** 23g
Total Fat 15g	**Sodium** 160mg	Dietary Fiber 0g
Saturated Fat 9g	**Protein** 3g	Sugars 23g

Straus Family Creamery, Organic Coffee Ice Cream

1/2 cup (91g)

Amount per serving	Amount per serving	Amount per serving
Calories 240	**Cholesterol** 70mg	**Total Carbohydrate** 19g
Total Fat 15g	**Sodium** 55mg	Dietary Fiber 0g
Saturated Fat 10g	**Protein** 4g	Sugars 19g

Straus Family Creamery, Organic Cookies & Cream Ice Cream

1/2 cup (91g)

Amount per serving	Amount per serving	Amount per serving
Calories 220	**Cholesterol** 60mg	**Total Carbohydrate** 25g
Total Fat 12g	**Sodium** 100mg	Dietary Fiber <1g
Saturated Fat 8g	**Protein** 3g	Sugars 19g

Straus Family Creamery, Organic Dutch Chocolate Ice Cream

1/2 cup (91g)

Amount per serving	Amount per serving	Amount per serving
Calories 230	**Cholesterol** 70mg	**Total Carbohydrate** 21g
Total Fat 15g	**Sodium** 55mg	Dietary Fiber 1g
Saturated Fat 10g	**Protein** 4g	Sugars 19g

Straus Family Creamery, Organic Mint Chocolate Chip Ice Cream

1/2 cup (91g)

Amount per serving	Amount per serving	Amount per serving
Calories 250	**Cholesterol** 65mg	**Total Carbohydrate** 22g
Total Fat 16g	**Sodium** 50mg	Dietary Fiber 0g
Saturated Fat 10g	**Protein** 4g	Sugars 22g

Straus Family Creamery, Organic Raspberry Ice Cream

1/2 cup (91g)

Amount per serving	Amount per serving	Amount per serving
Calories 230	**Cholesterol** 65mg	**Total Carbohydrate** 19g
Total Fat 14g	**Sodium** 50mg	Dietary Fiber 1g
Saturated Fat 9g	**Protein** 4g	Sugars 19g

Straus Family Creamery, Organic Vanilla Bean Ice Cream

1/2 cup (91g)

Amount per serving	Amount per serving	Amount per serving
Calories 240	**Cholesterol** 70mg	**Total Carbohydrate** 19g
Total Fat 15g	**Sodium** 55mg	Dietary Fiber 0g
Saturated Fat 10g	**Protein** 4g	Sugars 19g

Straus Family Creamery, Vanilla Chocolate Chip Ice Cream

1/2 cup (91g)

Amount per serving	Amount per serving	Amount per serving
Calories 230	**Cholesterol** 65mg	**Total Carbohydrate** 24g
Total Fat 14g	**Sodium** 40mg	Dietary Fiber 1g
Saturated Fat 9g	**Protein** 3g	Sugars 19g

Three Twins Ice Cream, Organic Bittersweet Chocolate Ice Cream

1/2 cup (85g)

Amount per serving	Amount per serving	Amount per serving
Calories 190	**Cholesterol** 60mg	**Total Carbohydrate** 21g
Total Fat 11g	**Sodium** 30mg	Dietary Fiber 3g
Saturated Fat 7g	**Protein** 4g	Sugars 17g

Three Twins Ice Cream, Organic Chocolate Orange Confetti Ice Cream

1/2 cup (85g)

Amount per serving	Amount per serving	Amount per serving
Calories 240	**Cholesterol** 70mg	**Total Carbohydrate** 22g
Total Fat 16g	**Sodium** 90mg	Dietary Fiber 0g
Saturated Fat 10g	**Protein** 3g	Sugars 17g

Three Twins Ice Cream, Organic Chocolate Peanut Butter Ice Cream

1/2 cup (85g)

Amount per serving	Amount per serving	Amount per serving
Calories 190	**Cholesterol** 60mg	**Total Carbohydrate** 21g
Total Fat 11g	**Sodium** 30mg	Dietary Fiber 3g
Saturated Fat 7g	**Protein** 4g	Sugars 17g

Three Twins Ice Cream, Organic Cookies and Cream Ice Cream

1/2 cup (85g)

Amount per serving	Amount per serving	Amount per serving
Calories 190	**Cholesterol** 60mg	**Total Carbohydrate** 21g
Total Fat 11g	**Sodium** 30mg	Dietary Fiber 3g
Saturated Fat 7g	**Protein** 4g	Sugars 17g

Three Twins Ice Cream, Organic Dad's Cardamom Ice Cream

1/2 cup (85g)

Amount per serving	Amount per serving	Amount per serving
Calories 190	**Cholesterol** 60mg	**Total Carbohydrate** 21g
Total Fat 11g	**Sodium** 30mg	Dietary Fiber 3g
Saturated Fat 7g	**Protein** 4g	Sugars 17g

Three Twins Ice Cream, Organic Fair Trade Vanilla Bean Speck Ice Cream

1/2 cup (85g)

Amount per serving	Amount per serving	Amount per serving
Calories 180	**Cholesterol** 65mg	**Total Carbohydrate** 16g
Total Fat 12g	**Sodium** 30mg	Dietary Fiber 0g
Saturated Fat 7g	**Protein** 2g	Sugars 15g

Three Twins Ice Cream, Organic Lemon Cookie Ice Cream

1/2 cup (85g)

Amount per serving	Amount per serving	Amount per serving
Calories 210	**Cholesterol** 55mg	**Total Carbohydrate** 23g
Total Fat 12g	**Sodium** 85mg	Dietary Fiber 0g
Saturated Fat 7g	**Protein** 3g	Sugars 18g

Three Twins Ice Cream, Organic Madagascar Vanilla Ice Cream

1/2 cup (85g)

Amount per serving	Amount per serving	Amount per serving
Calories 180	**Cholesterol** 65mg	**Total Carbohydrate** 16g
Total Fat 12g	**Sodium** 30mg	Dietary Fiber 0g
Saturated Fat 7g	**Protein** 2g	Sugars 15g

Three Twins Ice Cream, Organic Mint Confetti Ice Cream

1/2 cup (85g)

Amount per serving	Amount per serving	Amount per serving
Calories 210	**Cholesterol** 65mg	**Total Carbohydrate** 20g
Total Fat 13g	**Sodium** 30mg	Dietary Fiber 0g
Saturated Fat 8g	**Protein** 2g	Sugars 18g

Three Twins Ice Cream, Organic Mocha Difference Ice Cream

1/2 cup (85g)

Amount per serving	Amount per serving	Amount per serving
Calories 190	**Cholesterol** 60mg	**Total Carbohydrate** 21g
Total Fat 11g	**Sodium** 30mg	Dietary Fiber 3g
Saturated Fat 7g	**Protein** 4g	Sugars 17g

Three Twins Ice Cream, Organic Sea Salt Caramel Ice Cream

1/2 cup (85g)

Amount per serving	Amount per serving	Amount per serving
Calories 200	**Cholesterol** 60mg	**Total Carbohydrate** 24g
Total Fat 12g	**Sodium** 40mg	Dietary Fiber 0g
Saturated Fat 8g	**Protein** 3g	Sugars 17g

Three Twins Ice Cream, Organic Strawberry Je Ne Sais Quoi Ice Cream

1/2 cup (85g)

Amount per serving	Amount per serving	Amount per serving
Calories 150	**Cholesterol** 40mg	**Total Carbohydrate** 17g
Total Fat 8g	**Sodium** 30mg	Dietary Fiber 0g
Saturated Fat 5g	**Protein** 2g	Sugars 16g

Three Twins Ice Cream, Organic Vanilla Chocolate Chip Ice Cream

1/2 cup (85g)

Amount per serving	Amount per serving	Amount per serving
Calories 190	**Cholesterol** 60mg	**Total Carbohydrate** 21g
Total Fat 11g	**Sodium** 30mg	Dietary Fiber 3g
Saturated Fat 7g	**Protein** 4g	Sugars 17g

Milk

Horizon®, Fat-Free Milk plus DHA Omega-3

1 cup (240 ml)

Amount per serving	Amount per serving	Amount per serving
Calories 90	**Cholesterol** 5mg	**Total Carbohydrate** 13g
Total Fat 0g	**Sodium** 130mg	Dietary Fiber 0g
Saturated Fat 0g	**Protein** 8g	Sugars 12g

Horizon®, Lowfat Chocolate Milk Box

1 container

Amount per serving	Amount per serving	Amount per serving
Calories 150	**Cholesterol** 10mg	**Total Carbohydrate** 24g
Total Fat 2.5g	**Sodium** 200mg	Dietary Fiber <1g
Saturated Fat 1.5g	**Protein** 8g	Sugars 22g

Horizon®, Lowfat Chocolate Milk Box plus DHA Omega-3

1 container

Amount per serving	Amount per serving	Amount per serving
Calories 150	**Cholesterol** 15mg	**Total Carbohydrate** 24g
Total Fat 2.5g	**Sodium** 200mg	Dietary Fiber 0g
Saturated Fat 1.5g	**Protein** 8g	Sugars 22g

Horizon®, Lowfat Chocolate Milk plus DHA Omega-3

1 cup (240 ml)

Amount per serving	Amount per serving	Amount per serving
Calories 160	**Cholesterol** 10mg	**Total Carbohydrate** 26g
Total Fat 2.5g	**Sodium** 140mg	Dietary Fiber 0g
Saturated Fat 1.5g	**Protein** 8g	Sugars 26g

Horizon®, Lowfat Plain Milk Box

1 container

Amount per serving	Amount per serving	Amount per serving
Calories 110	**Cholesterol** 10mg	**Total Carbohydrate** 13g
Total Fat 2.5g	**Sodium** 130mg	Dietary Fiber 0g
Saturated Fat 1.5g	**Protein** 8g	Sugars 12g

Horizon®, Lowfat Strawberry Milk Box

1 container

Amount per serving	Amount per serving	Amount per serving
Calories 150	**Cholesterol** 15mg	**Total Carbohydrate** 24g
Total Fat 2.5g	**Sodium** 140mg	Dietary Fiber 0g
Saturated Fat 1.5g	**Protein** 8g	Sugars 23g

Horizon®, Lowfat Vanilla Milk Box

1 container

Amount per serving	Amount per serving	Amount per serving
Calories 150	**Cholesterol** 10mg	**Total Carbohydrate** 22g
Total Fat 2.5g	**Sodium** 115mg	Dietary Fiber 0g
Saturated Fat 1.5g	**Protein** 8g	Sugars 22g

Horizon®, Lowfat Vanilla Milk Box plus DHA Omega-3

1 container

Amount per serving	Amount per serving	Amount per serving
Calories 150	**Cholesterol** 15mg	**Total Carbohydrate** 23g
Total Fat 2.5g	**Sodium** 190mg	Dietary Fiber 0g
Saturated Fat 1.5g	**Protein** 8g	Sugars 21g

Horizon®, Organic Fat-Free Milk

1 cup (240 ml)

Amount per serving	Amount per serving	Amount per serving
Calories 90	**Cholesterol** 5mg	**Total Carbohydrate** 13g
Total Fat 0g	**Sodium** 130mg	Dietary Fiber 0g
Saturated Fat 0g	**Protein** 8g	Sugars 12g

Horizon®, Organic Half & Half

2 tbsp (30 ml)

Amount per serving	Amount per serving	Amount per serving
Calories 40	**Cholesterol** 15mg	**Total Carbohydrate** 1g
Total Fat 3.5g	**Sodium** 15mg	Dietary Fiber 0g
Saturated Fat 2g	**Protein** 1g	Sugars 1g

Horizon®, Organic Heavy Whipping Cream

1 tbsp (15 ml)

Amount per serving	Amount per serving	Amount per serving
Calories 50	**Cholesterol** 20mg	**Total Carbohydrate** 0g
Total Fat 5g	**Sodium** 5mg	Dietary Fiber 0g
Saturated Fat 3.5g	**Protein** 0g	Sugars 0g

Horizon®, Organic Lowfat Eggnog

1/2 cup (120 ml)

Amount per serving	Amount per serving	Amount per serving
Calories 140	**Cholesterol** 40mg	**Total Carbohydrate** 23g
Total Fat 3g	**Sodium** 85mg	Dietary Fiber 0g
Saturated Fat 1.5g	**Protein** 6g	Sugars 22g

Horizon®, Organic Lowfat Milk

1 cup (240 ml)

Amount per serving	Amount per serving	Amount per serving
Calories 110	**Cholesterol** 10mg	**Total Carbohydrate** 13g
Total Fat 2.5g	**Sodium** 130mg	Dietary Fiber 0g
Saturated Fat 1.5g	**Protein** 8g	Sugars 12g

Horizon®, Organic Lowfat Sour Cream

2 tbsp (30g)

Amount per serving	Amount per serving	Amount per serving
Calories 35	**Cholesterol** 10mg	**Total Carbohydrate** 3g
Total Fat 2g	**Sodium** 30mg	Dietary Fiber 0g
Saturated Fat 1g	**Protein** 2g	Sugars 2g

Horizon®, Organic Milk plus DHA Omega-3

1 cup (240 ml)

Amount per serving	Amount per serving	Amount per serving
Calories 150	**Cholesterol** 35mg	**Total Carbohydrate** 12g
Total Fat 8g	**Sodium** 120mg	Dietary Fiber 0g
Saturated Fat 5g	**Protein** 8g	Sugars 11g

Horizon®, Organic Reduced Fat Milk

1 cup (240 ml)

Amount per serving	Amount per serving	Amount per serving
Calories 130	**Cholesterol** 20mg	**Total Carbohydrate** 12g
Total Fat 5g	**Sodium** 130mg	Dietary Fiber 0g
Saturated Fat 3g	**Protein** 8g	Sugars 12g

Horizon®, Organic Sour Cream

2 tbsp (30g)

Amount per serving	Amount per serving	Amount per serving
Calories 60	**Cholesterol** 20mg	**Total Carbohydrate** 2g
Total Fat 5g	**Sodium** 20mg	Dietary Fiber 0g
Saturated Fat 3.5g	**Protein** 1g	Sugars 1g

Horizon®, Organic Whole Milk

1 cup (240 ml)

Amount per serving	Amount per serving	Amount per serving
Calories 150	**Cholesterol** 35mg	**Total Carbohydrate** 12g
Total Fat 8g	**Sodium** 120mg	Dietary Fiber 0g
Saturated Fat 5g	**Protein** 8g	Sugars 11g

Horizon®, Reduced Fat Milk with DHA Omega-3

1 cup (240 ml)

Amount per serving	Amount per serving	Amount per serving
Calories 130	**Cholesterol** 20mg	**Total Carbohydrate** 12g
Total Fat 5g	**Sodium** 130mg	Dietary Fiber 0g
Saturated Fat 3g	**Protein** 8g	Sugars 12g

Organic Valley, 1% Lowfat Chocolate Milk

8 fl oz (240 ml)

Amount per serving	Amount per serving	Amount per serving
Calories 150	**Cholesterol** 15mg	**Total Carbohydrate** 24g
Total Fat 2.5g	**Sodium** 220mg	Dietary Fiber 1g
Saturated Fat 1.5g	**Protein** 9g	Sugars 22g

Organic Valley, 2% Reduced Fat, Chocolate Milk

1 cup (240 ml)

Amount per serving	Amount per serving	Amount per serving
Calories 170	**Cholesterol** 20mg	**Total Carbohydrate** 24g
Total Fat 5g	**Sodium** 250mg	Dietary Fiber <1g
Saturated Fat 3g	**Protein** 8g	Sugars 23g

Organic Valley, Buttermilk Powder

3 tbsp (28g)

Amount per serving	Amount per serving	Amount per serving
Calories 110	**Cholesterol** 20mg	**Total Carbohydrate** 14g
Total Fat 1.5g	**Sodium** 130mg	Dietary Fiber 0g
Saturated Fat 1g	**Protein** 9g	Sugars 14g

Organic Valley, Buttermilk, Lowfat 1%, Pasteurized

1 cup (240 ml)

Amount per serving	Amount per serving	Amount per serving
Calories 100	**Cholesterol** 15mg	**Total Carbohydrate** 12g
Total Fat 2.5g	**Sodium** 250mg	Dietary Fiber 0g
Saturated Fat 1.5g	**Protein** 8g	Sugars 12g

Organic Valley, Chocolate, 2% Shelf-Stable Milk

1 cup (240 ml)

Amount per serving	Amount per serving	Amount per serving
Calories 170	**Cholesterol** 20mg	**Total Carbohydrate** 24g
Total Fat 5g	**Sodium** 250mg	Dietary Fiber <1g
Saturated Fat 3g	**Protein** 8g	Sugars 23g

Organic Valley, Chocolate, Single Serve, 1% Lowfat Milk

8 fl oz (240 ml)

Amount per serving	Amount per serving	Amount per serving
Calories 150	**Cholesterol** 15mg	**Total Carbohydrate** 24g
Total Fat 2.5g	**Sodium** 220mg	Dietary Fiber 1g
Saturated Fat 1.5g	**Protein** 9g	Sugars 22g

Organic Valley, Eggnog, Ultra Pasteurized

1/2 cup (120 ml)

Amount per serving	Amount per serving	Amount per serving
Calories 180	Cholesterol 90mg	Total Carbohydrate 18g
Total Fat 10g	Sodium 85mg	Dietary Fiber 0g
Saturated Fat 6g	Protein 5g	Sugars 17g

Organic Valley, Fat Free, Skim, Milk, Lactose Free, Ultra Pasteurized

1 cup (240 ml)

Amount per serving	Amount per serving	Amount per serving
Calories 90	Cholesterol 5mg	Total Carbohydrate 14g
Total Fat 0g	Sodium 130mg	Dietary Fiber 0g
Saturated Fat 0g	Protein 8g	Sugars 13g

Organic Valley, Fat Free, Skim, Milk, Pasteurized

1 cup (240 ml)

Amount per serving	Amount per serving	Amount per serving
Calories 90	Cholesterol 5mg	Total Carbohydrate 12g
Total Fat 0g	Sodium 125mg	Dietary Fiber 0g
Saturated Fat 0g	Protein 8g	Sugars 12g

Organic Valley, Fat Free, Skim, Milk, Ultra Pasteurized

1 cup (240 ml)

Amount per serving	Amount per serving	Amount per serving
Calories 90	Cholesterol 5mg	Total Carbohydrate 12g
Total Fat 0g	Sodium 125mg	Dietary Fiber 0g
Saturated Fat 0g	Protein 8g	Sugars 12g

Organic Valley, Grassmilk, 100% Grass-Fed, Fat Free, Non-Homogenized, Pasteurized

1 cup (240 ml)

Amount per serving	Amount per serving	Amount per serving
Calories 90	Cholesterol 5mg	Total Carbohydrate 12g
Total Fat 0g	Sodium 125mg	Dietary Fiber 0g
Saturated Fat 0g	Protein 8g	Sugars 12g

Organic Valley, Grassmilk, 100% Grass-Fed, Reduced Fat 2% Milk

1 cup (240 ml)

Amount per serving	Amount per serving	Amount per serving
Calories 130	Cholesterol 20mg	Total Carbohydrate 13g
Total Fat 5g	Sodium 140mg	Dietary Fiber 0g
Saturated Fat 3g	Protein 10g	Sugars 13g

Organic Valley, Grassmilk, 100% Grass-Fed, Whole Milk

1 cup (240 ml)

Amount per serving	Amount per serving	Amount per serving
Calories 150	**Cholesterol** 30mg	**Total Carbohydrate** 12g
Total Fat 8g	**Sodium** 120mg	Dietary Fiber 0g
Saturated Fat 5g	**Protein** 8g	Sugars 11g

Organic Valley, Half & Half, French Vanilla, Ultra Pasteurized

2 tbsp (30 ml)

Amount per serving	Amount per serving	Amount per serving
Calories 70	**Cholesterol** 10mg	**Total Carbohydrate** 10g
Total Fat 3.5g	**Sodium** 10mg	Dietary Fiber 0g
Saturated Fat 2g	**Protein** 1g	Sugars 9g

Organic Valley, Half & Half, Hazelnut, Ultra Pasteurized

2 tbsp (30 ml)

Amount per serving	Amount per serving	Amount per serving
Calories 70	**Cholesterol** 10mg	**Total Carbohydrate** 10g
Total Fat 3.5g	**Sodium** 10mg	Dietary Fiber 0g
Saturated Fat 2g	**Protein** 1g	Sugars 9g

Organic Valley, Half & Half, Ultra Pasteurized

2 tbsp (30 ml)

Amount per serving	Amount per serving	Amount per serving
Calories 40	**Cholesterol** 10mg	**Total Carbohydrate** 1g
Total Fat 3.5g	**Sodium** 10mg	Dietary Fiber 0g
Saturated Fat 2g	**Protein** <1g	Sugars 1g

Organic Valley, Lactose Free, Lowfat 1% Ultra Pasteurized Milk

1 cup (240 ml)

Amount per serving	Amount per serving	Amount per serving
Calories 110	**Cholesterol** 10mg	**Total Carbohydrate** 14g
Total Fat 2.5g	**Sodium** 125mg	Dietary Fiber 0g
Saturated Fat 1.5g	**Protein** 8g	Sugars 13g

Organic Valley, Lactose Free, Reduced Fat 2%, Ultra Pasteurized Milk

1 cup (240 ml)

Amount per serving	Amount per serving	Amount per serving
Calories 130	**Cholesterol** 20mg	**Total Carbohydrate** 13g
Total Fat 5g	**Sodium** 120mg	Dietary Fiber 0g
Saturated Fat 3g	**Protein** 8g	Sugars 12g

Organic Valley, Lactose Free, Ultra Pasteurized Half & Half

2 tbsp (30 ml)

Amount per serving	Amount per serving	Amount per serving
Calories 40	**Cholesterol** 10mg	**Total Carbohydrate** 1g
Total Fat 3.5g	**Sodium** 10mg	Dietary Fiber 0g
Saturated Fat 2g	**Protein** <1g	Sugars 1g

Organic Valley, Lactose Free, Whole, Ultra Pasteurized Milk

1 cup (240 ml)

Amount per serving	Amount per serving	Amount per serving
Calories 150	**Cholesterol** 30mg	**Total Carbohydrate** 12g
Total Fat 8g	**Sodium** 120mg	Dietary Fiber 0g
Saturated Fat 5g	**Protein** 8g	Sugars 11g

Organic Valley, Lowfat 1% Milk, Pasteurized

1 cup (240 ml)

Amount per serving	Amount per serving	Amount per serving
Calories 110	**Cholesterol** 15mg	**Total Carbohydrate** 13g
Total Fat 2.5g	**Sodium** 125mg	Dietary Fiber 0g
Saturated Fat 1.5g	**Protein** 8g	Sugars 12g

Organic Valley, Nonfat Dry Milk

3 tbsp (26g)

Amount per serving	Amount per serving	Amount per serving
Calories 90	**Cholesterol** <5mg	**Total Carbohydrate** 13g
Total Fat 0g	**Sodium** 130mg	Dietary Fiber 0g
Saturated Fat 0g	**Protein** 9g	Sugars 13g

Organic Valley, Omega-3 Ultra Pasteurized Whole Milk

1 cup (240 ml)

Amount per serving	Amount per serving	Amount per serving
Calories 150	**Cholesterol** 30mg	**Total Carbohydrate** 12g
Total Fat 8g	**Sodium** 120mg	Dietary Fiber 0g
Saturated Fat 5g	**Protein** 8g	Sugars 11g

Organic Valley, Organic Balance, Milk Protein Shake, Dark Chocolate

1 bottle (325 ml)

Amount per serving	Amount per serving	Amount per serving
Calories 190	**Cholesterol** 20mg	**Total Carbohydrate** 24g
Total Fat 3.5g	**Sodium** 210mg	Dietary Fiber 1g
Saturated Fat 2g	**Protein** 16g	Sugars 23g

Organic Valley, Organic Balance, Milk Protein Shake, Vanilla Bean

1 bottle (325 ml)

Amount per serving	Amount per serving	Amount per serving
Calories 190	**Cholesterol** 20mg	**Total Carbohydrate** 24g
Total Fat 3.5g	**Sodium** 210mg	Dietary Fiber 1g
Saturated Fat 2g	**Protein** 16g	Sugars 23g

Organic Valley, Organic Fuel, High Protein Milk Shake, Vanilla

1 bottle (325 ml)

Amount per serving	Amount per serving	Amount per serving
Calories 260	**Cholesterol** 35mg	**Total Carbohydrate** 27g
Total Fat 6g	**Sodium** 190mg	Dietary Fiber 1g
Saturated Fat 3g	**Protein** 26g	Sugars 26g

Organic Valley, Pasteurized Whole Milk

1 cup (240 ml)

Amount per serving	Amount per serving	Amount per serving
Calories 150	**Cholesterol** 35mg	**Total Carbohydrate** 12g
Total Fat 8g	**Sodium** 125mg	Dietary Fiber 0g
Saturated Fat 5g	**Protein** 8g	Sugars 12g

Organic Valley, Reduced Fat 2% Milk, Pasteurized

1 cup (240 ml)

Amount per serving	Amount per serving	Amount per serving
Calories 130	**Cholesterol** 20mg	**Total Carbohydrate** 12g
Total Fat 5g	**Sodium** 120mg	Dietary Fiber 0g
Saturated Fat 3g	**Protein** 8g	Sugars 11g

Organic Valley, Reduced Fat 2% Milk, Ultra Pasteurized

1 cup (240 ml)

Amount per serving	Amount per serving	Amount per serving
Calories 130	**Cholesterol** 20mg	**Total Carbohydrate** 12g
Total Fat 5g	**Sodium** 120mg	Dietary Fiber 0g
Saturated Fat 3g	**Protein** 8g	Sugars 11g

Organic Valley, Reduced Fat 2%, Ultra Pasteurized Omega-3 Milk

1 cup (240 ml)

Amount per serving	Amount per serving	Amount per serving
Calories 130	**Cholesterol** 20mg	**Total Carbohydrate** 12g
Total Fat 5g	**Sodium** 120mg	Dietary Fiber 0g
Saturated Fat 3g	**Protein** 8g	Sugars 11g

Organic Valley, Reduced Fat, Shelf-Stable Milk

1 cup (240 ml)

Amount per serving	Amount per serving	Amount per serving
Calories 135	**Cholesterol** 20mg	**Total Carbohydrate** 12g
Total Fat 5g	**Sodium** 120mg	Dietary Fiber 0g
Saturated Fat 3g	**Protein** 8g	Sugars 11g

Organic Valley, Strawberry Lowfat 1%, Shelf-Stable Milk

8 fl oz (240 ml) (242g)

Amount per serving	Amount per serving	Amount per serving
Calories 150	**Cholesterol** 15mg	**Total Carbohydrate** 27g
Total Fat 2.5g	**Sodium** 120mg	Dietary Fiber 2g
Saturated Fat 1.5g	**Protein** 8g	Sugars 24g

Organic Valley, Strawberry Lowfat 1%, Single Serve

8 fl oz (240 ml) (242g)

Amount per serving	Amount per serving	Amount per serving
Calories 150	**Cholesterol** 15mg	**Total Carbohydrate** 27g
Total Fat 2.5g	**Sodium** 120mg	Dietary Fiber 2g
Saturated Fat 1.5g	**Protein** 8g	Sugars 24g

Organic Valley, Ultra Pasteurized Whole Milk

1 cup (240 ml)

Amount per serving	Amount per serving	Amount per serving
Calories 150	**Cholesterol** 30mg	**Total Carbohydrate** 12g
Total Fat 8g	**Sodium** 120mg	Dietary Fiber 0g
Saturated Fat 5g	**Protein** 8g	Sugars 11g

Organic Valley, Vanilla Lowfat 1%, Shelf-Stable Milk

8 fl oz (240 ml) (242g)

Amount per serving	Amount per serving	Amount per serving
Calories 150	**Cholesterol** 15mg	**Total Carbohydrate** 26g
Total Fat 2.5g	**Sodium** 120mg	Dietary Fiber 2g
Saturated Fat 1.5g	**Protein** 8g	Sugars 23g

Organic Valley, Vanilla Lowfat 1%, Single Serve

8 fl oz (240 ml) (242g)

Amount per serving	Amount per serving	Amount per serving
Calories 150	**Cholesterol** 15mg	**Total Carbohydrate** 26g
Total Fat 2.5g	**Sodium** 120mg	Dietary Fiber 2g
Saturated Fat 1.5g	**Protein** 8g	Sugars 23g

Organic Valley, Whole Milk, Single Serve

8 fl oz (240 ml)

Amount per serving	Amount per serving	Amount per serving
Calories 150	**Cholesterol** 30mg	**Total Carbohydrate** 12g
Total Fat 8g	**Sodium** 120mg	Dietary Fiber 0g
Saturated Fat 5g	**Protein** 8g	Sugars 11g

Organic Valley, Whole, Ultra Pasteurized Omega-3 Milk

1 cup (240 ml)

Amount per serving	Amount per serving	Amount per serving
Calories 150	**Cholesterol** 30mg	**Total Carbohydrate** 12g
Total Fat 8g	**Sodium** 120mg	Dietary Fiber 0g
Saturated Fat 5g	**Protein** 8g	Sugars 11g

Stonyfield Organic, 1% Milk Fat Organic Lowfat Milk, Half Gallon Size

1 cup (240 ml)

Amount per serving	Amount per serving	Amount per serving
Calories 110	**Cholesterol** 15mg	**Total Carbohydrate** 12g
Total Fat 2.5g	**Sodium** 125mg	Dietary Fiber 0g
Saturated Fat 1.5g	**Protein** 8g	Sugars 12g

Stonyfield Organic, 2% Milk Fat Organic Reduced Fat Milk, Half Gallon Size

1 cup

Amount per serving	Amount per serving	Amount per serving
Calories 130	**Cholesterol** 20mg	**Total Carbohydrate** 12g
Total Fat 5g	**Sodium** 120mg	Dietary Fiber 0g
Saturated Fat 3g	**Protein** 8g	Sugars 11g

Stonyfield Organic, 2% Milk Fat, Organic Omega-3 Milk

1 cup

Amount per serving	Amount per serving	Amount per serving
Calories 130	**Cholesterol** 20mg	**Total Carbohydrate** 12g
Total Fat 5g	**Sodium** 120mg	Dietary Fiber 0g
Saturated Fat 3g	**Protein** 8g	Sugars 11g

Stonyfield Organic, Chocolate Lowfat Milk & Omega-3s, 1% Milkfat

1 cup

Amount per serving	Amount per serving	Amount per serving
Calories 150	**Cholesterol** 15mg	**Total Carbohydrate** 23g
Total Fat 3g	**Sodium** 170mg	Dietary Fiber 0g
Saturated Fat 1.5g	**Protein** 8g	Sugars 22g

Stonyfield Organic, Fat Free Organic Milk, Half Gallon Size

1 cup (240 ml)

Amount per serving	Amount per serving	Amount per serving
Calories 90	**Cholesterol** 5mg	**Total Carbohydrate** 12g
Total Fat 0g	**Sodium** 125mg	Dietary Fiber 0g
Saturated Fat 0g	**Protein** 8g	Sugars 12g

Stonyfield Organic, Organic Half & Half

2 tbsp (30 ml)

Amount per serving	Amount per serving	Amount per serving
Calories 40	**Cholesterol** 10mg	**Total Carbohydrate** 1g
Total Fat 3.5g	**Sodium** 10mg	Dietary Fiber 0g
Saturated Fat 2g	**Protein** <1g	Sugars 1g

Stonyfield Organic, Organic Heavy Whipping Cream

1 tbsp (15 ml)

Amount per serving	Amount per serving	Amount per serving
Calories 50	**Cholesterol** 20mg	**Total Carbohydrate** 0g
Total Fat 6g	**Sodium** 5mg	Dietary Fiber 0g
Saturated Fat 3.5g	**Protein** 0g	Sugars 0g

Stonyfield Organic, Whole Milk Organic Milk, Half Gallon Size

1 cup

Amount per serving	Amount per serving	Amount per serving
Calories 150	**Cholesterol** 30mg	**Total Carbohydrate** 12g
Total Fat 8g	**Sodium** 120mg	Dietary Fiber 0g
Saturated Fat 5g	**Protein** 8g	Sugars 11g

Stonyfield Organic, Whole Milk Organic Omega-3 Milk

1 cup

Amount per serving	Amount per serving	Amount per serving
Calories 150	**Cholesterol** 30mg	**Total Carbohydrate** 12g
Total Fat 8g	**Sodium** 120mg	Dietary Fiber 0g
Saturated Fat 5g	**Protein** 8g	Sugars 11g

Straus Family Creamery, Organic Half & Half

2 tbsp (30 ml)

Amount per serving	Amount per serving	Amount per serving
Calories 35	**Cholesterol** 15mg	**Total Carbohydrate** 1g
Total Fat 3g	**Sodium** 15mg	Dietary Fiber 0g
Saturated Fat 2g	**Protein** 1g	Sugars 1g

Straus Family Creamery, Organic Lowfat Milk, Cream-Top

1 cup (240 ml)

Amount per serving	Amount per serving	Amount per serving
Calories 100	**Cholesterol** 15mg	**Total Carbohydrate** 15g
Total Fat 2.5g	**Sodium** 160mg	Dietary Fiber 0g
Saturated Fat 1.5g	**Protein** 11g	Sugars 15g

Straus Family Creamery, Organic Nonfat Milk

1 cup (240 ml)

Amount per serving	Amount per serving	Amount per serving
Calories 90	**Cholesterol** <5mg	**Total Carbohydrate** 12g
Total Fat 0g	**Sodium** 140mg	Dietary Fiber 0g
Saturated Fat 0g	**Protein** 10g	Sugars 12g

Straus Family Creamery, Organic Reduced Fat Milk, Cream-Top

1 cup (240 ml)

Amount per serving	Amount per serving	Amount per serving
Calories 130	**Cholesterol** 25mg	**Total Carbohydrate** 13g
Total Fat 5g	**Sodium** 130mg	Dietary Fiber 0g
Saturated Fat 3g	**Protein** 10g	Sugars 13g

Straus Family Creamery, Organic Sour Cream

2 tbsp (30g)

Amount per serving	Amount per serving	Amount per serving
Calories 50	**Cholesterol** 15mg	**Total Carbohydrate** 1g
Total Fat 5g	**Sodium** 15mg	Dietary Fiber 0g
Saturated Fat 3.5g	**Protein** 1g	Sugars 1g

Straus Family Creamery, Organic Whipping Cream

1 tbsp (15 ml)

Amount per serving	Amount per serving	Amount per serving
Calories 50	**Cholesterol** 15mg	**Total Carbohydrate** <1g
Total Fat 5g	**Sodium** 10mg	Dietary Fiber 0g
Saturated Fat 3.5g	**Protein** 0g	Sugars 0g

Straus Family Creamery, Organic Whole Milk, Cream-Top

1 cup (240 ml)

Amount per serving	Amount per serving	Amount per serving
Calories 150	**Cholesterol** 35mg	**Total Carbohydrate** 11g
Total Fat 8g	**Sodium** 120mg	Dietary Fiber 0g
Saturated Fat 5g	**Protein** 8g	Sugars 11g

Stremicks Heritage Foods, Omega-3 DHA Organic Lowfat Milk

1 cup (240 ml)

Amount per serving	Amount per serving	Amount per serving
Calories 120	**Cholesterol** 10mg	**Total Carbohydrate** 14g
Total Fat 2.5g	**Sodium** 150mg	Dietary Fiber 0g
Saturated Fat 1.5g	**Protein** 11g	Sugars 14g

Stremicks Heritage Foods, Omega-3 DHA Organic Reduced Fat Milk

1 cup (240 ml)

Amount per serving	Amount per serving	Amount per serving
Calories 130	**Cholesterol** 25mg	**Total Carbohydrate** 13g
Total Fat 5g	**Sodium** 130mg	Dietary Fiber 0g
Saturated Fat 3g	**Protein** 10g	Sugars 13g

Stremicks Heritage Foods, Omega-3 DHA Organic Vitamin D Milk

1 cup (240 ml)

Amount per serving	Amount per serving	Amount per serving
Calories 150	**Cholesterol** 35mg	**Total Carbohydrate** 11g
Total Fat 8g	**Sodium** 115mg	Dietary Fiber 0g
Saturated Fat 5g	**Protein** 8g	Sugars 11g

Stremicks Heritage Foods, Organic Fat Free Milk

1 cup (240 ml)

Amount per serving	Amount per serving	Amount per serving
Calories 90	**Cholesterol** <5mg	**Total Carbohydrate** 12g
Total Fat 0g	**Sodium** 120mg	Dietary Fiber 0g
Saturated Fat 0g	**Protein** 9g	Sugars 12g

Stremicks Heritage Foods, Organic Lowfat Milk

1 cup (240 ml)

Amount per serving	Amount per serving	Amount per serving
Calories 120	**Cholesterol** 10mg	**Total Carbohydrate** 14g
Total Fat 2.5g	**Sodium** 150mg	Dietary Fiber 0g
Saturated Fat 1.5g	**Protein** 11g	Sugars 14g

Stremicks Heritage Foods, Organic Reduced Fat Milk

1 cup (240 ml)

Amount per serving	Amount per serving	Amount per serving
Calories 130	**Cholesterol** 25mg	**Total Carbohydrate** 13g
Total Fat 5g	**Sodium** 130mg	Dietary Fiber 0g
Saturated Fat 3g	**Protein** 10g	Sugars 13g

Stremicks Heritage Foods, Organic Vitamin D Milk

1 cup (240 ml)

Amount per serving	Amount per serving	Amount per serving
Calories 150	Cholesterol 35mg	Total Carbohydrate 11g
Total Fat 8g	Sodium 115mg	Dietary Fiber 0g
Saturated Fat 5g	Protein 8g	Sugars 11g

Yogurt

Green Valley Organics, Lactose Free Blueberry Pomegranate Acai Kefir

1 cup, 8 fl oz (240 ml)

Amount per serving	Amount per serving	Amount per serving
Calories 150	Cholesterol 10mg	Total Carbohydrate 25g
Total Fat 2.5g	Sodium 70mg	Dietary Fiber 0g
Saturated Fat 1.5g	Protein 7g	Sugars 23g

Green Valley Organics, Lactose Free Blueberry Yogurt

6 oz (170g)

Amount per serving	Amount per serving	Amount per serving
Calories 140	Cholesterol 10mg	Total Carbohydrate 23g
Total Fat 2g	Sodium 70mg	Dietary Fiber 0g
Saturated Fat 1g	Protein 7g	Sugars 19g

Green Valley Organics, Lactose Free Honey Yogurt

6 oz (170g)

Amount per serving	Amount per serving	Amount per serving
Calories 140	Cholesterol 10mg	Total Carbohydrate 24g
Total Fat 2g	Sodium 79mg	Dietary Fiber 0g
Saturated Fat 1.5g	Protein 7g	Sugars 17g

Green Valley Organics, Lactose Free Peach Yogurt

6 oz (170g)

Amount per serving	Amount per serving	Amount per serving
Calories 140	Cholesterol 10mg	Total Carbohydrate 23g
Total Fat 2g	Sodium 70mg	Dietary Fiber 0g
Saturated Fat 1g	Protein 7g	Sugars 19g

Green Valley Organics, Lactose Free Plain Kefir

1 cup, 8 fl oz (240 ml)

Amount per serving	Amount per serving	Amount per serving
Calories 90	Cholesterol 10mg	Total Carbohydrate 10g
Total Fat 2.5g	Sodium 75mg	Dietary Fiber 0g
Saturated Fat 1.5g	Protein 8g	Sugars 9g

Green Valley Organics, Lactose Free Plain Yogurt

6 oz (170g)

Amount per serving	Amount per serving	Amount per serving
Calories 100	**Cholesterol** 10mg	**Total Carbohydrate** 11g
Total Fat 2.5g	**Sodium** 85mg	Dietary Fiber 0g
Saturated Fat 1.5g	**Protein** 8g	Sugars 8g

Green Valley Organics, Lactose Free Strawberry Pomegranate Acai Kefir

1 cup, 8 fl oz (240 ml)

Amount per serving	Amount per serving	Amount per serving
Calories 150	**Cholesterol** 10mg	**Total Carbohydrate** 25g
Total Fat 2.5g	**Sodium** 65mg	Dietary Fiber 0g
Saturated Fat 1.5g	**Protein** 7g	Sugars 23g

Green Valley Organics, Lactose Free Strawberry Yogurt

6 oz (170g)

Amount per serving	Amount per serving	Amount per serving
Calories 140	**Cholesterol** 10mg	**Total Carbohydrate** 23g
Total Fat 2g	**Sodium** 70mg	Dietary Fiber 0g
Saturated Fat 1g	**Protein** 7g	Sugars 19g

Green Valley Organics, Lactose Free Vanilla Yogurt

6 oz (170g)

Amount per serving	Amount per serving	Amount per serving
Calories 120	**Cholesterol** 10mg	**Total Carbohydrate** 17g
Total Fat 3g	**Sodium** 84mg	Dietary Fiber 0g
Saturated Fat 2g	**Protein** 7g	Sugars 12g

Horizon®, Cream-on-Top Whole Milk Yogurt Vanilla

1 cup (227g)

Amount per serving	Amount per serving	Amount per serving
Calories 230	**Cholesterol** 30mg	**Total Carbohydrate** 33g
Total Fat 6g	**Sodium** 140mg	Dietary Fiber 0g
Saturated Fat 4g	**Protein** 9g	Sugars 31g

Horizon®, Organic Cream-on-Top Whole Milk Yogurt Plain

1 cup (227g)

Amount per serving	Amount per serving	Amount per serving
Calories 170	**Cholesterol** 35mg	**Total Carbohydrate** 16g
Total Fat 8g	**Sodium** 180mg	Dietary Fiber 0g
Saturated Fat 5g	**Protein** 10g	Sugars 14g

Horizon®, Organic Fat-Free Plain Yogurt

1 cup (227g)

Amount per serving	Amount per serving	Amount per serving
Calories 110	**Cholesterol** 5mg	**Total Carbohydrate** 17g
Total Fat 0g	**Sodium** 190mg	Dietary Fiber 0g
Saturated Fat 0g	**Protein** 11g	Sugars 15g

Horizon®, Organic Fat-Free Vanilla Yogurt

1 cup (227g)

Amount per serving	Amount per serving	Amount per serving
Calories 190	**Cholesterol** 5mg	**Total Carbohydrate** 35g
Total Fat 0g	**Sodium** 180mg	Dietary Fiber 0g
Saturated Fat 0g	**Protein** 10g	Sugars 34g

Horizon®, Tuberz®, Blueberry Wave

1 tube (57g)

Amount per serving	Amount per serving	Amount per serving
Calories 60	**Cholesterol** <5mg	**Total Carbohydrate** 11g
Total Fat 0.5g	**Sodium** 40mg	Dietary Fiber 0g
Saturated Fat 0g	**Protein** 2g	Sugars 10g

Horizon®, Tuberz®, Sour Apple Spray

1 tube (57g)

Amount per serving	Amount per serving	Amount per serving
Calories 60	**Cholesterol** <5mg	**Total Carbohydrate** 12g
Total Fat 0.5g	**Sodium** 50mg	Dietary Fiber 0g
Saturated Fat 0g	**Protein** 2g	Sugars 11g

Horizon®, Tuberz®, Strawberry Lemonade Squeeze

1 tube (57g)

Amount per serving	Amount per serving	Amount per serving
Calories 60	**Cholesterol** <5mg	**Total Carbohydrate** 12g
Total Fat 0.5g	**Sodium** 50mg	Dietary Fiber 0g
Saturated Fat 0g	**Protein** 2g	Sugars 11g

Horizon®, Tuberz®, Surfin' Strawberry

1 tube (57g)

Amount per serving	Amount per serving	Amount per serving
Calories 60	**Cholesterol** <5mg	**Total Carbohydrate** 11g
Total Fat 0.5g	**Sodium** 40mg	Dietary Fiber 0g
Saturated Fat 0g	**Protein** 2g	Sugars 10g

Lifeway Foods, Helios Organic Nonfat–Coconut Kefir

1 cup (240 ml)

Amount per serving	Amount per serving	Amount per serving
Calories 160	**Cholesterol** 5mg	**Total Carbohydrate** 29g
Total Fat 0g	**Sodium** 125mg	Dietary Fiber 2g
Saturated Fat 0g	**Protein** 11g	Sugars 27g

Lifeway Foods, Helios Organic Nonfat–Original Kefir

1 cup (240 ml)

Amount per serving	Amount per serving	Amount per serving
Calories 100	**Cholesterol** 5mg	**Total Carbohydrate** 14g
Total Fat 0g	**Sodium** 120mg	Dietary Fiber 2g
Saturated Fat 0g	**Protein** 12g	Sugars 12g

Lifeway Foods, Helios Organic Nonfat–Passion Fruit Kefir

1 cup (240 ml)

Amount per serving	Amount per serving	Amount per serving
Calories 120	**Cholesterol** 15mg	**Total Carbohydrate** 23g
Total Fat 0g	**Sodium** 85mg	Dietary Fiber 0g
Saturated Fat 0g	**Protein** 8g	Sugars 23g

Lifeway Foods, Helios Organic Nonfat–Plain Kefir

1 cup (240 ml)

Amount per serving	Amount per serving	Amount per serving
Calories 80	**Cholesterol** 18mg	**Total Carbohydrate** 10g
Total Fat 0g	**Sodium** 90mg	Dietary Fiber 0g
Saturated Fat 0g	**Protein** 9g	Sugars 10g

Lifeway Foods, Helios Organic Nonfat–Pomegranate/Acai Kefir

1 cup (240 ml)

Amount per serving	Amount per serving	Amount per serving
Calories 120	**Cholesterol** 15mg	**Total Carbohydrate** 23g
Total Fat 0g	**Sodium** 85mg	Dietary Fiber 0g
Saturated Fat 0g	**Protein** 8g	Sugars 23g

Lifeway Foods, Helios Organic Nonfat–Pomegranate/Blueberry Kefir

1 cup (240 ml)

Amount per serving	Amount per serving	Amount per serving
Calories 160	**Cholesterol** 5mg	**Total Carbohydrate** 29g
Total Fat 0g	**Sodium** 125mg	Dietary Fiber 2g
Saturated Fat 0g	**Protein** 11g	Sugars 27g

Lifeway Foods, Helios Organic Nonfat–Raspberry Kefir

1 cup (240 ml)

Amount per serving	Amount per serving	Amount per serving
Calories 160	**Cholesterol** 5mg	**Total Carbohydrate** 29g
Total Fat 0g	**Sodium** 125mg	Dietary Fiber 2g
Saturated Fat 0g	**Protein** 11g	Sugars 27g

Lifeway Foods, Helios Organic Nonfat–Strawberry Kefir

1 cup (240 ml)

Amount per serving	Amount per serving	Amount per serving
Calories 160	**Cholesterol** 5mg	**Total Carbohydrate** 29g
Total Fat 0g	**Sodium** 125mg	Dietary Fiber 2g
Saturated Fat 0g	**Protein** 11g	Sugars 27g

Lifeway Foods, Helios Organic Nonfat–Vanilla Kefir

1 cup (240 ml)

Amount per serving	Amount per serving	Amount per serving
Calories 160	**Cholesterol** 5mg	**Total Carbohydrate** 29g
Total Fat 0g	**Sodium** 125mg	Dietary Fiber 2g
Saturated Fat 0g	**Protein** 11g	Sugars 27g

Lifeway Foods, Organic Green Kefir–Kiwi Passion Fruit

1 cup (240 ml)

Amount per serving	Amount per serving	Amount per serving
Calories 170	**Cholesterol** NA	**Total Carbohydrate** 25g
Total Fat 2g	**Sodium** 137mg	Dietary Fiber 4g
Saturated Fat 0g	**Protein** 12g	Sugars 21g

Lifeway Foods, Organic Green Kefir–Pomegranate Acai Blueberry

1 cup (240 ml)

Amount per serving	Amount per serving	Amount per serving
Calories 170	**Cholesterol** NA	**Total Carbohydrate** 25g
Total Fat 2g	**Sodium** 137mg	Dietary Fiber 4g
Saturated Fat 0g	**Protein** 12g	Sugars 21g

Lifeway Foods, Organic Low Fat Blueberry Kefir

1 cup (240 ml)

Amount per serving	Amount per serving	Amount per serving
Calories 140	**Cholesterol** 10mg	**Total Carbohydrate** 20g
Total Fat 2g	**Sodium** 125mg	Dietary Fiber NA
Saturated Fat 1.5g	**Protein** 11g	Sugars 20g

Lifeway Foods, Organic Low Fat Low Carb Plain Kefir

1 cup (240 ml)

Amount per serving	Amount per serving	Amount per serving
Calories 110	**Cholesterol** 10mg	**Total Carbohydrate** 12g
Total Fat 2g	**Sodium** 125mg	Dietary Fiber NA
Saturated Fat 1.5g	**Protein** 11g	Sugars 12g

Lifeway Foods, Organic Low Fat Peach Kefir

1 cup (240 ml)

Amount per serving	Amount per serving	Amount per serving
Calories 140	**Cholesterol** 10mg	**Total Carbohydrate** 20g
Total Fat 2g	**Sodium** 125mg	Dietary Fiber NA
Saturated Fat 1.5g	**Protein** 11g	Sugars 20g

Lifeway Foods, Organic Low Fat Plain Kefir

1 cup (240 ml)

Amount per serving	Amount per serving	Amount per serving
Calories 110	**Cholesterol** 10mg	**Total Carbohydrate** 12g
Total Fat 2g	**Sodium** 125mg	Dietary Fiber NA
Saturated Fat 1.5g	**Protein** 11g	Sugars 12g

Lifeway Foods, Organic Low Fat Pomegranate/Acai Kefir

1 cup (240 ml)

Amount per serving	Amount per serving	Amount per serving
Calories 140	**Cholesterol** 10mg	**Total Carbohydrate** 20g
Total Fat 2g	**Sodium** 125mg	Dietary Fiber NA
Saturated Fat 1.5g	**Protein** 11g	Sugars 20g

Lifeway Foods, Organic Low Fat Raspberry Kefir

1 cup (240 ml)

Amount per serving	Amount per serving	Amount per serving
Calories 140	**Cholesterol** 10mg	**Total Carbohydrate** 20g
Total Fat 2g	**Sodium** 125mg	Dietary Fiber NA
Saturated Fat 1.5g	**Protein** 11g	Sugars 20g

Lifeway Foods, Organic Low Fat Strawberries n' Cream Kefir

1 cup (240 ml)

Amount per serving	Amount per serving	Amount per serving
Calories 140	**Cholesterol** 10mg	**Total Carbohydrate** 20g
Total Fat 2g	**Sodium** 125mg	Dietary Fiber NA
Saturated Fat 1.5g	**Protein** 11g	Sugars 20g

Lifeway Foods, Organic Whole Milk Plain Kefir

1 cup (240 ml)

Amount per serving	Amount per serving	Amount per serving
Calories 160	**Cholesterol** 30mg	**Total Carbohydrate** 12g
Total Fat 8g	**Sodium** 125mg	Dietary Fiber NA
Saturated Fat 5g	**Protein** 10g	Sugars 12g

Lifeway Foods, Organic Whole Milk Strawberries n' Cream Kefir

1 cup (240 ml)

Amount per serving	Amount per serving	Amount per serving
Calories 190	**Cholesterol** 30mg	**Total Carbohydrate** 20g
Total Fat 8g	**Sodium** 125mg	Dietary Fiber NA
Saturated Fat 5g	**Protein** 10g	Sugars 20g

Lifeway Foods, Organic Whole Milk Wildberries Kefir

1 cup (240 ml)

Amount per serving	Amount per serving	Amount per serving
Calories 190	**Cholesterol** 30mg	**Total Carbohydrate** 20g
Total Fat 8g	**Sodium** 125mg	Dietary Fiber NA
Saturated Fat 5g	**Protein** 10g	Sugars 20g

Stonyfield Organic, Black Cherry Petite Lowfat Crème

1 container (150g)

Amount per serving	Amount per serving	Amount per serving
Calories 130	**Cholesterol** 10mg	**Total Carbohydrate** 18g
Total Fat 2.5g	**Sodium** 50mg	Dietary Fiber 0g
Saturated Fat 1.5g	**Protein** 10g	Sugars 16g

Stonyfield Organic, Blends, Fat Free, Black Cherry Yogurt

1 container (170g)

Amount per serving	Amount per serving	Amount per serving
Calories 170	**Cholesterol** 15mg	**Total Carbohydrate** 27g
Total Fat 3g	**Sodium** 110mg	Dietary Fiber <1g
Saturated Fat 1.5g	**Protein** 8g	Sugars 27g

Stonyfield Organic, Blends, Fat Free, Blackberry Yogurt

1 container (170g)

Amount per serving	Amount per serving	Amount per serving
Calories 150	**Cholesterol** 5mg	**Total Carbohydrate** 28g
Total Fat 0g	**Sodium** 120mg	Dietary Fiber <1g
Saturated Fat 0g	**Protein** 8g	Sugars 28g

Stonyfield Organic, Blends, Fat Free, Blueberry Yogurt

1 container (170g)

Amount per serving	Amount per serving	Amount per serving
Calories 150	**Cholesterol** 5mg	**Total Carbohydrate** 28g
Total Fat 0g	**Sodium** 120mg	Dietary Fiber <1g
Saturated Fat 0g	**Protein** 8g	Sugars 28g

Stonyfield Organic, Blends, Fat Free, French Vanilla Yogurt

1 container (170g)

Amount per serving	Amount per serving	Amount per serving
Calories 140	**Cholesterol** 5mg	**Total Carbohydrate** 28g
Total Fat 0g	**Sodium** 120mg	Dietary Fiber 0g
Saturated Fat 0g	**Protein** 8g	Sugars 27g

Stonyfield Organic, Blends, Fat Free, Lemon Yogurt

1 container (170g)

Amount per serving	Amount per serving	Amount per serving
Calories 140	**Cholesterol** 5mg	**Total Carbohydrate** 28g
Total Fat 0g	**Sodium** 120mg	Dietary Fiber 0g
Saturated Fat 0g	**Protein** 8g	Sugars 27g

Stonyfield Organic, Blends, Fat Free, Peach Mango Yogurt

1 container (170g)

Amount per serving	Amount per serving	Amount per serving
Calories 140	**Cholesterol** 5mg	**Total Carbohydrate** 28g
Total Fat 0g	**Sodium** 130mg	Dietary Fiber 0g
Saturated Fat 0g	**Protein** 8g	Sugars 28g

Stonyfield Organic, Blends, Fat Free, Peach Yogurt

1 container (170g)

Amount per serving	Amount per serving	Amount per serving
Calories 170	**Cholesterol** 15mg	**Total Carbohydrate** 27g
Total Fat 3g	**Sodium** 120mg	Dietary Fiber <1g
Saturated Fat 1.5g	**Protein** 8g	Sugars 26g

Stonyfield Organic, Blends, Fat Free, Raspberry Yogurt

1 container (170g)

Amount per serving	Amount per serving	Amount per serving
Calories 170	**Cholesterol** 15mg	**Total Carbohydrate** 27g
Total Fat 3g	**Sodium** 110mg	Dietary Fiber <1g
Saturated Fat 1.5g	**Protein** 8g	Sugars 27g

Stonyfield Organic, Blends, Fat Free, Strawberry Banana Yogurt

1 container (170g)

Amount per serving	Amount per serving	Amount per serving
Calories 140	**Cholesterol** 5mg	**Total Carbohydrate** 28g
Total Fat 0g	**Sodium** 120mg	Dietary Fiber <1g
Saturated Fat 0g	**Protein** 8g	Sugars 28g

Stonyfield Organic, Blends, Fat Free, Strawberry Yogurt

1 container (170g)

Amount per serving	Amount per serving	Amount per serving
Calories 170	**Cholesterol** 15mg	**Total Carbohydrate** 27g
Total Fat 3g	**Sodium** 120mg	Dietary Fiber <1g
Saturated Fat 1.5g	**Protein** 8g	Sugars 27g

Stonyfield Organic, Blueberry Petite Lowfat Crème

1 container (150g)

Amount per serving	Amount per serving	Amount per serving
Calories 130	**Cholesterol** 10mg	**Total Carbohydrate** 17g
Total Fat 2.5g	**Sodium** 55mg	Dietary Fiber 1g
Saturated Fat 1.5g	**Protein** 10g	Sugars 15g

Stonyfield Organic, Fruit on the Bottom, Fat Free, Blueberry Yogurt

1 container (170g)

Amount per serving	Amount per serving	Amount per serving
Calories 110	**Cholesterol** <5mg	**Total Carbohydrate** 22g
Total Fat 0g	**Sodium** 120mg	Dietary Fiber <1g
Saturated Fat 0g	**Protein** 6g	Sugars 22g

Stonyfield Organic, Fruit on the Bottom, Fat Free, Chocolate Underground Yogurt

1 container (170g)

Amount per serving	Amount per serving	Amount per serving
Calories 170	**Cholesterol** 5mg	**Total Carbohydrate** 36g
Total Fat 0g	**Sodium** 100mg	Dietary Fiber <1g
Saturated Fat 0g	**Protein** 7g	Sugars 35g

Stonyfield Organic, Fruit on the Bottom, Fat Free, Strawberry Yogurt

1 container (170g)

Amount per serving	Amount per serving	Amount per serving
Calories 120	**Cholesterol** <5mg	**Total Carbohydrate** 23g
Total Fat 0g	**Sodium** 140mg	Dietary Fiber <1g
Saturated Fat 0g	**Protein** 6g	Sugars 22g

Stonyfield Organic, Fruit on the Bottom, Pomegranate Raspberry Acai Yogurt

1 container (170g)

Amount per serving	Amount per serving	Amount per serving
Calories 110	**Cholesterol** <5mg	**Total Carbohydrate** 22g
Total Fat 0g	**Sodium** 130mg	Dietary Fiber <1g
Saturated Fat 0g	**Protein** 6g	Sugars 22g

Stonyfield Organic, Greek and Chia, Blood Orange Yogurt

1 container (150g)

Amount per serving	Amount per serving	Amount per serving
Calories 130	**Cholesterol** <5mg	**Total Carbohydrate** 19g
Total Fat 1g	**Sodium** 75mg	Dietary Fiber 1g
Saturated Fat 0g	**Protein** 12g	Sugars 17g

Stonyfield Organic, Greek and Chia, Blueberry Yogurt

1 container (150g)

Amount per serving	Amount per serving	Amount per serving
Calories 140	**Cholesterol** <5mg	**Total Carbohydrate** 20g
Total Fat 1g	**Sodium** 80mg	Dietary Fiber 1g
Saturated Fat 0g	**Protein** 12g	Sugars 18g

Stonyfield Organic, Greek and Chia, Strawberry Raspberry Cranberry Yogurt

1 container (150g)

Amount per serving	Amount per serving	Amount per serving
Calories 130	**Cholesterol** <5mg	**Total Carbohydrate** 18g
Total Fat 1g	**Sodium** 80mg	Dietary Fiber 1g
Saturated Fat 0g	**Protein** 12g	Sugars 16g

Stonyfield Organic, Greek, 0% Fat Black Cherry Yogurt

1 container (150g)

Amount per serving	Amount per serving	Amount per serving
Calories 120	**Cholesterol** <5mg	**Total Carbohydrate** 18g
Total Fat 0g	**Sodium** 55mg	Dietary Fiber 0g
Saturated Fat 0g	**Protein** 13g	Sugars 17g

Stonyfield Organic, Greek, 0% Fat Blueberry Yogurt

1 container (150g)

Amount per serving	Amount per serving	Amount per serving
Calories 120	**Cholesterol** <5mg	**Total Carbohydrate** 17g
Total Fat 0g	**Sodium** 60mg	Dietary Fiber 0g
Saturated Fat 0g	**Protein** 12g	Sugars 15g

Stonyfield Organic, Greek, 0% Fat Café Latte Yogurt

1 container (150g)

Amount per serving	Amount per serving	Amount per serving
Calories 130	Cholesterol <5mg	Total Carbohydrate 20g
Total Fat 0g	Sodium 60mg	Dietary Fiber 0g
Saturated Fat 0g	Protein 12g	Sugars 18g

Stonyfield Organic, Greek, 0% Fat Chocolate Yogurt

1 container (150g)

Amount per serving	Amount per serving	Amount per serving
Calories 140	Cholesterol <5mg	Total Carbohydrate 23g
Total Fat 0g	Sodium 60mg	Dietary Fiber <1g
Saturated Fat 0g	Protein 13g	Sugars 21g

Stonyfield Organic, Greek, 0% Fat Honey Yogurt

1 container (150g)

Amount per serving	Amount per serving	Amount per serving
Calories 120	Cholesterol <5mg	Total Carbohydrate 18g
Total Fat 0g	Sodium 50mg	Dietary Fiber 0g
Saturated Fat 0g	Protein 13g	Sugars 17g

Stonyfield Organic, Greek, 0% Fat Lemon Yogurt

1 container (150g)

Amount per serving	Amount per serving	Amount per serving
Calories 130	Cholesterol <5mg	Total Carbohydrate 19g
Total Fat 0g	Sodium 100mg	Dietary Fiber 0g
Saturated Fat 0g	Protein 13g	Sugars 19g

Stonyfield Organic, Greek, 0% Fat Peach Yogurt

1 container (150g)

Amount per serving	Amount per serving	Amount per serving
Calories 120	Cholesterol <5mg	Total Carbohydrate 18g
Total Fat 0g	Sodium 65mg	Dietary Fiber 0g
Saturated Fat 0g	Protein 12g	Sugars 17g

Stonyfield Organic, Greek, 0% Fat Pineapple Yogurt

1 container (150g)

Amount per serving	Amount per serving	Amount per serving
Calories 130	Cholesterol <5mg	Total Carbohydrate 19g
Total Fat 0g	Sodium 70mg	Dietary Fiber 0g
Saturated Fat 0g	Protein 13g	Sugars 18g

Stonyfield Organic, Greek, 0% Fat Plain Yogurt

1 container (150g)

Amount per serving

Calories 80
Total Fat 0g
    Saturated Fat 0g

Amount per serving

Cholesterol <5mg
Sodium 60mg
Protein 15g

Amount per serving

Total Carbohydrate 6g
    Dietary Fiber 0g
    Sugars 6g

Stonyfield Organic, Greek, 0% Fat Raspberry Yogurt

1 container (150g)

Amount per serving

Calories 120
Total Fat 0g
    Saturated Fat 0g

Amount per serving

Cholesterol <5mg
Sodium 90mg
Protein 13g

Amount per serving

Total Carbohydrate 17g
    Dietary Fiber <1g
    Sugars 16g

Stonyfield Organic, Greek, 0% Fat Salted Caramel Yogurt

1 container (150g)

Amount per serving

Calories 140
Total Fat 0g
    Saturated Fat 0g

Amount per serving

Cholesterol <5mg
Sodium 160mg
Protein 13g

Amount per serving

Total Carbohydrate 22g
    Dietary Fiber <1g
    Sugars 22g

Stonyfield Organic, Greek, 0% Fat Super Fruits Yogurt

1 container (150g)

Amount per serving

Calories 120
Total Fat 0g
    Saturated Fat 0g

Amount per serving

Cholesterol <5mg
Sodium 35mg
Protein 12g

Amount per serving

Total Carbohydrate 19g
    Dietary Fiber 0g
    Sugars 17g

Stonyfield Organic, Greek, 0% Fat Vanilla Yogurt

1 container (150g)

Amount per serving

Calories 130
Total Fat 0g
    Saturated Fat 0g

Amount per serving

Cholesterol <5mg
Sodium 50mg
Protein 12g

Amount per serving

Total Carbohydrate 20g
    Dietary Fiber 0g
    Sugars 19g

Stonyfield Organic, O'Soy, Soy Yogurt, Blueberry on the Bottom

6 oz / 1 container

Amount per serving

Calories 170
Total Fat 2.5g
    Saturated Fat 0g

Amount per serving

Cholesterol 0mg
Sodium 30mg
Protein 7g

Amount per serving

Total Carbohydrate 29g
    Dietary Fiber 2g
    Sugars 26g

Stonyfield Organic, O'Soy, Soy Yogurt, Raspberry on the Bottom

6 oz / 1 container

Amount per serving	Amount per serving	Amount per serving
Calories 170	**Cholesterol** 0mg	**Total Carbohydrate** 29g
Total Fat 2.5g	**Sodium** 75mg	Dietary Fiber 2g
Saturated Fat 0g	**Protein** 7g	Sugars 27g

Stonyfield Organic, O'Soy, Soy Yogurt, Strawberry & Peach on the Bottom

6 oz / 1 container

Amount per serving	Amount per serving	Amount per serving
Calories 100	**Cholesterol** 0mg	**Total Carbohydrate** 15g
Total Fat 2g	**Sodium** 25mg	Dietary Fiber 1g
Saturated Fat 0g	**Protein** 5g	Sugars 13g

Stonyfield Organic, O'Soy, Soy Yogurt, Strawberry on the Bottom

6 oz / 1 container

Amount per serving	Amount per serving	Amount per serving
Calories 170	**Cholesterol** 0mg	**Total Carbohydrate** 29g
Total Fat 2.5g	**Sodium** 55mg	Dietary Fiber 2g
Saturated Fat 0g	**Protein** 7g	Sugars 26g

Stonyfield Organic, O'Soy, Soy Yogurt, Vanilla on the Bottom

6 oz / 1 container

Amount per serving	Amount per serving	Amount per serving
Calories 150	**Cholesterol** 0mg	**Total Carbohydrate** 24g
Total Fat 3g	**Sodium** 40mg	Dietary Fiber 1g
Saturated Fat 0g	**Protein** 7g	Sugars 21g

Stonyfield Organic, Peach Petite Lowfat Crème

1 container (150g)

Amount per serving	Amount per serving	Amount per serving
Calories 130	**Cholesterol** 10mg	**Total Carbohydrate** 17g
Total Fat 2.5g	**Sodium** 65mg	Dietary Fiber 1g
Saturated Fat 1.5g	**Protein** 10g	Sugars 15g

Stonyfield Organic, Plain Petite Lowfat Crème

1 container (150g)

Amount per serving	Amount per serving	Amount per serving
Calories 100	**Cholesterol** 10mg	**Total Carbohydrate** 7g
Total Fat 3g	**Sodium** 60mg	Dietary Fiber 0g
Saturated Fat 2g	**Protein** 12g	Sugars 5g

Stonyfield Organic, Smooth & Creamy, Fat Free, French Vanilla Yogurt, 32 oz

1 cup (227g)

Amount per serving	Amount per serving	Amount per serving
Calories 170	**Cholesterol** 5mg	**Total Carbohydrate** 33g
Total Fat 0g	**Sodium** 140mg	Dietary Fiber 0g
Saturated Fat 0g	**Protein** 9g	Sugars 33g

Stonyfield Organic, Smooth & Creamy, Fat Free, Plain Yogurt, 32 oz

1 cup (227g)

Amount per serving	Amount per serving	Amount per serving
Calories 120	**Cholesterol** 15mg	**Total Carbohydrate** 15g
Total Fat 2g	**Sodium** 140mg	Dietary Fiber 0g
Saturated Fat 1.5g	**Protein** 10g	Sugars 15g

Stonyfield Organic, Smooth & Creamy, Fat Free, Plain Yogurt, 6 oz

1 container (170g)

Amount per serving	Amount per serving	Amount per serving
Calories 80	**Cholesterol** <5mg	**Total Carbohydrate** 12g
Total Fat 0g	**Sodium** 115mg	Dietary Fiber 0g
Saturated Fat 0g	**Protein** 8g	Sugars 12g

Stonyfield Organic, Smooth & Creamy, Low Fat, Banilla Yogurt, 32 oz

1 cup (227g)

Amount per serving	Amount per serving	Amount per serving
Calories 190	**Cholesterol** 15mg	**Total Carbohydrate** 35g
Total Fat 2g	**Sodium** 125mg	Dietary Fiber 0g
Saturated Fat 1.5g	**Protein** 9g	Sugars 35g

Stonyfield Organic, Smooth & Creamy, Low Fat, Blueberry Yogurt, 32 oz

1 cup (227g)

Amount per serving	Amount per serving	Amount per serving
Calories 180	**Cholesterol** 10mg	**Total Carbohydrate** 31g
Total Fat 2g	**Sodium** 160mg	Dietary Fiber 0g
Saturated Fat 1.5g	**Protein** 9g	Sugars 30g

Stonyfield Organic, Smooth & Creamy, Low Fat, French Vanilla Yogurt, 32 oz

1 cup (227g)

Amount per serving	Amount per serving	Amount per serving
Calories 170	**Cholesterol** 10mg	**Total Carbohydrate** 29g
Total Fat 2g	**Sodium** 130mg	Dietary Fiber 0g
Saturated Fat 1.5g	**Protein** 9g	Sugars 29g

Stonyfield Organic, Smooth & Creamy, Low Fat, Plain Yogurt, 32 oz

1 cup (227g)

Amount per serving	Amount per serving	Amount per serving
Calories 120	**Cholesterol** 15mg	**Total Carbohydrate** 15g
Total Fat 2g	**Sodium** 140mg	Dietary Fiber 0g
Saturated Fat 1.5g	**Protein** 10g	Sugars 15g

Stonyfield Organic, Smooth & Creamy, Low Fat, Plain Yogurt, 6 oz

1 container (170g)

Amount per serving	Amount per serving	Amount per serving
Calories 90	**Cholesterol** 10mg	**Total Carbohydrate** 11g
Total Fat 1.5g	**Sodium** 105mg	Dietary Fiber 0g
Saturated Fat 1g	**Protein** 8g	Sugars 11g

Stonyfield Organic, Smooth & Creamy, Low Fat, Strawberry Yogurt, 32 oz

1 cup (227g)

Amount per serving	Amount per serving	Amount per serving
Calories 200	**Cholesterol** 15mg	**Total Carbohydrate** 36g
Total Fat 2g	**Sodium** 125mg	Dietary Fiber 0g
Saturated Fat 1.5g	**Protein** 9g	Sugars 35g

Stonyfield Organic, Smooth & Creamy, Whole Milk, French Vanilla Yogurt, 32 oz

1 cup (227g)

Amount per serving	Amount per serving	Amount per serving
Calories 230	**Cholesterol** 30mg	**Total Carbohydrate** 31g
Total Fat 8g	**Sodium** 120mg	Dietary Fiber 0g
Saturated Fat 4.5g	**Protein** 8g	Sugars 30g

Stonyfield Organic, Smooth & Creamy, Whole Milk, Plain Yogurt, 32 oz

1 cup (227g)

Amount per serving	Amount per serving	Amount per serving
Calories 170	**Cholesterol** 35mg	**Total Carbohydrate** 13g
Total Fat 9g	**Sodium** 125mg	Dietary Fiber 0g
Saturated Fat 5g	**Protein** 9g	Sugars 12g

Stonyfield Organic, Smoothies, Peach

10 oz / 1 bottle

Amount per serving	Amount per serving	Amount per serving
Calories 230	**Cholesterol** 10mg	**Total Carbohydrate** 41g
Total Fat 3g	**Sodium** 140mg	Dietary Fiber <1g
Saturated Fat 2g	**Protein** 10g	Sugars 40g

Stonyfield Organic, Smoothies, Raspberry

10 oz / 1 bottle

Amount per serving	Amount per serving	Amount per serving
Calories 230	**Cholesterol** 10mg	**Total Carbohydrate** 40g
Total Fat 3g	**Sodium** 150mg	Dietary Fiber <1g
Saturated Fat 2g	**Protein** 10g	Sugars 39g

Stonyfield Organic, Smoothies, Strawberry

10 oz / 1 bottle

Amount per serving	Amount per serving	Amount per serving
Calories 230	**Cholesterol** 10mg	**Total Carbohydrate** 39g
Total Fat 3g	**Sodium** 150mg	Dietary Fiber <1g
Saturated Fat 2g	**Protein** 10g	Sugars 38g

Stonyfield Organic, Smoothies, Strawberry Banana

10 oz / 1 bottle

Amount per serving	Amount per serving	Amount per serving
Calories 230	**Cholesterol** 10mg	**Total Carbohydrate** 40g
Total Fat 3g	**Sodium** 150mg	Dietary Fiber <1g
Saturated Fat 2g	**Protein** 10g	Sugars 38g

Stonyfield Organic, Smoothies, Vanilla

10 oz / 1 bottle

Amount per serving	Amount per serving	Amount per serving
Calories 240	**Cholesterol** 10mg	**Total Carbohydrate** 40g
Total Fat 3g	**Sodium** 140mg	Dietary Fiber <1g
Saturated Fat 2g	**Protein** 10g	Sugars 37g

Stonyfield Organic, Smoothies, Wild Berry

10 oz / 1 bottle

Amount per serving	Amount per serving	Amount per serving
Calories 230	**Cholesterol** 10mg	**Total Carbohydrate** 39g
Total Fat 3g	**Sodium** 150mg	Dietary Fiber <1g
Saturated Fat 2g	**Protein** 10g	Sugars 38g

Stonyfield Organic, Strawberry Banana Petite Lowfat Crème

1 container (150g)

Amount per serving	Amount per serving	Amount per serving
Calories 130	**Cholesterol** 10mg	**Total Carbohydrate** 18g
Total Fat 2.5g	**Sodium** 50mg	Dietary Fiber 1g
Saturated Fat 1.5g	**Protein** 10g	Sugars 15g

Stonyfield Organic, Strawberry Petite Lowfat Crème

1 container (150g)

Amount per serving	Amount per serving	Amount per serving
Calories 130	**Cholesterol** 10mg	**Total Carbohydrate** 17g
Total Fat 2.5g	**Sodium** 60mg	Dietary Fiber 1g
Saturated Fat 1.5g	**Protein** 10g	Sugars 15g

Stonyfield Organic, Vanilla Bean Petite Lowfat Crème

1 container (150g)

Amount per serving	Amount per serving	Amount per serving
Calories 140	**Cholesterol** 10mg	**Total Carbohydrate** 20g
Total Fat 2.5g	**Sodium** 50mg	Dietary Fiber 0g
Saturated Fat 1.5g	**Protein** 10g	Sugars 18g

Straus Family Creamery, Organic Blueberry Pomegranate Whole Milk Yofurt

1 cup (227g)

Amount per serving	Amount per serving	Amount per serving
Calories 220	**Cholesterol** 30mg	**Total Carbohydrate** 31g
Total Fat 6g	**Sodium** 110mg	Dietary Fiber 0g
Saturated Fat 4g	**Protein** 11g	Sugars 25g

Straus Family Creamery, Organic Greek Nonfat Yogurt

1 cup (227g)

Amount per serving	Amount per serving	Amount per serving
Calories 160	**Cholesterol** 10mg	**Total Carbohydrate** 19g
Total Fat 0g	**Sodium** 125mg	Dietary Fiber 0g
Saturated Fat 0g	**Protein** 20g	Sugars 12g

Straus Family Creamery, Organic Greek Plain Yogurt

1 cup (227g)

Amount per serving	Amount per serving	Amount per serving
Calories 240	**Cholesterol** 70mg	**Total Carbohydrate** 15g
Total Fat 12g	**Sodium** 105mg	Dietary Fiber 0g
Saturated Fat 8g	**Protein** 19g	Sugars 9g

Straus Family Creamery, Organic Lowfat Yogurt

1 cup (227g)

Amount per serving	Amount per serving	Amount per serving
Calories 150	**Cholesterol** 15mg	**Total Carbohydrate** 21g
Total Fat 1.5g	**Sodium** 140mg	Dietary Fiber 0g
Saturated Fat 0g	**Protein** 12g	Sugars 10g

Straus Family Creamery, Organic Maple Yogurt

1 cup (227g)

Amount per serving	Amount per serving	Amount per serving
Calories 220	**Cholesterol** 15mg	**Total Carbohydrate** 28g
Total Fat 7g	**Sodium** 170mg	Dietary Fiber 0g
Saturated Fat 4.5g	**Protein** 12g	Sugars 27g

Straus Family Creamery, Organic Nonfat Vanilla Yogurt

1 cup (227g)

Amount per serving	Amount per serving	Amount per serving
Calories 190	**Cholesterol** 0mg	**Total Carbohydrate** 34g
Total Fat 0g	**Sodium** 180mg	Dietary Fiber 0g
Saturated Fat 0g	**Protein** 12g	Sugars 33g

Straus Family Creamery, Organic Nonfat Yogurt

1 cup (227g)

Amount per serving	Amount per serving	Amount per serving
Calories 120	**Cholesterol** 10mg	**Total Carbohydrate** 17g
Total Fat 0g	**Sodium** 160mg	Dietary Fiber 0g
Saturated Fat 0g	**Protein** 14g	Sugars 10g

Straus Family Creamery, Organic Plain Yogurt

1 cup (227g)

Amount per serving	Amount per serving	Amount per serving
Calories 170	**Cholesterol** 35mg	**Total Carbohydrate** 14g
Total Fat 7g	**Sodium** 125mg	Dietary Fiber 0g
Saturated Fat 4.5g	**Protein** 12g	Sugars 7g

Straus Family Creamery, Organic Vanilla Yogurt

1 cup (227g)

Amount per serving	Amount per serving	Amount per serving
Calories 240	**Cholesterol** 15mg	**Total Carbohydrate** 33g
Total Fat 7g	**Sodium** 170mg	Dietary Fiber 0g
Saturated Fat 4.5g	**Protein** 11g	Sugars 32g

Protein Foods

Why Eat Protein?

Protein foods include both animal and plant proteins (meat, poultry, fish, eggs, beans, nuts, and seeds) and provide vital nutrients, including B vitamins (niacin, thiamin, riboflavin, and B6), vitamin E, iron, zinc, and magnesium. Proteins also provide the building blocks needed by the body to grow and maintain and repair bones, muscles, cartilage, skin and blood. B vitamins help the body release energy, play a vital role in the function of the nervous system, aid in the formation of red blood cells, and help build tissues. Iron is used to carry oxygen in the blood.

Eggs and dairy products are good protein sources, and you don't need to eat large amounts to meet your protein needs. Vegetarians can easily obtain protein from plant-based foods such as soy products and legumes, lentils, nuts, seeds, and whole grains. Diets that do not include fish and eggs may be low in active forms of omega-3 fatty acids. Walnuts, ground flaxseed, and soybeans are good sources of essential fatty acids. Seafood contains a range of nutrients, notably the omega-3 fatty acids EPA (eicosapentanoic acid) and DHA (docosahexaenoic acid). Eating about 8 ounces per week of a variety of seafood contributes to the prevention of heart disease.

The USDA emphasizes the importance of choosing lean or low-fat protein foods since consuming protein foods that are high in saturated fat and cholesterol may have health implications. Examples of low-fat protein foods include lean beef, pork or ham, chicken or turkey served without skin, fish and shellfish as well as beans, which includes soy products such as tofu and peas.

Why Choose Organic Protein Foods?

Eating humanely raised organic meat confirms the relationship between the health of an animal and the health of the human who consumes it. The animals from which organic protein foods are derived are raised in clean, healthy environments. They are fed certified organic feed and are not given antibiotics or growth hormones to fatten them up quickly.

Similarly, choosing organic plant protein foods affirms the relationship between the health of the land and the health of the people who consume the plants grown on that land. Organic produce is grown and cultivated without the use of synthetic pesticides, chemical fertilizers, sewage sludge, bioengineering, or ionizing radiation. Organic plant protein foods are processed without the use of chemical food additives. In addition, USDA-certified 100% organic food products do not contain genetically modified organisms.

Daily Goal

5 ½ ounces for an adult on a 2,000-calorie diet
8 ounces per week of fish

1 oz. equivalents:
- 1 oz. lean meat, poultry, or fish
- 1 egg (listed in the dairy section)
- ½ oz. nuts or seeds (listed in the fats/oils section)
- 1 Tbsp. peanut butter (listed in the fats/oils section)
- ¼ cup cooked dried beans or peas
- ¼ cup tofu/roasted soybeans

When choosing protein, look for only certified USDA organic lean meats, fish, or other foods with high levels of protein. MyPlate recommends that only ¼ of your plate should be a protein.

Beans / Peas / Legumes

Amy's, Organic Black Bean Chili

1 cup

Amount per serving	Amount per serving	Amount per serving
Calories 200	**Cholesterol** 0mg	**Total Carbohydrate** 31g
Total Fat 3g	**Sodium** 680mg	Dietary Fiber 13g
Saturated Fat 0g	**Protein** 13g	Sugars 3g

Amy's, Organic Light in Sodium, Medium Chili

1 cup

Amount per serving	Amount per serving	Amount per serving
Calories 280	**Cholesterol** 0mg	**Total Carbohydrate** 35g
Total Fat 9g	**Sodium** 340mg	Dietary Fiber 7g
Saturated Fat 1g	**Protein** 15g	Sugars 5g

Amy's, Organic Light in Sodium, Refried Black Beans

1/2 cup

Amount per serving	Amount per serving	Amount per serving
Calories 140	**Cholesterol** 0mg	**Total Carbohydrate** 21g
Total Fat 3g	**Sodium** 220mg	Dietary Fiber 6g
Saturated Fat 0g	**Protein** 8g	Sugars 1g

Amy's, Organic Light in Sodium, Traditional Refried Beans

1/2 cup

Amount per serving	Amount per serving	Amount per serving
Calories 140	**Cholesterol** 0mg	**Total Carbohydrate** 22g
Total Fat 3g	**Sodium** 190mg	Dietary Fiber 6g
Saturated Fat 0g	**Protein** 7g	Sugars 1g

Amy's, Organic, Medium Chili

1 cup

Amount per serving	Amount per serving	Amount per serving
Calories 280	**Cholesterol** 0mg	**Total Carbohydrate** 35g
Total Fat 9g	**Sodium** 680mg	Dietary Fiber 7g
Saturated Fat 1g	**Protein** 15g	Sugars 5g

Amy's, Organic, Medium Chili with Vegetables

1 cup

Amount per serving	Amount per serving	Amount per serving
Calories 230	**Cholesterol** 0mg	**Total Carbohydrate** 34g
Total Fat 6g	**Sodium** 590mg	Dietary Fiber 9g
Saturated Fat 0.5g	**Protein** 10g	Sugars 6g

Amy's, Organic, Refried Beans with Green Chiles

1/2 cup

Amount per serving	Amount per serving	Amount per serving
Calories 130	**Cholesterol** 0mg	**Total Carbohydrate** 20g
Total Fat 3g	**Sodium** 440mg	Dietary Fiber 6g
Saturated Fat 0g	**Protein** 7g	Sugars 1g

Amy's, Organic, Refried Black Beans

1/2 cup

Amount per serving	Amount per serving	Amount per serving
Calories 140	**Cholesterol** 0mg	**Total Carbohydrate** 21g
Total Fat 3g	**Sodium** 440mg	Dietary Fiber 6g
Saturated Fat 0g	**Protein** 8g	Sugars 1g

Amy's, Organic, Spicy Chili

1 cup

Amount per serving	Amount per serving	Amount per serving
Calories 280	**Cholesterol** 0mg	**Total Carbohydrate** 35g
Total Fat 9g	**Sodium** 680mg	Dietary Fiber 7g
Saturated Fat 1g	**Protein** 15g	Sugars 5g

Amy's, Organic, Traditional Refried Beans

1/2 cup

Amount per serving	Amount per serving	Amount per serving
Calories 140	**Cholesterol** 0mg	**Total Carbohydrate** 22g
Total Fat 3g	**Sodium** 390mg	Dietary Fiber 6g
Saturated Fat 0g	**Protein** 7g	Sugars 1g

Amy's, Organic, Vegetarian Baked Beans

1/2 cup

Amount per serving	Amount per serving	Amount per serving
Calories 140	**Cholesterol** 0mg	**Total Carbohydrate** 28g
Total Fat 0.5g	**Sodium** 480mg	Dietary Fiber 6g
Saturated Fat 0g	**Protein** 7g	Sugars 9g

Eden Foods, Aduki Beans, Dry, Organic

3 tbsp

Amount per serving	Amount per serving	Amount per serving
Calories 120	**Cholesterol** 0mg	**Total Carbohydrate** 22g
Total Fat 0g	**Sodium** 0mg	Dietary Fiber 5g
Saturated Fat 0g	**Protein** 7g	Sugars 0g

Eden Foods, Baked Beans with Sorghum & Mustard, Organic

1/2 cup

Amount per serving	Amount per serving	Amount per serving
Calories 150	**Cholesterol** NA	**Total Carbohydrate** 27g
Total Fat 0g	**Sodium** 130mg	Dietary Fiber 7g
Saturated Fat 0g	**Protein** 8g	Sugars 6g

Eden Foods, Black Beans, Organic

1/2 cup

Amount per serving	Amount per serving	Amount per serving
Calories 110	**Cholesterol** NA	**Total Carbohydrate** 18g
Total Fat 1g	**Sodium** 15mg	Dietary Fiber 6g
Saturated Fat 0g	**Protein** 7g	Sugars NA

Eden Foods, Black Eyed Peas, Organic

1/2 cup

Amount per serving	Amount per serving	Amount per serving
Calories 90	**Cholesterol** 0mg	**Total Carbohydrate** 16g
Total Fat 1g	**Sodium** 25mg	Dietary Fiber 4g
Saturated Fat 0g	**Protein** 6g	Sugars <1g

Eden Foods, Black Soybean, Dry, Organic

3 tbsp

Amount per serving	Amount per serving	Amount per serving
Calories 140	**Cholesterol** 0mg	**Total Carbohydrate** 11g
Total Fat 5g	**Sodium** 0mg	Dietary Fiber 8g
Saturated Fat 0.5g	**Protein** 13g	Sugars NA

Eden Foods, Black Soybeans, Organic

1/2 cup

Amount per serving	Amount per serving	Amount per serving
Calories 120	**Cholesterol** 0mg	**Total Carbohydrate** 8g
Total Fat 6g	**Sodium** 30mg	Dietary Fiber 7g
Saturated Fat 1g	**Protein** 11g	Sugars 1g

Eden Foods, Black Turtle Beans, Dry, Organic

3 tbsp

Amount per serving	Amount per serving	Amount per serving
Calories 110	**Cholesterol** NA	**Total Carbohydrate** 18g
Total Fat 1g	**Sodium** 15mg	Dietary Fiber 6g
Saturated Fat 0g	**Protein** 7g	Sugars NA

Eden Foods, Brown Rice & Kidney Beans, Organic

1/2 cup

Amount per serving	Amount per serving	Amount per serving
Calories 110	**Cholesterol** NA	**Total Carbohydrate** 23g
Total Fat 1g	**Sodium** 135mg	Dietary Fiber 3g
Saturated Fat 0g	**Protein** 3g	Sugars 0g

Eden Foods, Brown Rice & Lentils, Organic

1/2 cup

Amount per serving	Amount per serving	Amount per serving
Calories 120	**Cholesterol** NA	**Total Carbohydrate** 23g
Total Fat 1g	**Sodium** 120mg	Dietary Fiber 2g
Saturated Fat 0g	**Protein** 4g	Sugars 0g

Eden Foods, Brown Rice & Pinto Beans, Organic

1/2 cup

Amount per serving	Amount per serving	Amount per serving
Calories 120	**Cholesterol** NA	**Total Carbohydrate** 24g
Total Fat 1g	**Sodium** 140mg	Dietary Fiber 3g
Saturated Fat 0g	**Protein** 4g	Sugars <1g

Eden Foods, Butter Beans (Baby Lima), Organic

1/2 cup

Amount per serving	Amount per serving	Amount per serving
Calories 100	**Cholesterol** 0mg	**Total Carbohydrate** 17g
Total Fat 1g	**Sodium** 35mg	Dietary Fiber 4g
Saturated Fat 0g	**Protein** 5g	Sugars NA

Eden Foods, Cannellini (White Kidney) Beans, Organic

1/2 cup

Amount per serving	Amount per serving	Amount per serving
Calories 100	**Cholesterol** 0mg	**Total Carbohydrate** 17g
Total Fat 1g	**Sodium** 40mg	Dietary Fiber 5g
Saturated Fat 0g	**Protein** 6g	Sugars 1g

Eden Foods, Caribbean Black Beans, Organic

1/2 cup

Amount per serving	Amount per serving	Amount per serving
Calories 90	**Cholesterol** NA	**Total Carbohydrate** 20g
Total Fat 0.5g	**Sodium** 135mg	Dietary Fiber 7g
Saturated Fat 0g	**Protein** 7g	Sugars 1g

Eden Foods, Dark Red Kidney Beans, Dry, Organic

3 tbsp

Amount per serving	Amount per serving	Amount per serving
Calories 120	**Cholesterol** 0mg	**Total Carbohydrate** 21g
Total Fat 0g	**Sodium** 0mg	Dietary Fiber 5g
Saturated Fat 0g	**Protein** 8g	Sugars <1g

Eden Foods, Garbanzo Beans (chick peas), Organic

1/2 cup

Amount per serving	Amount per serving	Amount per serving
Calories 120	**Cholesterol** 0mg	**Total Carbohydrate** 19g
Total Fat 1.5g	**Sodium** 110mg	Dietary Fiber 5g
Saturated Fat 0g	**Protein** 7g	Sugars NA

Eden Foods, Great Northern Beans, Organic

1/2 cup

Amount per serving	Amount per serving	Amount per serving
Calories 110	**Cholesterol** 0mg	**Total Carbohydrate** 20g
Total Fat 1g	**Sodium** 45mg	Dietary Fiber 8g
Saturated Fat 0g	**Protein** 5g	Sugars 1g

Eden Foods, Green Lentils, Dry, Organic

3 tbsp

Amount per serving	Amount per serving	Amount per serving
Calories 120	**Cholesterol** 0mg	**Total Carbohydrate** 21g
Total Fat 0g	**Sodium** 0mg	Dietary Fiber 11g
Saturated Fat 0g	**Protein** 9g	Sugars <1g

Eden Foods, Green Split Peas, Dry, Organic

3 tbsp

Amount per serving	Amount per serving	Amount per serving
Calories 120	**Cholesterol** 0mg	**Total Carbohydrate** 21g
Total Fat 0g	**Sodium** 5mg	Dietary Fiber 9g
Saturated Fat 0g	**Protein** 9g	Sugars 3g

Eden Foods, Kidney (dark red) Beans, Organic

1/2 cup

Amount per serving	Amount per serving	Amount per serving
Calories 100	**Cholesterol** NA	**Total Carbohydrate** 18g
Total Fat 0g	**Sodium** 15mg	Dietary Fiber 10g
Saturated Fat 0g	**Protein** 8g	Sugars <1g

Eden Foods, Lentils with Onion & Bay Leaf, Organic

1/2 cup

Amount per serving	Amount per serving	Amount per serving
Calories 90	Cholesterol NA	Total Carbohydrate 13g
Total Fat 0g	Sodium 210mg	Dietary Fiber 4g
Saturated Fat 0g	Protein 8g	Sugars 0g

Eden Foods, Navy Beans, Dry, Organic

3 tbsp

Amount per serving	Amount per serving	Amount per serving
Calories 120	Cholesterol 0mg	Total Carbohydrate 21g
Total Fat 0.5g	Sodium 0mg	Dietary Fiber 9g
Saturated Fat 0g	Protein 8g	Sugars 1g

Eden Foods, Navy Beans, Organic

1/2 cup

Amount per serving	Amount per serving	Amount per serving
Calories 110	Cholesterol 0mg	Total Carbohydrate 20g
Total Fat 0g	Sodium 15mg	Dietary Fiber 7g
Saturated Fat 0g	Protein 7g	Sugars NA

Eden Foods, Organic Shiro Miso (Aged and Fermented Rice and Soybeans)

1 tbsp

Amount per serving	Amount per serving	Amount per serving
Calories 30	Cholesterol 0mg	Total Carbohydrate 6g
Total Fat 0.5g	Sodium 330mg	Dietary Fiber <1g
Saturated Fat 0g	Protein 1g	Sugars 4g

Eden Foods, Pinto Beans, Dry, Organic

3 tbsp

Amount per serving	Amount per serving	Amount per serving
Calories 120	Cholesterol 0mg	Total Carbohydrate 22g
Total Fat 0g	Sodium 0mg	Dietary Fiber 5g
Saturated Fat 0g	Protein 7g	Sugars <1g

Eden Foods, Pinto Beans, Organic

1/2 cup

Amount per serving	Amount per serving	Amount per serving
Calories 100	Cholesterol 0mg	Total Carbohydrate 18g
Total Fat 0g	Sodium 110mg	Dietary Fiber 6g
Saturated Fat 0g	Protein 6g	Sugars 0g

Eden Foods, Refried Black Beans, Organic

1/2 cup

Amount per serving	Amount per serving	Amount per serving
Calories 110	**Cholesterol** NA	**Total Carbohydrate** 18g
Total Fat 1.5g	**Sodium** 180mg	Dietary Fiber 7g
Saturated Fat 0g	**Protein** 6g	Sugars NA

Eden Foods, Refried Black Soy & Black Beans, Organic

1/2 cup

Amount per serving	Amount per serving	Amount per serving
Calories 90	**Cholesterol** NA	**Total Carbohydrate** 13g
Total Fat 3g	**Sodium** 170mg	Dietary Fiber 6g
Saturated Fat 0.5g	**Protein** 8g	Sugars 1g

Eden Foods, Refried Kidney Beans, Organic

1/2 cup

Amount per serving	Amount per serving	Amount per serving
Calories 80	**Cholesterol** 15mg	**Total Carbohydrate** 15g
Total Fat 1g	**Sodium** 180mg	Dietary Fiber 6g
Saturated Fat 0g	**Protein** 7g	Sugars NA

Eden Foods, Refried Pinto Beans, Organic

1/2 cup

Amount per serving	Amount per serving	Amount per serving
Calories 90	**Cholesterol** NA	**Total Carbohydrate** 19g
Total Fat 1g	**Sodium** 180mg	Dietary Fiber 7g
Saturated Fat 0g	**Protein** 6g	Sugars 1g

Eden Foods, Small Red Beans, Dry, Organic

3 tbsp

Amount per serving	Amount per serving	Amount per serving
Calories 120	**Cholesterol** 0mg	**Total Carbohydrate** 22g
Total Fat 0g	**Sodium** 5mg	Dietary Fiber 3g
Saturated Fat 0g	**Protein** 8g	Sugars <1g

Eden Foods, Small Red Beans, Organic

1/2 cup

Amount per serving	Amount per serving	Amount per serving
Calories 100	**Cholesterol** 0mg	**Total Carbohydrate** 17g
Total Fat 0.5g	**Sodium** 25mg	Dietary Fiber 5g
Saturated Fat 0g	**Protein** 6g	Sugars <1g

Eden Foods, Spicy Refried Black Beans, Organic

1/2 cup

Amount per serving	Amount per serving	Amount per serving
Calories 110	**Cholesterol** NA	**Total Carbohydrate** 18g
Total Fat 1.5g	**Sodium** 180mg	Dietary Fiber 7g
Saturated Fat 0g	**Protein** 6g	Sugars NA

Health Valley Organic, Vegetarian Chili, 40% Less Sodium, 3 Bean Chipotle

1 cup (245g)

Amount per serving	Amount per serving	Amount per serving
Calories 200	**Cholesterol** 0mg	**Total Carbohydrate** 37g
Total Fat 3g	**Sodium** 470mg	Dietary Fiber 8g
Saturated Fat 0g	**Protein** 11g	Sugars 8g

Health Valley Organic, Vegetarian Chili, 40% Less Sodium, Black Bean Molé

1 cup (245g)

Amount per serving	Amount per serving	Amount per serving
Calories 200	**Cholesterol** 0mg	**Total Carbohydrate** 36g
Total Fat 3g	**Sodium** 470mg	Dietary Fiber 7g
Saturated Fat 0g	**Protein** 11g	Sugars 7g

Health Valley Organic, Vegetarian Chili, 40% Less Sodium, Santa Fe White Bean

1 cup (245g)

Amount per serving	Amount per serving	Amount per serving
Calories 200	**Cholesterol** 0mg	**Total Carbohydrate** 39g
Total Fat 3g	**Sodium** 470mg	Dietary Fiber 9g
Saturated Fat 0g	**Protein** 10g	Sugars 9g

Health Valley Organic, Vegetarian Chili, 40% Less Sodium, Spicy Tomato

1 cup

Amount per serving	Amount per serving	Amount per serving
Calories 190	**Cholesterol** 0mg	**Total Carbohydrate** 36g
Total Fat 3g	**Sodium** 470mg	Dietary Fiber 8g
Saturated Fat 0g	**Protein** 10g	Sugars 9g

Health Valley Organic, Vegetarian Chili, No Salt Added Tame Tomato

1 cup (245g)

Amount per serving	Amount per serving	Amount per serving
Calories 210	**Cholesterol** 0mg	**Total Carbohydrate** 41g
Total Fat 2.5g	**Sodium** 70mg	Dietary Fiber 8g
Saturated Fat 0g	**Protein** 10g	Sugars 11g

Health Vally Organic, Vegetarian Chili, 40% Less Sodium, Black Bean Mango

1 cup (245g)

Amount per serving	Amount per serving	Amount per serving
Calories 210	**Cholesterol** 0mg	**Total Carbohydrate** 41g
Total Fat 3g	**Sodium** 460mg	Dietary Fiber 7g
Saturated Fat 0g	**Protein** 9g	Sugars 9g

Westbrae Natural, Organic Black Beans

1/2 cup (130g)

Amount per serving	Amount per serving	Amount per serving
Calories 100	**Cholesterol** 0mg	**Total Carbohydrate** 19g
Total Fat 0g	**Sodium** 140mg	Dietary Fiber 5g
Saturated Fat 0g	**Protein** 6g	Sugars 4g

Westbrae Natural, Organic Chili Beans

1/2 cup (130g)

Amount per serving	Amount per serving	Amount per serving
Calories 100	**Cholesterol** 0mg	**Total Carbohydrate** 19g
Total Fat 0g	**Sodium** 150mg	Dietary Fiber 5g
Saturated Fat 0g	**Protein** 7g	Sugars 2g

Westbrae Natural, Organic Garbanzo Beans

1/2 cup (130g)

Amount per serving	Amount per serving	Amount per serving
Calories 110	**Cholesterol** 0mg	**Total Carbohydrate** 18g
Total Fat 2g	**Sodium** 140mg	Dietary Fiber 5g
Saturated Fat 0g	**Protein** 6g	Sugars 3g

Westbrae Natural, Organic Great Northern Beans

1/2 cup (130g)

Amount per serving	Amount per serving	Amount per serving
Calories 100	**Cholesterol** 0mg	**Total Carbohydrate** 19g
Total Fat 0g	**Sodium** 140mg	Dietary Fiber 6g
Saturated Fat 0g	**Protein** 7g	Sugars 2g

Westbrae Natural, Organic Kidney Beans

1/2 cup (130g)

Amount per serving	Amount per serving	Amount per serving
Calories 100	**Cholesterol** 0mg	**Total Carbohydrate** 18g
Total Fat 0g	**Sodium** 140mg	Dietary Fiber 5g
Saturated Fat 0g	**Protein** 7g	Sugars 2g

Westbrae Natural, Organic Lentils

1/2 cup (130g)

Amount per serving	Amount per serving	Amount per serving
Calories 100	**Cholesterol** 0mg	**Total Carbohydrate** 17g
Total Fat 0g	**Sodium** 150mg	Dietary Fiber 9g
Saturated Fat 0g	**Protein** 8g	Sugars 2g

Westbrae Natural, Organic Pinto Beans

1/2 cup (130g)

Amount per serving	Amount per serving	Amount per serving
Calories 100	**Cholesterol** 0mg	**Total Carbohydrate** 19g
Total Fat 0g	**Sodium** 140mg	Dietary Fiber 7g
Saturated Fat 0g	**Protein** 6g	Sugars 2g

Westbrae Natural, Organic Red Beans

1/2 cup (130g)

Amount per serving	Amount per serving	Amount per serving
Calories 100	**Cholesterol** 0mg	**Total Carbohydrate** 19g
Total Fat 0g	**Sodium** 140mg	Dietary Fiber 7g
Saturated Fat 0g	**Protein** 6g	Sugars 2g

Westbrae Natural, Organic Salad Beans

1/2 cup (130g)

Amount per serving	Amount per serving	Amount per serving
Calories 100	**Cholesterol** 0mg	**Total Carbohydrate** 19g
Total Fat 0.5g	**Sodium** 150mg	Dietary Fiber 5g
Saturated Fat 0g	**Protein** 7g	Sugars 2g

Westbrae Natural, Organic Soup Beans

1/2 cup (130g)

Amount per serving	Amount per serving	Amount per serving
Calories 100	**Cholesterol** 0mg	**Total Carbohydrate** 19g
Total Fat 0g	**Sodium** 140mg	Dietary Fiber 6g
Saturated Fat 0g	**Protein** 6g	Sugars 2g

Westbrae Natural, Organic Soy Beans

1/2 cup (130g)

Amount per serving	Amount per serving	Amount per serving
Calories 150	**Cholesterol** 0mg	**Total Carbohydrate** 11g
Total Fat 7g	**Sodium** 140mg	Dietary Fiber 3g
Saturated Fat 1g	**Protein** 13g	Sugars 3g

Frankfurters / Hot Dogs

Applegate Farms, Great Organic Beef Hot Dog

1 hot dog

Amount per serving	Amount per serving	Amount per serving
Calories 110	**Cholesterol** 30mg	**Total Carbohydrate** 0g
Total Fat 8g	**Sodium** 330mg	Dietary Fiber 0g
Saturated Fat 3g	**Protein** 7g	Sugars 0g

Applegate Farms, Great Organic Chicken Hot Dog

1 hot dog

Amount per serving	Amount per serving	Amount per serving
Calories 70	**Cholesterol** 35mg	**Total Carbohydrate** 0g
Total Fat 3.5g	**Sodium** 360mg	Dietary Fiber 0g
Saturated Fat 1g	**Protein** 8g	Sugars 0g

Applegate Farms, Great Organic Hotdog, Original Beef

1 hot dog

Amount per serving	Amount per serving	Amount per serving
Calories 90	**Cholesterol** 25mg	**Total Carbohydrate** 0g
Total Fat 6g	**Sodium** 380mg	Dietary Fiber 0g
Saturated Fat 2.5g	**Protein** 6g	Sugars 0g

Applegate Farms, Great Organic Stadium Hot Dog

1 hot dog

Amount per serving	Amount per serving	Amount per serving
Calories 110	**Cholesterol** 30mg	**Total Carbohydrate** 0g
Total Fat 8g	**Sodium** 330mg	Dietary Fiber 0g
Saturated Fat 3g	**Protein** 7g	Sugars 0g

Applegate Farms, Great Organic Turkey Hot Dog

1 hot dog

Amount per serving	Amount per serving	Amount per serving
Calories 60	**Cholesterol** 25mg	**Total Carbohydrate** 1g
Total Fat 3.5g	**Sodium** 370mg	Dietary Fiber 0g
Saturated Fat 1g	**Protein** 7g	Sugars 0g

Applegate Farms, Greatest Little Organic Uncured Smoky Cocktail Pork Franks

7 links

Amount per serving	Amount per serving	Amount per serving
Calories 120	**Cholesterol** 35mg	**Total Carbohydrate** 1g
Total Fat 9g	**Sodium** 390mg	Dietary Fiber 0g
Saturated Fat 3.5g	**Protein** 8g	Sugars 1g

Meats, Beef

Applegate Farms, Organic Roast Beef

2 oz

Amount per serving	Amount per serving	Amount per serving
Calories 80	Cholesterol 35mg	Total Carbohydrate 0g
Total Fat 3g	Sodium 320mg	Dietary Fiber 0g
Saturated Fat 1g	Protein 12g	Sugars 0g

Organic Grassfed 85% Lean Ground Beef

4 oz (113g)

Amount per serving	Amount per serving	Amount per serving
Calories 240	Cholesterol 75mg	Total Carbohydrate 0g
Total Fat 17g	Sodium 75mg	Dietary Fiber 0g
Saturated Fat 7g	Protein 21g	Sugars 0g

Organic Prairie, Organic 85% Lean Ground Beef

4 oz (113g)

Amount per serving	Amount per serving	Amount per serving
Calories 240	Cholesterol 75mg	Total Carbohydrate 0g
Total Fat 17g	Sodium 75mg	Dietary Fiber 0g
Saturated Fat 7g	Protein 21g	Sugars 0g

Organic Prairie, Organic Beef Chuck Pot Roast

4 oz (113g)

Amount per serving	Amount per serving	Amount per serving
Calories 210	Cholesterol 95mg	Total Carbohydrate 0g
Total Fat 9g	Sodium 60mg	Dietary Fiber 0g
Saturated Fat 3.5g	Protein 31g	Sugars 0g

Organic Prairie, Organic Beef Liver Steak

2 oz (56g)

Amount per serving	Amount per serving	Amount per serving
Calories 80	Cholesterol 155mg	Total Carbohydrate 2g
Total Fat 2g	Sodium 40mg	Dietary Fiber 0g
Saturated Fat 0.5g	Protein 11g	Sugars 0g

Organic Prairie, Organic Diced Beef

4 oz (113g)

Amount per serving	Amount per serving	Amount per serving
Calories 240	Cholesterol 85mg	Total Carbohydrate 0g
Total Fat 9g	Sodium 60mg	Dietary Fiber 0g
Saturated Fat 3.5g	Protein 38g	Sugars 0g

Organic Prairie, Organic Short Ribs

4 oz (113g)

Amount per serving	Amount per serving	Amount per serving
Calories 320	**Cholesterol** 100mg	**Total Carbohydrate** 0g
Total Fat 24g	**Sodium** 70mg	Dietary Fiber 0g
Saturated Fat 11g	**Protein** 25g	Sugars 0g

Organic Prairie, Organic Uncured Beef Cocktail Franks

3 links (53g)

Amount per serving	Amount per serving	Amount per serving
Calories 150	**Cholesterol** 40mg	**Total Carbohydrate** 1g
Total Fat 13g	**Sodium** 500mg	Dietary Fiber 0g
Saturated Fat 5g	**Protein** 8g	Sugars 1g

Organic Prairie, Organic Uncured Beef Summer Sausage

2 oz (56g)

Amount per serving	Amount per serving	Amount per serving
Calories 200	**Cholesterol** 40mg	**Total Carbohydrate** 1g
Total Fat 18g	**Sodium** 510mg	Dietary Fiber 0g
Saturated Fat 7g	**Protein** 9g	Sugars 0g

Organic Prairie, Organic Uncured Grassfed Beef Hot Dogs

1 hot dog/2 oz (57g)

Amount per serving	Amount per serving	Amount per serving
Calories 160	**Cholesterol** 40mg	**Total Carbohydrate** 1g
Total Fat 13g	**Sodium** 450mg	Dietary Fiber 0g
Saturated Fat 5g	**Protein** 8g	Sugars 1g

Organic Prairie, Premium Organic Boneless New York Strip Steak

1 steak (187g)

Amount per serving	Amount per serving	Amount per serving
Calories 450	**Cholesterol** 150mg	**Total Carbohydrate** 0g
Total Fat 28g	**Sodium** 110mg	Dietary Fiber 0g
Saturated Fat 11g	**Protein** 50g	Sugars 0g

Organic Prairie, Premium Organic Boneless Ribeye Steak

1 steak (173g)

Amount per serving	Amount per serving	Amount per serving
Calories 470	**Cholesterol** 160mg	**Total Carbohydrate** 0g
Total Fat 31g	**Sodium** 100mg	Dietary Fiber 0g
Saturated Fat 12g	**Protein** 47g	Sugars 0g

Organic Prairie, Premium Organic Filet Mignon Steak

1 steak (113g)

Amount per serving	Amount per serving	Amount per serving
Calories 280	**Cholesterol** 75mg	**Total Carbohydrate** 0g
Total Fat 21g	**Sodium** 55mg	Dietary Fiber 0g
Saturated Fat 8g	**Protein** 22g	Sugars 0g

Organic Prairie, Premium Organic Sirloin Steak

1 steak (227g)

Amount per serving	Amount per serving	Amount per serving
Calories 430	**Cholesterol** 163mg	**Total Carbohydrate** 0g
Total Fat 25g	**Sodium** 120mg	Dietary Fiber 0g
Saturated Fat 10g	**Protein** 47g	Sugars 0g

Organic Prairie, Premium Organic Steak Burger Patties

1 patty (150g)

Amount per serving	Amount per serving	Amount per serving
Calories 320	**Cholesterol** 100mg	**Total Carbohydrate** 0g
Total Fat 22g	**Sodium** 100mg	Dietary Fiber 0g
Saturated Fat 9g	**Protein** 28g	Sugars 0g

Organic Prairie, Premium Organic Tenderloin Steak Tips

4 oz raw (113g)

Amount per serving	Amount per serving	Amount per serving
Calories 280	**Cholesterol** 100mg	**Total Carbohydrate** 0g
Total Fat 21g	**Sodium** 55mg	Dietary Fiber 0g
Saturated Fat 8g	**Protein** 22g	Sugars 0g

Meats, Pork

Applegate Farms, Organic Sunday Bacon

2 pan fried slices

Amount per serving	Amount per serving	Amount per serving
Calories 60	**Cholesterol** 10mg	**Total Carbohydrate** 0g
Total Fat 5g	**Sodium** 290mg	Dietary Fiber 0g
Saturated Fat 2g	**Protein** 4g	Sugars 0g

Applegate Farms, Organic Uncured Ham

2 oz

Amount per serving	Amount per serving	Amount per serving
Calories 50	**Cholesterol** 35mg	**Total Carbohydrate** 0g
Total Fat 1.5g	**Sodium** 530mg	Dietary Fiber 0g
Saturated Fat 0.5g	**Protein** 10g	Sugars 0g

Organic Prairie, Organic Boneless Hardwood Smoked Ham

3 oz (85g)

Amount per serving	Amount per serving	Amount per serving
Calories 110	**Cholesterol** 40mg	**Total Carbohydrate** <1g
Total Fat 3g	**Sodium** 940mg	Dietary Fiber 0g
Saturated Fat 1g	**Protein** 19g	Sugars <1g

Organic Prairie, Organic Boneless Pork Loin Roast

4 oz (113g)

Amount per serving	Amount per serving	Amount per serving
Calories 220	**Cholesterol** 65mg	**Total Carbohydrate** 0g
Total Fat 13g	**Sodium** 50mg	Dietary Fiber 0g
Saturated Fat 4.5g	**Protein** 23g	Sugars 1g

Organic Prairie, Organic Brown-n-Serve Pork Breakfast Links

2 links (50g)

Amount per serving	Amount per serving	Amount per serving
Calories 150	**Cholesterol** 40mg	**Total Carbohydrate** 0g
Total Fat 13g	**Sodium** 500mg	Dietary Fiber 0g
Saturated Fat 4g	**Protein** 9g	Sugars 0g

Organic Prairie, Organic Center Cut Boneless Pork Chops

1 chop (113g)

Amount per serving	Amount per serving	Amount per serving
Calories 240	**Cholesterol** 70mg	**Total Carbohydrate** 0g
Total Fat 16g	**Sodium** 50mg	Dietary Fiber 0g
Saturated Fat 6g	**Protein** 23g	Sugars 1g

Organic Prairie, Organic Country Style Boneless Pork Ribs

1 rib (113g)

Amount per serving	Amount per serving	Amount per serving
Calories 160	**Cholesterol** 75mg	**Total Carbohydrate** 0g
Total Fat 7g	**Sodium** 55mg	Dietary Fiber 0g
Saturated Fat 2.5g	**Protein** 23g	Sugars 1g

Organic Prairie, Organic Ground Pork

4 oz (113g)

Amount per serving	Amount per serving	Amount per serving
Calories 300	**Cholesterol** 80mg	**Total Carbohydrate** 0g
Total Fat 24g	**Sodium** 65mg	Dietary Fiber 0g
Saturated Fat 9g	**Protein** 19g	Sugars 0g

Organic Prairie, Organic Hardwood Smoked Bone-In Spiral Cut Sliced Ham

3 oz (85g)

Amount per serving	Amount per serving	Amount per serving
Calories 110	**Cholesterol** 40mg	**Total Carbohydrate** <1g
Total Fat 3g	**Sodium** 940mg	Dietary Fiber 0g
Saturated Fat 1g	**Protein** 19g	Sugars <1g

Organic Prairie, Organic Hardwood Smoked Uncured Bacon

2 slices (54g)

Amount per serving	Amount per serving	Amount per serving
Calories 270	**Cholesterol** 35mg	**Total Carbohydrate** 1g
Total Fat 27g	**Sodium** 620mg	Dietary Fiber 0g
Saturated Fat 10g	**Protein** 5g	Sugars 1g

Organic Prairie, Organic Italian Pork Sausage

1 link (84g)

Amount per serving	Amount per serving	Amount per serving
Calories 200	**Cholesterol** 55mg	**Total Carbohydrate** 1g
Total Fat 18g	**Sodium** 580mg	Dietary Fiber 0g
Saturated Fat 6g	**Protein** 13g	Sugars 0g

Organic Prairie, Organic Pork Bratwurst

1 link (84g)

Amount per serving	Amount per serving	Amount per serving
Calories 210	**Cholesterol** 50mg	**Total Carbohydrate** 1g
Total Fat 19g	**Sodium** 720mg	Dietary Fiber 0g
Saturated Fat 6g	**Protein** 13g	Sugars 1g

Organic Prairie, Organic Pork Breakfast Sausage

4 oz (113g)

Amount per serving	Amount per serving	Amount per serving
Calories 280	**Cholesterol** 75mg	**Total Carbohydrate** 1g
Total Fat 23g	**Sodium** 930mg	Dietary Fiber 0g
Saturated Fat 8g	**Protein** 18g	Sugars 0g

Organic Prairie, Organic Pork Chops Bone-In

1 chop (93g)

Amount per serving	Amount per serving	Amount per serving
Calories 220	**Cholesterol** 80mg	**Total Carbohydrate** 0g
Total Fat 13g	**Sodium** 55mg	Dietary Fiber 0g
Saturated Fat 5g	**Protein** 26g	Sugars 1g

Organic Prairie, Organic Pork Tenderloin

4 oz (113g)

Amount per serving	Amount per serving	Amount per serving
Calories 150	Cholesterol 75mg	Total Carbohydrate 0g
Total Fat 6g	Sodium 55mg	Dietary Fiber 0g
Saturated Fat 2g	Protein 23g	Sugars 1g

Poultry

Applegate Farms, Organic Chicken Strips

3 strips (84g)

Amount per serving	Amount per serving	Amount per serving
Calories 170	Cholesterol 40mg	Total Carbohydrate 12g
Total Fat 8g	Sodium 350mg	Dietary Fiber 0g
Saturated Fat 1g	Protein 12g	Sugars 1g

Applegate Farms, Organic Herb Turkey Breast

2 oz (56g)

Amount per serving	Amount per serving	Amount per serving
Calories 50	Cholesterol 25mg	Total Carbohydrate 0g
Total Fat 0g	Sodium 360mg	Dietary Fiber 0g
Saturated Fat 0g	Protein 10g	Sugars 0g

Applegate Farms, Organic Roasted Chicken Breast

2 oz (56g)

Amount per serving	Amount per serving	Amount per serving
Calories 60	Cholesterol 30mg	Total Carbohydrate 1g
Total Fat 1.5g	Sodium 360mg	Dietary Fiber 0g
Saturated Fat 0.5g	Protein 10g	Sugars 1g

Applegate Farms, Organic Roasted Turkey Breast

2 oz (56g)

Amount per serving	Amount per serving	Amount per serving
Calories 50	Cholesterol 25mg	Total Carbohydrate 0g
Total Fat 0g	Sodium 360mg	Dietary Fiber 0g
Saturated Fat 0g	Protein 10g	Sugars 0g

Applegate Farms, Organic Smoked Chicken Breast

2 oz (56g)

Amount per serving	Amount per serving	Amount per serving
Calories 60	Cholesterol 30mg	Total Carbohydrate 1g
Total Fat 1.5g	Sodium 360mg	Dietary Fiber 0g
Saturated Fat 0.5g	Protein 10g	Sugars 1g

Applegate Farms, Organic Smoked Turkey Breast

2 oz (56g)

Amount per serving	Amount per serving	Amount per serving
Calories 50	**Cholesterol** 25mg	**Total Carbohydrate** 0g
Total Fat 0g	**Sodium** 360mg	Dietary Fiber 0g
Saturated Fat 0g	**Protein** 10g	Sugars 0g

Applegate Farms, Organic Turkey Bacon

1 pan fried slice

Amount per serving	Amount per serving	Amount per serving
Calories 35	**Cholesterol** 25mg	**Total Carbohydrate** 0g
Total Fat 1.5g	**Sodium** 200mg	Dietary Fiber 0g
Saturated Fat 0g	**Protein** 6g	Sugars 0g

Applegate Farms, Organic Turkey Burgers

1 cooked burger (85g)

Amount per serving	Amount per serving	Amount per serving
Calories 140	**Cholesterol** 60mg	**Total Carbohydrate** 0g
Total Fat 7g	**Sodium** 55mg	Dietary Fiber 0g
Saturated Fat 2g	**Protein** 17g	Sugars 0g

Bell&Evans, Fresh Freeze Organic Boneless Skinless Chicken Breasts

4 oz (113g)

Amount per serving	Amount per serving	Amount per serving
Calories 120	**Cholesterol** 75mg	**Total Carbohydrate** 0g
Total Fat 1.5g	**Sodium** 70mg	Dietary Fiber 0g
Saturated Fat 0g	**Protein** 27g	Sugars 0g

Bell&Evans, Fresh, Organic Boneless Skinless Chicken Breasts

4 oz (113g)

Amount per serving	Amount per serving	Amount per serving
Calories 120	**Cholesterol** 75mg	**Total Carbohydrate** 0g
Total Fat 1.5g	**Sodium** 70mg	Dietary Fiber 0g
Saturated Fat 0g	**Protein** 27g	Sugars 0g

Bell&Evans, Fresh, Organic Boneless Skinless Thighs

4 oz (113g)

Amount per serving	Amount per serving	Amount per serving
Calories 160	**Cholesterol** 105mg	**Total Carbohydrate** 1g
Total Fat 8g	**Sodium** 65mg	Dietary Fiber 0g
Saturated Fat 2g	**Protein** 21g	Sugars 0g

Bell&Evans, Fresh, Organic Buffalo Wings

4 oz (113g)

Amount per serving	Amount per serving	Amount per serving
Calories 190	**Cholesterol** 120mg	**Total Carbohydrate** 0g
Total Fat 11g	**Sodium** 106mg	Dietary Fiber 0g
Saturated Fat 3g	**Protein** 22g	Sugars 0g

Bell&Evans, Fresh, Organic Drumsticks

4 oz (113g)

Amount per serving	Amount per serving	Amount per serving
Calories 120	**Cholesterol** 110mg	**Total Carbohydrate** 1g
Total Fat 3g	**Sodium** 136mg	Dietary Fiber 0g
Saturated Fat 1g	**Protein** 22g	Sugars 0g

Bell&Evans, Fresh, Organic Split Halves Breasts

4 oz (113g)

Amount per serving	Amount per serving	Amount per serving
Calories 140	**Cholesterol** 80mg	**Total Carbohydrate** 1g
Total Fat 3.5g	**Sodium** 50mg	Dietary Fiber 0g
Saturated Fat 1g	**Protein** 26g	Sugars 0g

Bell&Evans, Fresh, Organic Thighs

4 oz (113g)

Amount per serving	Amount per serving	Amount per serving
Calories 140	**Cholesterol** 85mg	**Total Carbohydrate** 2g
Total Fat 5g	**Sodium** 90mg	Dietary Fiber 0g
Saturated Fat 1g	**Protein** 22g	Sugars 0g

Bell&Evans, Fresh, Organic Whole Broiler Chicken

4 oz (113g)

Amount per serving	Amount per serving	Amount per serving
Calories 160	**Cholesterol** 90mg	**Total Carbohydrate** 0g
Total Fat 7g	**Sodium** 75mg	Dietary Fiber 0g
Saturated Fat 2.5g	**Protein** 23g	Sugars 0g

Bell&Evans, Fresh, Organic Whole Legs

4 oz (113g)

Amount per serving	Amount per serving	Amount per serving
Calories 170	**Cholesterol** 100mg	**Total Carbohydrate** 0g
Total Fat 11g	**Sodium** 80mg	Dietary Fiber 0g
Saturated Fat 3g	**Protein** 19g	Sugars 0g

Bell&Evans, Fully Cooked, Organic Chicken Franks

1 frank (65g)

Amount per serving	Amount per serving	Amount per serving
Calories 90	**Cholesterol** 35mg	**Total Carbohydrate** 1g
Total Fat 5g	**Sodium** 440mg	Dietary Fiber 0g
Saturated Fat 1.5g	**Protein** 10g	Sugars 0g

FreeBird Chicken, Bagged Whole Bird

4 oz (112g)

Amount per serving	Amount per serving	Amount per serving
Calories 240	**Cholesterol** 85mg	**Total Carbohydrate** 0g
Total Fat 17g	**Sodium** 80mg	Dietary Fiber NA
Saturated Fat 5g	**Protein** 21g	Sugars NA

FreeBird Chicken, Boneless, Skinless Chicken Thighs

1 thigh (69g)

Amount per serving	Amount per serving	Amount per serving
Calories 80	**Cholesterol** 55mg	**Total Carbohydrate** 0g
Total Fat 2.5g	**Sodium** 60mg	Dietary Fiber NA
Saturated Fat 0.5g	**Protein** 14g	Sugars NA

FreeBird Chicken, Chicken Thighs

1 thigh (94g)

Amount per serving	Amount per serving	Amount per serving
Calories 200	**Cholesterol** 80mg	**Total Carbohydrate** 0g
Total Fat 14g	**Sodium** 70mg	Dietary Fiber NA
Saturated Fat 4g	**Protein** 16g	Sugars NA

FreeBird Chicken, Chicken Wings

5 pieces (120g)

Amount per serving	Amount per serving	Amount per serving
Calories 270	**Cholesterol** 90mg	**Total Carbohydrate** 0g
Total Fat 19g	**Sodium** 90mg	Dietary Fiber NA
Saturated Fat 5g	**Protein** 22g	Sugars NA

FreeBird Chicken, Drumsticks

1 drumstick (73g)

Amount per serving	Amount per serving	Amount per serving
Calories 120	**Cholesterol** 60mg	**Total Carbohydrate** 0g
Total Fat 6g	**Sodium** 60mg	Dietary Fiber NA
Saturated Fat 1.5g	**Protein** 14g	Sugars NA

FreeBird Chicken, Party Wings (1st and 2nd Joints, Tips Removed)

5 pieces (120g)

Amount per serving	Amount per serving	Amount per serving
Calories 270	**Cholesterol** 90mg	**Total Carbohydrate** 0g
Total Fat 19g	**Sodium** 90mg	Dietary Fiber NA
Saturated Fat 5g	**Protein** 22g	Sugars NA

FreeBird Chicken, Split Chicken Breast with Ribs

1 breast (145g)

Amount per serving	Amount per serving	Amount per serving
Calories 250	**Cholesterol** 95mg	**Total Carbohydrate** 0g
Total Fat 13g	**Sodium** 90mg	Dietary Fiber NA
Saturated Fat 4g	**Protein** 30g	Sugars NA

FreeBird Chicken, Whole Chicken Legs

1 leg (167g)

Amount per serving	Amount per serving	Amount per serving
Calories 310	**Cholesterol** 140mg	**Total Carbohydrate** 0g
Total Fat 20g	**Sodium** 130mg	Dietary Fiber NA
Saturated Fat 6g	**Protein** 30g	Sugars NA

Organic Prairie, Organic Bone-In, Skin-On Turkey Breast

4 oz (113g)

Amount per serving	Amount per serving	Amount per serving
Calories 180	**Cholesterol** 75mg	**Total Carbohydrate** 0g
Total Fat 8g	**Sodium** 65mg	Dietary Fiber 0g
Saturated Fat 2g	**Protein** 25g	Sugars 0g

Organic Prairie, Organic Boneless and Skinless Chicken Breast (Whole)

4 oz (113g)

Amount per serving	Amount per serving	Amount per serving
Calories 130	**Cholesterol** 80mg	**Total Carbohydrate** 0g
Total Fat 3.5g	**Sodium** 55mg	Dietary Fiber 0g
Saturated Fat 1g	**Protein** 25g	Sugars 0g

Organic Prairie, Organic Boneless Skinless Turkey Breast

4 oz (113g)

Amount per serving	Amount per serving	Amount per serving
Calories 130	**Cholesterol** 70mg	**Total Carbohydrate** 0g
Total Fat 0.5g	**Sodium** 55mg	Dietary Fiber 0g
Saturated Fat 0g	**Protein** 28g	Sugars 0g

Organic Prairie, Organic Chicken Wings Split & Tipped

2–3 wings (114g)

Amount per serving	Amount per serving	Amount per serving
Calories 250	**Cholesterol** 90mg	**Total Carbohydrate** 0g
Total Fat 18g	**Sodium** 85mg	Dietary Fiber 0g
Saturated Fat 5g	**Protein** 21g	Sugars 0g

Organic Prairie, Organic Extra Lean Ground Turkey Breast

2–4 oz (113g)

Amount per serving	Amount per serving	Amount per serving
Calories 130	**Cholesterol** 70mg	**Total Carbohydrate** 0g
Total Fat 0.5g	**Sodium** 55mg	Dietary Fiber 0g
Saturated Fat 0g	**Protein** 28g	Sugars 0g

Organic Prairie, Organic Ground Chicken

4 oz (113g)

Amount per serving	Amount per serving	Amount per serving
Calories 200	**Cholesterol** 95mg	**Total Carbohydrate** 1g
Total Fat 12g	**Sodium** 90mg	Dietary Fiber 0g
Saturated Fat 3g	**Protein** 21g	Sugars 0g

Organic Prairie, Organic Ground Turkey

4 oz (113g)

Amount per serving	Amount per serving	Amount per serving
Calories 180	**Cholesterol** 70mg	**Total Carbohydrate** 0g
Total Fat 9g	**Sodium** 75mg	Dietary Fiber 0g
Saturated Fat 2.5g	**Protein** 23g	Sugars 0g

Organic Prairie, Organic Hardwood Smoked Uncured Turkey Bacon

2 slices (28g)

Amount per serving	Amount per serving	Amount per serving
Calories 40	**Cholesterol** 25mg	**Total Carbohydrate** 0g
Total Fat 1g	**Sodium** 160mg	Dietary Fiber 0g
Saturated Fat 0g	**Protein** 7g	Sugars 0g

Organic Prairie, Organic Italian Chicken Sausage

1 link (85g)

Amount per serving	Amount per serving	Amount per serving
Calories 140	**Cholesterol** 85mg	**Total Carbohydrate** 1g
Total Fat 7g	**Sodium** 480mg	Dietary Fiber 0g
Saturated Fat 2g	**Protein** 18g	Sugars 0g

Organic Prairie, Organic Whole Chicken

4 oz (113g)

Amount per serving	Amount per serving	Amount per serving
Calories 160	**Cholesterol** 85mg	**Total Carbohydrate** 0g
Total Fat 7g	**Sodium** 65mg	Dietary Fiber 0g
Saturated Fat 2g	**Protein** 23g	Sugars 0g

Organic Prairie, Organic Whole Young Turkey

4 oz (113g)

Amount per serving	Amount per serving	Amount per serving
Calories 190	**Cholesterol** 70mg	**Total Carbohydrate** 0g
Total Fat 10g	**Sodium** 70mg	Dietary Fiber 0g
Saturated Fat 3g	**Protein** 23g	Sugars 0g

Protein Alternatives

Bob's Red Mill, Organic Textured Soy Protein

1/4 cup

Amount per serving	Amount per serving	Amount per serving
Calories 80	**Cholesterol** 0mg	**Total Carbohydrate** 5g
Total Fat 1.5g	**Sodium** 0mg	Dietary Fiber 3g
Saturated Fat 0g	**Protein** 7g	Sugars 1.5g

Mori-Nu, Organic Silken Tofu–Firm

3 oz (84g/about 1")

Amount per serving	Amount per serving	Amount per serving
Calories 50	**Cholesterol** 0mg	**Total Carbohydrate** 2g
Total Fat 2.5g	**Sodium** 15mg	Dietary Fiber NA
Saturated Fat 0g	**Protein** 6g	Sugars NA

Wildwood Organic, Organic Meatless Crumbles—Italian Inspired

1/3 cup (55g)

Amount per serving	Amount per serving	Amount per serving
Calories 100	**Cholesterol** 0mg	**Total Carbohydrate** 5g
Total Fat 4g	**Sodium** 360mg	Dietary Fiber 2g
Saturated Fat 0g	**Protein** 9g	Sugars 2g

Wildwood Organic, Organic Meatless Crumbles—Mexican Inspired Mild

1/3 cup (55g)

Amount per serving	Amount per serving	Amount per serving
Calories 60	**Cholesterol** 0mg	**Total Carbohydrate** 7g
Total Fat 2g	**Sodium** 180mg	Dietary Fiber 2g
Saturated Fat 0g	**Protein** 6g	Sugars 2g

Wildwood Organic, Organic Original Meatless Meatballs

6 meatballs (85g)

Amount per serving	Amount per serving	Amount per serving
Calories 220	**Cholesterol** 0mg	**Total Carbohydrate** 17g
Total Fat 13g	**Sodium** 240mg	Dietary Fiber 4g
Saturated Fat 1g	**Protein** 11g	Sugars 3g

Wildwood Organic, Organic SprouTofu® Aloha Baked

3 oz (85g)

Amount per serving	Amount per serving	Amount per serving
Calories 150	**Cholesterol** 0mg	**Total Carbohydrate** 13g
Total Fat 4.5g	**Sodium** 200mg	Dietary Fiber 3g
Saturated Fat 1g	**Protein** 17g	Sugars 2g

Wildwood Organic, Organic SprouTofu® Extra Firm Two Pack

3 oz (85g)

Amount per serving	Amount per serving	Amount per serving
Calories 90	**Cholesterol** 0mg	**Total Carbohydrate** 1g
Total Fat 5g	**Sodium** 15mg	Dietary Fiber 1g
Saturated Fat 1g	**Protein** 9g	Sugars 0g

Wildwood Organic, Organic SprouTofu® Extra Firm Water Pack

3 oz (85g)

Amount per serving	Amount per serving	Amount per serving
Calories 90	**Cholesterol** 0mg	**Total Carbohydrate** 1g
Total Fat 5g	**Sodium** 15mg	Dietary Fiber 1g
Saturated Fat 1g	**Protein** 9g	Sugars 0g

Wildwood Organic, Organic SprouTofu® Firm Two Pack

3 oz (85g)

Amount per serving	Amount per serving	Amount per serving
Calories 80	**Cholesterol** 0mg	**Total Carbohydrate** 1g
Total Fat 5g	**Sodium** 20mg	Dietary Fiber 1g
Saturated Fat 1g	**Protein** 8g	Sugars 0g

Wildwood Organic, Organic SprouTofu® Firm Water Pack

3 oz (85g)

Amount per serving	Amount per serving	Amount per serving
Calories 80	**Cholesterol** 0mg	**Total Carbohydrate** 1g
Total Fat 5g	**Sodium** 20mg	Dietary Fiber 1g
Saturated Fat 1g	**Protein** 8g	Sugars 0g

Wildwood Organic, Organic SprouTofu® Garlic Teriyaki Smoked

3 oz (85g)

Amount per serving	Amount per serving	Amount per serving
Calories 150	**Cholesterol** 0mg	**Total Carbohydrate** 11g
Total Fat 6g	**Sodium** 438mg	Dietary Fiber 2g
Saturated Fat 1g	**Protein** 14g	Sugars 4g

Wildwood Organic, Organic SprouTofu® Hickory BBQ Smoked

3 oz (85g)

Amount per serving	Amount per serving	Amount per serving
Calories 150	**Cholesterol** 0mg	**Total Carbohydrate** 14g
Total Fat 4g	**Sodium** 310mg	Dietary Fiber 3g
Saturated Fat 1g	**Protein** 15g	Sugars 5g

Wildwood Organic, Organic SprouTofu® Hi-Protein, 10 oz

3 oz (85g)

Amount per serving	Amount per serving	Amount per serving
Calories 130	**Cholesterol** 0mg	**Total Carbohydrate** 3g
Total Fat 7g	**Sodium** 15mg	Dietary Fiber <1g
Saturated Fat 1g	**Protein** 14g	Sugars 0g

Wildwood Organic, Organic SprouTofu® Hi-Protein, 20 oz

3 oz (85g)

Amount per serving	Amount per serving	Amount per serving
Calories 130	**Cholesterol** 0mg	**Total Carbohydrate** 3g
Total Fat 7g	**Sodium** 15mg	Dietary Fiber <1g
Saturated Fat 1g	**Protein** 14g	Sugars 0g

Wildwood Organic, Organic SprouTofu® Hi-Protein, 30 oz

3 oz (85g)

Amount per serving	Amount per serving	Amount per serving
Calories 130	**Cholesterol** 0mg	**Total Carbohydrate** 3g
Total Fat 7g	**Sodium** 15mg	Dietary Fiber <1g
Saturated Fat 1g	**Protein** 14g	Sugars 0g

Wildwood Organic, Organic SprouTofu® Medium-Soft Two Pack

3 oz (85g)

Amount per serving	Amount per serving	Amount per serving
Calories 80	**Cholesterol** 0mg	**Total Carbohydrate** 1g
Total Fat 4.5g	**Sodium** 25mg	Dietary Fiber 1g
Saturated Fat 0.5g	**Protein** 8g	Sugars 0g

Wildwood Organic, Organic SprouTofu® Medium-Soft Water Pack

3 oz (85g)

Amount per serving	Amount per serving	Amount per serving
Calories 80	**Cholesterol** 0mg	**Total Carbohydrate** 1g
Total Fat 4.5g	**Sodium** 25mg	Dietary Fiber 1g
Saturated Fat 0.5g	**Protein** 8g	Sugars 0g

Wildwood Organic, Organic SprouTofu® Mild Szechuan Smoked

3 oz (85g)

Amount per serving	Amount per serving	Amount per serving
Calories 150	**Cholesterol** 0mg	**Total Carbohydrate** 11g
Total Fat 6g	**Sodium** 368mg	Dietary Fiber 2g
Saturated Fat 1g	**Protein** 14g	Sugars 4g

Wildwood Organic, Organic SprouTofu® Pineapple Teriyaki Golden

3 oz (85g)

Amount per serving	Amount per serving	Amount per serving
Calories 160	**Cholesterol** 0mg	**Total Carbohydrate** 5g
Total Fat 12g	**Sodium** 230mg	Dietary Fiber 1g
Saturated Fat 1.5g	**Protein** 13g	Sugars 3g

Wildwood Organic, Organic SprouTofu® Royal Thai Baked

3 oz (85g)

Amount per serving	Amount per serving	Amount per serving
Calories 150	**Cholesterol** 0mg	**Total Carbohydrate** 15g
Total Fat 5g	**Sodium** 290mg	Dietary Fiber 3g
Saturated Fat 1g	**Protein** 15g	Sugars 3g

Wildwood Organic, Organic SprouTofu® Savory Baked

3 oz (85g)

Amount per serving	Amount per serving	Amount per serving
Calories 150	**Cholesterol** 0mg	**Total Carbohydrate** 3g
Total Fat 9g	**Sodium** 390mg	Dietary Fiber 1g
Saturated Fat 1.5g	**Protein** 14g	Sugars <1g

Wildwood Organic, Organic SprouTofu® Shiitake Veggie Burger

1 patty (85g)

Amount per serving	Amount per serving	Amount per serving
Calories 170	**Cholesterol** 0mg	**Total Carbohydrate** 8g
Total Fat 11g	**Sodium** 240mg	Dietary Fiber 2g
Saturated Fat 1.5g	**Protein** 8g	Sugars 2g

Wildwood Organic, Organic SprouTofu® Silken Water Pack

3 oz (85g)

Amount per serving	Amount per serving	Amount per serving
Calories 50	**Cholesterol** 0mg	**Total Carbohydrate** 2g
Total Fat 3g	**Sodium** 25mg	Dietary Fiber 0g
Saturated Fat 0g	**Protein** 6g	Sugars 0g

Wildwood Organic, Organic SprouTofu® Southwest Veggie Burger

1 patty (85g)

Amount per serving	Amount per serving	Amount per serving
Calories 180	**Cholesterol** 0mg	**Total Carbohydrate** 8g
Total Fat 12g	**Sodium** 300mg	Dietary Fiber 2g
Saturated Fat 1.5g	**Protein** 10g	Sugars 1g

Wildwood Organic, Organic SprouTofu® Super Firm Water Pack

3 oz (85g)

Amount per serving	Amount per serving	Amount per serving
Calories 130	**Cholesterol** 0mg	**Total Carbohydrate** 3g
Total Fat 7g	**Sodium** 15mg	Dietary Fiber <1g
Saturated Fat 1g	**Protein** 14g	Sugars 0g

Wildwood Organic, Organic SprouTofu® Teriyaki Baked

3 oz (85g)

Amount per serving	Amount per serving	Amount per serving
Calories 140	**Cholesterol** 0mg	**Total Carbohydrate** 13g
Total Fat 4.5g	**Sodium** 450mg	Dietary Fiber 3g
Saturated Fat 1g	**Protein** 14g	Sugars 2g

Wildwood Organic, Organic SprouTofu® Veggie Burger Original

3 oz (85g)

Amount per serving	Amount per serving	Amount per serving
Calories 170	**Cholesterol** 0mg	**Total Carbohydrate** 7g
Total Fat 12g	**Sodium** 300mg	Dietary Fiber 1g
Saturated Fat 1.5g	**Protein** 11g	Sugars 1g

Wildwood Organic, Organic SprouTofu® Veggie Burger Reduced Fat Original

1 patty (85g)

Amount per serving	Amount per serving	Amount per serving
Calories 120	**Cholesterol** 0mg	**Total Carbohydrate** 10g
Total Fat 4.5g	**Sodium** 280mg	Dietary Fiber 3g
Saturated Fat 0.5g	**Protein** 12g	Sugars 2g

Sausages

Aidell's, Organic Cajun Style Andouille Sausage

1 link

Amount per serving	Amount per serving	Amount per serving
Calories 160	**Cholesterol** 90mg	**Total Carbohydrate** 2g
Total Fat 10g	**Sodium** 700mg	Dietary Fiber 0g
Saturated Fat 3g	**Protein** 13g	Sugars 2g

Aidell's, Organic Chicken & Apple Breakfast Links Sausage

2 oz

Amount per serving	Amount per serving	Amount per serving
Calories 120	**Cholesterol** 50mg	**Total Carbohydrate** 2g
Total Fat 8g	**Sodium** 440mg	Dietary Fiber <1g
Saturated Fat 2.5g	**Protein** 9g	Sugars 1g

Aidell's, Organic Chicken & Apple Sausage

1 link

Amount per serving	Amount per serving	Amount per serving
Calories 150	**Cholesterol** 85mg	**Total Carbohydrate** 3g
Total Fat 10g	**Sodium** 680mg	Dietary Fiber <1g
Saturated Fat 3g	**Protein** 13g	Sugars 2g

Aidell's, Organic Chicken and Apple Breakfast Sausage Links

2 oz

Amount per serving	Amount per serving	Amount per serving
Calories 120	**Cholesterol** 50mg	**Total Carbohydrate** 2g
Total Fat 8g	**Sodium** 440mg	Dietary Fiber <1g
Saturated Fat 2.5g	**Protein** 9g	Sugars 1g

Aidell's, Organic Spinach & Feta Sausage

1 link

Amount per serving	Amount per serving	Amount per serving
Calories 140	**Cholesterol** 90mg	**Total Carbohydrate** 2g
Total Fat 9g	**Sodium** 600mg	Dietary Fiber <1g
Saturated Fat 2.5g	**Protein** 13g	Sugars <1g

Aidell's, Organic Sun-Dried Tomato Sausage

1 link

Amount per serving	Amount per serving	Amount per serving
Calories 150	**Cholesterol** 85mg	**Total Carbohydrate** 3g
Total Fat 9g	**Sodium** 770mg	Dietary Fiber <1g
Saturated Fat 2.5g	**Protein** 13g	Sugars 2g

Aidell's, Organic Sweet Basil & Roasted Garlic Sausage

1 link

Amount per serving | Amount per serving | Amount per serving

Calories 160
Total Fat 11g
  Saturated Fat 3g

Cholesterol 65mg
Sodium 700mg
Protein 13g

Total Carbohydrate 2g
  Dietary Fiber <1g
  Sugars 1g

Applegate Farms, Organic Andouille Poultry Sausage

1 link

Amount per serving | Amount per serving | Amount per serving

Calories 140
Total Fat 6g
  Saturated Fat 2g

Cholesterol 60mg
Sodium 620mg
Protein 13g

Total Carbohydrate 3g
  Dietary Fiber 1g
  Sugars 1g

Applegate Farms, Organic Chicken & Apple Sausage

1 link

Amount per serving | Amount per serving | Amount per serving

Calories 140
Total Fat 7g
  Saturated Fat 1.5g

Cholesterol 65mg
Sodium 500mg
Protein 14g

Total Carbohydrate 6g
  Dietary Fiber 1g
  Sugars 3g

Applegate Farms, Organic Fire Roasted Red Pepper Poultry Sausage

1 link

Amount per serving | Amount per serving | Amount per serving

Calories 120
Total Fat 6g
  Saturated Fat 1.5g

Cholesterol 65mg
Sodium 500mg
Protein 14g

Total Carbohydrate 2g
  Dietary Fiber 1g
  Sugars 0g

Applegate Farms, Organic Genoa Salami

1 oz

Amount per serving | Amount per serving | Amount per serving

Calories 100
Total Fat 7g
  Saturated Fat 3g

Cholesterol 20mg
Sodium 480mg
Protein 8g

Total Carbohydrate 0g
  Dietary Fiber 0g
  Sugars 0g

Applegate Farms, Organic Spinach & Feta Poultry Sausage

1 link

Amount per serving | Amount per serving | Amount per serving

Calories 120
Total Fat 7g
  Saturated Fat 2.5g

Cholesterol 60mg
Sodium 470mg
Protein 13g

Total Carbohydrate 2g
  Dietary Fiber 0g
  Sugars 0g

Applegate Farms, Organic Sweet Italian Poultry Sausage

1 link

Amount per serving	Amount per serving	Amount per serving
Calories 130	**Cholesterol** 70mg	**Total Carbohydrate** 2g
Total Fat 6g	**Sodium** 500mg	Dietary Fiber 1g
Saturated Fat 2g	**Protein** 15g	Sugars 0g

Fats and Oils

Why Eat Fats and Oils?

Technically, fats and oils are not a food group, but they do provide important nutrients. So if you've been avoiding fats and oils because you think they all are bad for your health, then it's time to rethink your diet. Some fats are actually essential for health, which is why they are termed "essential fatty acids." Chief among these are the omega-3 fatty acids in nuts, fruits and vegetables, and coldwater fish. Omega-3s are crucial for the health of cell membranes and can help to reduce inflammation throughout the body. They help to reduce the risk of developing cardiovascular disease, joint pain, and inflammation, and they support a healthy immune system.

Omega-6 fatty acids found in eggs, poultry, cereal, and vegetable oils are also considered essential—they act to reduce cholesterol and support blood clotting and healthy skin. But the balance between omega-3s and omega-6s is also important. Experts advise aiming for a four to one ratio, that is, four times as many omega-3s as omega-6s. Since the typical American diet usually contains more omega-6s than omega-3s, most people benefit from reducing omega-6s, especially those found in baked goods and margarine, and increasing consumption of omega-3s.

Learn About Lipids

Lipids—the molecular family consisting of fats, oils, and waxes (though we don't typically eat much wax)—are long chains of carbon atoms, hooking left and right with neighboring carbon atoms. Each carbon atom can also hook above and below with a hydrogen atom. That's why lipid molecules are also referred to as hydrocarbon chains. In some lipids, every possible carbon hook is attached to a hydrogen atom. This makes the chain rigid, like solid animal fats and butter. These lipids are referred to as *saturated fats* because all the places a hydrogen atom can attach to a carbon atom are occupied, or "saturated."

But some lipids have gaps—places where, instead of being filled with a hydrogen atom, the carbon doubles back on itself to create a flexible joint. These *unsaturated lipids* are typically liquid at room temperature, like corn oil and olive oil. In oils that are omega-3s, the very first gap in the hydrocarbon chain, the first place that *isn't* filled up with a hydrogen atom, occurs three positions back from the far end of the chain, which is known as the *omega* end after the last letter in the Greek alphabet. An omega-6 oil has its first gap located six positions back from the omega end of the molecular chain. The specific structure of an oil or fat—namely, the length of the carbon chain, how many unsaturated gaps exist, and where the gaps are located—can radically change its properties. This is something you may want to learn more about if you want to incorporate more healthy fats in your diet.

While the body needs some saturated fats, most of the lipids in our diet should consist of unsaturated fats and oils. Different healthful lipids from different sources provide an array of health benefits. Some help to protect cells and build healthy membranes, while others contribute directly to building the insulating layers wrapped around nerve cells. Even though fats and oils are considered macronutrients, different forms can have a different impact on the body, from wonderful benefits to outright harm.

Avoid Unhealthy Fats

Practically everyone has heard about the problem with trans fats. These are lipids where adjacent gaps in the hydrocarbon molecule are on opposite sides of the chain. The opposite of a trans fat is a cis-fat, meaning that adjacent gaps are on the same side of the chain. In general, trans fats are unhealthy. This is particularly significant since artificial hydrogenation processes, like the ones that turn liquid corn oil into solid margarine, wind up generating unhealthy trans fats as a byproduct. (There are some naturally occurring forms of trans fats that may be healthy to consume in moderation, including CLA or conjugated linoleic acid. CLA is sometimes purified and sold as a nutritional supplement, particularly for weight loss. But healthy trans fats are definitely the exception and not the rule.)

Consumption of trans fats poses a risk to health—it is linked to elevated blood cholesterol and increased risk of heart disease. Trans fats are produced when liquid fat (oil) is turned into solid fat when heated to high temperatures or through a process called partial or complete hydrogenation. Partially hydrogenated oil is a common source of trans fats and is often used in commercially prepared baked goods, margarine, snack foods, and many processed foods.

Nutritionists advise eliminating trans fats and sharply limiting or avoiding saturated fats in favor of a diet including the healthy unsaturated fats. In recent years, we've grown accustomed to hearing trans fats and saturated fat criticized as equally unhealthy. In general, saturated fats are animal fats—butter, cream, bacon, cheese, lard, and shortening—are all high in saturated fats, while unsaturated fats come from plants—olive, corn, soy, safflower, sunflower, and canola oils. But not all saturated fats are equally unhealthy. Some, like coconut oil, with its high saturated fat content—92%—have many health benefits and can be heated to moderately high temperatures without forming unhealthy trans fats.

Choose Healthy Fats

Olive oil and other vegetable oils are high in healthy monounsaturated fats (meaning they have exactly one gap in the hydrocarbon chain), are good for your heart, and taste terrific. Used sparingly, butter, which contains about 50% saturated fat, can also be part of a healthy diet. It's rich in vitamin A and helps the body absorb fat-soluble vitamins from other foods. Other plant-derived oils—safflower, sunflower, canola, peanut, sesame, avocado, and grapessed oils, also contain healthy fats. Even lard—rendered pork fat—that is nearly half monounsaturated fat and contains just 35% saturated fat may, in moderation, be considered a healthy fat. It can substitute for vegetable shortening, which contains unhealthy trans fats. Duck fat is also high in monounsaturated fats and contains just 14% saturated fats, making it another better-for-you fat.

Why Choose Organic Fats and Oils?

Organic oils come from plants grown under the USDA National Organic Program (NOP) standard of organic farming. Organic crops are grown without the use of synthetic pesticides, synthetic nitrogen fertilizers, or GMOs. Organic oils are naturally pressed, expeller-pressed, or cold-pressed—mechanical processes that extract oil in a way that preserves their flavor, aroma, and nutrients, rather than chemical extraction, which often involves the use of the petrochemical hexane.

Daily Goal

Six teaspoons for an adult on a 2,000-calorie diet.

1 teaspoon equivalents:
    1 tbsp. oil = 2.5 teaspoons
    1 tbsp. mayonnaise = 2.5 teaspoons
    4 large olives = ½ teaspoon
    1 oz. nuts = 3 teaspoons
    2 tbsp. peanut butter = 4 teaspoons

Dips

Muir Glen Organic, Black Bean & Corn Salsa, 16 oz

2 tbsp (31g)

Amount per serving	Amount per serving	Amount per serving
Calories 15	**Cholesterol** 0mg	**Total Carbohydrate** 3g
Total Fat 0g	**Sodium** 100mg	Dietary Fiber <1g
Saturated Fat 0g	**Protein** <1g	Sugars 1g

Muir Glen Organic, Chipotle Salsa, 16 oz

2 tbsp (31g)

Amount per serving	Amount per serving	Amount per serving
Calories 10	**Cholesterol** 0mg	**Total Carbohydrate** 2g
Total Fat 0g	**Sodium** 100mg	Dietary Fiber 0g
Saturated Fat 0g	**Protein** 0g	Sugars 1g

Muir Glen Organic, Garlic Cilantro Salsa, 16 oz

2 tbsp (31g)

Amount per serving	Amount per serving	Amount per serving
Calories 10	**Cholesterol** 0mg	**Total Carbohydrate** 2g
Total Fat 0g	**Sodium** 100mg	Dietary Fiber 0g
Saturated Fat 0g	**Protein** 0g	Sugars 1g

Muir Glen Organic, Medium Salsa, 16 oz

2 tbsp (31g)

Amount per serving	Amount per serving	Amount per serving
Calories 10	**Cholesterol** 0mg	**Total Carbohydrate** 2g
Total Fat 0g	**Sodium** 100mg	Dietary Fiber 0g
Saturated Fat 0g	**Protein** 0g	Sugars 1g

Muir Glen Organic, Mild Salsa, 16 oz

2 tbsp (31g)

Amount per serving	Amount per serving	Amount per serving
Calories 10	**Cholesterol** 0mg	**Total Carbohydrate** 3g
Total Fat 0g	**Sodium** 130mg	Dietary Fiber 0g
Saturated Fat 0g	**Protein** 0g	Sugars 1g

OrganicVille®, Medium Organic Salsa

2 tbsp (30g)

Amount per serving	Amount per serving	Amount per serving
Calories 15	**Cholesterol** 0mg	**Total Carbohydrate** 3g
Total Fat 0g	**Sodium** 135mg	Dietary Fiber 0g
Saturated Fat 0g	**Protein** 0g	Sugars 1g

OrganicVille®, Mild Organic Salsa

2 tbsp (30g)

Amount per serving	Amount per serving	Amount per serving
Calories 15	**Cholesterol** 0mg	**Total Carbohydrate** 0g
Total Fat 0g	**Sodium** 135mg	Dietary Fiber 0g
Saturated Fat 0g	**Protein** 0g	Sugars 1g

OrganicVille®, Pineapple Organic Salsa

2 tbsp (30g)

Amount per serving	Amount per serving	Amount per serving
Calories 15	**Cholesterol** 0mg	**Total Carbohydrate** 4g
Total Fat 0g	**Sodium** 130mg	Dietary Fiber 0g
Saturated Fat 0g	**Protein** 0g	Sugars 3g

Simply Organic Foods, Chipotle Black Bean Dip

1 tsp

Amount per serving	Amount per serving	Amount per serving
Calories 15	**Cholesterol** 0mg	**Total Carbohydrate** 2g
Total Fat 0g	**Sodium** 140mg	Dietary Fiber 1g
Saturated Fat 0g	**Protein** 1g	Sugars 0g

Simply Organic Foods, Creamy Dill Dip

1/2 tsp

Amount per serving	Amount per serving	Amount per serving
Calories 5	**Cholesterol** 0mg	**Total Carbohydrate** <1g
Total Fat 0g	**Sodium** 90mg	Dietary Fiber 0g
Saturated Fat 0g	**Protein** 0g	Sugars 0g

Simply Organic Foods, Fruit Dip

2 tsp

Amount per serving	Amount per serving	Amount per serving
Calories 15	**Cholesterol** 0mg	**Total Carbohydrate** 4g
Total Fat 0g	**Sodium** 0mg	Dietary Fiber 0g
Saturated Fat 0g	**Protein** 0g	Sugars 3g

Simply Organic Foods, Guacamole Dip

1/2 tsp

Amount per serving	Amount per serving	Amount per serving
Calories 5	**Cholesterol** 0mg	**Total Carbohydrate** 1g
Total Fat 0g	**Sodium** 90mg	Dietary Fiber 0g
Saturated Fat 0g	**Protein** 0g	Sugars 0g

Simply Organic Foods, Ranch Dip

1 tsp

Amount per serving	Amount per serving	Amount per serving
Calories 10	**Cholesterol** 0mg	**Total Carbohydrate** 1g
Total Fat 0g	**Sodium** 140mg	Dietary Fiber 0g
Saturated Fat 0g	**Protein** 1g	Sugars 1g

Simply Organic Foods, Spinach Dip

3/4 tsp

Amount per serving	Amount per serving	Amount per serving
Calories 10	**Cholesterol** 0mg	**Total Carbohydrate** 2g
Total Fat 0g	**Sodium** 105mg	Dietary Fiber 0g
Saturated Fat 0g	**Protein** 0g	Sugars 0g

Wan Ja Shan, Organic Gluten Free Mild Sodium Dumpling Sauce, 6.7 oz

1 tbsp (15 ml)

Amount per serving	Amount per serving	Amount per serving
Calories 11	**Cholesterol** 0mg	**Total Carbohydrate** 2g
Total Fat 0g	**Sodium** 319mg	Dietary Fiber NA
Saturated Fat NA	**Protein** 0g	Sugars 1g

Wan Ja Shan, Organic Gluten Free Ponzu Viniagrette, 10 oz

1 tbsp (15 ml)

Amount per serving	Amount per serving	Amount per serving
Calories 16	**Cholesterol** 0mg	**Total Carbohydrate** 3g
Total Fat 0g	**Sodium** 235mg	Dietary Fiber 0g
Saturated Fat 0g	**Protein** 1g	Sugars 2g

Wan Ja Shan, Organic Gluten Free, Hot, Mild Sodium Dumpling Sauce, 6.7 oz

1 tbsp (15 ml)

Amount per serving	Amount per serving	Amount per serving
Calories 11	**Cholesterol** 0mg	**Total Carbohydrate** 2g
Total Fat 0g	**Sodium** 319mg	Dietary Fiber NA
Saturated Fat NA	**Protein** 0g	Sugars 1g

Wildwood Organic, Organic Hot Salsa

2 tbsp (30g)

Amount per serving	Amount per serving	Amount per serving
Calories 10	**Cholesterol** 0mg	**Total Carbohydrate** 2g
Total Fat 0g	**Sodium** 160mg	Dietary Fiber 1g
Saturated Fat 0g	**Protein** 0g	Sugars 1g

Wildwood Organic, Organic Medium Salsa

2 tbsp (30g)

Amount per serving	Amount per serving	Amount per serving
Calories 10	**Cholesterol** 0mg	**Total Carbohydrate** 2g
Total Fat 0g	**Sodium** 140mg	Dietary Fiber 0g
Saturated Fat 0g	**Protein** 0g	Sugars 1g

Wildwood Organic, Organic Mild Salsa

2 tbsp (30g)

Amount per serving	Amount per serving	Amount per serving
Calories 10	**Cholesterol** 0mg	**Total Carbohydrate** 2g
Total Fat 0g	**Sodium** 140mg	Dietary Fiber 0g
Saturated Fat 0g	**Protein** 0g	Sugars 1g

Oils

Bragg, Organic Extra Virgin Olive Oil

1 tbsp (15 ml)

Amount per serving	Amount per serving	Amount per serving
Calories 120	**Cholesterol** 0mg	**Total Carbohydrate** 0g
Total Fat 14g	**Sodium** 0mg	Dietary Fiber NA
Saturated Fat 2g	**Protein** 0g	Sugars NA

Eden Foods, Safflower Oil, High Oleic, Organic

1 tbsp

Amount per serving	Amount per serving	Amount per serving
Calories 120	**Cholesterol** 0mg	**Total Carbohydrate** 0g
Total Fat 14g	**Sodium** 0mg	Dietary Fiber 0g
Saturated Fat 1g	**Protein** 0g	Sugars 0g

Eden Foods, Sesame Oil, Extra Virgin, Organic

1 tbsp (15 ml)

Amount per serving	Amount per serving	Amount per serving
Calories 120	**Cholesterol** 0mg	**Total Carbohydrate** 0g
Total Fat 14g	**Sodium** 0mg	Dietary Fiber 0g
Saturated Fat 2g	**Protein** 0g	Sugars 0g

Jovial Foods, Jovial 100% Organic Olive Oil

1 tbsp (15 ml)

Amount per serving	Amount per serving	Amount per serving
Calories 120	**Cholesterol** NA	**Total Carbohydrate** 0g
Total Fat 14g	**Sodium** 0mg	Dietary Fiber NA
Saturated Fat 2g	**Protein** 0g	Sugars NA

Lucini, Limited Reserve, Premium Select Extra Virgin Olive Oil, 100% Organic

1 tbsp

Amount per serving	Amount per serving	Amount per serving
Calories 120	**Cholesterol** NA	**Total Carbohydrate** 0g
Total Fat 14g	**Sodium** 0mg	Dietary Fiber NA
Saturated Fat 2g	**Protein** 0g	Sugars NA

Newman's Own Organics, Organic Balsamic Vinegar

1 tbsp (15 ml)

Amount per serving	Amount per serving	Amount per serving
Calories 20	**Cholesterol** 0mg	**Total Carbohydrate** 5g
Total Fat 0g	**Sodium** 0mg	Dietary Fiber 0g
Saturated Fat NA	**Protein** 0g	Sugars 5g

Newman's Own Organics, Organic Extra Virgin Olive Oil

1 tbsp (15 ml)

Amount per serving	Amount per serving	Amount per serving
Calories 130	**Cholesterol** 0mg	**Total Carbohydrate** 0g
Total Fat 14g	**Sodium** 0mg	Dietary Fiber 0g
Saturated Fat NA	**Protein** 0g	Sugars 5g

Spectrum®, Canola Oil, Organic, Refined

1 tbsp (14g)

Amount per serving	Amount per serving	Amount per serving
Calories 120	**Cholesterol** 0mg	**Total Carbohydrate** 0g
Total Fat 14g	**Sodium** 0mg	Dietary Fiber NA
Saturated Fat 1g	**Protein** 0g	Sugars NA

Spectrum®, Coconut Oil, Organic, Refined

1 tbsp (14g)

Amount per serving	Amount per serving	Amount per serving
Calories 120	**Cholesterol** 0mg	**Total Carbohydrate** 0g
Total Fat 14g	**Sodium** 0mg	Dietary Fiber NA
Saturated Fat 12g	**Protein** 0g	Sugars NA

Spectrum®, Coconut Oil, Organic, Virgin Unrefined

1 tbsp (14g)

Amount per serving	Amount per serving	Amount per serving
Calories 120	**Cholesterol** 0mg	**Total Carbohydrate** 0g
Total Fat 14g	**Sodium** 0mg	Dietary Fiber NA
Saturated Fat 12g	**Protein** 0g	Sugars NA

Spectrum®, Mediterranean Olive Oil, Organic, Extra Virgin, Unrefined

1 tbsp (14g)

Amount per serving	Amount per serving	Amount per serving
Calories 120	Cholesterol 0mg	Total Carbohydrate 0g
Total Fat 14g	Sodium 0mg	Dietary Fiber NA
Saturated Fat 2.5g	Protein 0g	Sugars NA

Spectrum®, Olive Oil, Organic, Extra Virgin, Unrefined

1 tbsp (14g)

Amount per serving	Amount per serving	Amount per serving
Calories 120	Cholesterol 0mg	Total Carbohydrate 0g
Total Fat 14g	Sodium 0mg	Dietary Fiber NA
Saturated Fat 2.5g	Protein 0g	Sugars NA

Spectrum®, Organic Asian Stir Fry Oil

1 tbsp

Amount per serving	Amount per serving	Amount per serving
Calories 120	Cholesterol 0mg	Total Carbohydrate 0g
Total Fat 14g	Sodium 0mg	Dietary Fiber NA
Saturated Fat 2g	Protein 0g	Sugars NA

Spectrum®, Organic Extra Virgin Olive Oil Spray

1/3 second spray (0.25g)

Amount per serving	Amount per serving	Amount per serving
Calories 0	Cholesterol 0mg	Total Carbohydrate 0g
Total Fat 0g	Sodium 0mg	Dietary Fiber NA
Saturated Fat 0g	Protein 0g	Sugars NA

Spectrum®, Organic Shortening

1 tbsp (12g)

Amount per serving	Amount per serving	Amount per serving
Calories 110	Cholesterol 0mg	Total Carbohydrate 0g
Total Fat 12g	Sodium 0mg	Dietary Fiber 0g
Saturated Fat 6g	Protein 0g	Sugars 0g

Spectrum®, Organic Shortening, Butter Flavor

1 tbsp (12g)

Amount per serving	Amount per serving	Amount per serving
Calories 110	Cholesterol 0mg	Total Carbohydrate 0g
Total Fat 12g	Sodium 0mg	Dietary Fiber 0g
Saturated Fat 6g	Protein 0g	Sugars 0g

Spectrum®, Organic, High Heat, Sunflower Oil Spray

1/3 second spray (0.25g)

Amount per serving	Amount per serving	Amount per serving
Calories 0	**Cholesterol** 0mg	**Total Carbohydrate** 0g
Total Fat 0g	**Sodium** 0mg	Dietary Fiber NA
Saturated Fat 0g	**Protein** 0g	Sugars NA

Spectrum®, Peanut Oil, Organic, Hight Heat, Refined

1 tbsp

Amount per serving	Amount per serving	Amount per serving
Calories 120	**Cholesterol** 0mg	**Total Carbohydrate** 0g
Total Fat 14g	**Sodium** 0mg	Dietary Fiber NA
Saturated Fat 1.5g	**Protein** 0g	Sugars NA

Spectrum®, Safflower Oil, Organic, High Heat, Refined

1 tbsp (14g)

Amount per serving	Amount per serving	Amount per serving
Calories 120	**Cholesterol** 0mg	**Total Carbohydrate** 0g
Total Fat 14g	**Sodium** 0mg	Dietary Fiber NA
Saturated Fat 1g	**Protein** 0g	Sugars NA

Spectrum®, Sesame Oil, Organic, Unrefined

1 tbsp (14g)

Amount per serving	Amount per serving	Amount per serving
Calories 120	**Cholesterol** 0mg	**Total Carbohydrate** 0g
Total Fat 14g	**Sodium** 0mg	Dietary Fiber NA
Saturated Fat 2g	**Protein** 0g	Sugars NA

Spectrum®, Sesame Oil, Toasted, Organic, Unrefined

1 tbsp (14g)

Amount per serving	Amount per serving	Amount per serving
Calories 120	**Cholesterol** 0mg	**Total Carbohydrate** 0g
Total Fat 14g	**Sodium** 0mg	Dietary Fiber NA
Saturated Fat 2g	**Protein** 0g	Sugars NA

Spectrum®, Sunflower Oil, Organic, High Heat, Refined

1 tbsp (14g)

Amount per serving	Amount per serving	Amount per serving
Calories 120	**Cholesterol** 0mg	**Total Carbohydrate** 0g
Total Fat 14g	**Sodium** 0mg	Dietary Fiber NA
Saturated Fat 1g	**Protein** 0g	Sugars NA

Salad Dressings

Annie's, Organic Balsamic Vinaigrette

2 tbsp

Amount per serving	Amount per serving	Amount per serving
Calories 100	**Cholesterol** NA	**Total Carbohydrate** 1g
Total Fat 10g	**Sodium** 55mg	Dietary Fiber NA
Saturated Fat 1g	**Protein** 0g	Sugars 1g

Annie's, Organic Buttermilk Dressing

2 tbsp

Amount per serving	Amount per serving	Amount per serving
Calories 70	**Cholesterol** 250mg	**Total Carbohydrate** 1g
Total Fat 6g	**Sodium** 250mg	Dietary Fiber NA
Saturated Fat 1g	**Protein** 1g	Sugars 1g

Annie's, Organic Caesar Dressing

2 tbsp

Amount per serving	Amount per serving	Amount per serving
Calories 110	**Cholesterol** 10mg	**Total Carbohydrate** 3g
Total Fat 11g	**Sodium** 240mg	Dietary Fiber NA
Saturated Fat 1g	**Protein** 1g	Sugars 2g

Annie's, Organic Cowgirl Ranch Dressing

2 tbsp

Amount per serving	Amount per serving	Amount per serving
Calories 110	**Cholesterol** 10mg	**Total Carbohydrate** 3g
Total Fat 11g	**Sodium** 240mg	Dietary Fiber NA
Saturated Fat 1g	**Protein** 1g	Sugars 2g

Annie's, Organic Creamy Asiago Cheese Dressing

2 tbsp

Amount per serving	Amount per serving	Amount per serving
Calories 80	**Cholesterol** 5mg	**Total Carbohydrate** 1g
Total Fat 8g	**Sodium** 320mg	Dietary Fiber NA
Saturated Fat 1g	**Protein** 1g	Sugars NA

Annie's, Organic French Dressing

2 tbsp

Amount per serving	Amount per serving	Amount per serving
Calories 110	**Cholesterol** NA	**Total Carbohydrate** 3g
Total Fat 11g	**Sodium** 200mg	Dietary Fiber NA
Saturated Fat 1g	**Protein** 0g	Sugars 3g

Annie's, Organic Green Garlic Dressing

2 tbsp

Amount per serving	Amount per serving	Amount per serving
Calories 80	**Cholesterol** NA	**Total Carbohydrate** 2g
Total Fat 8g	**Sodium** 170mg	Dietary Fiber NA
Saturated Fat 0.5g	**Protein** 0g	Sugars 1g

Annie's, Organic Green Goddess Dressing

2 tbsp

Amount per serving	Amount per serving	Amount per serving
Calories 110	**Cholesterol** 5mg	**Total Carbohydrate** 1g
Total Fat 11g	**Sodium** 260mg	Dietary Fiber NA
Saturated Fat 1.5g	**Protein** 0g	Sugars 1g

Annie's, Organic Oil & Vinegar

2 tbsp

Amount per serving	Amount per serving	Amount per serving
Calories 120	**Cholesterol** NA	**Total Carbohydrate** 1g
Total Fat 13g	**Sodium** 220mg	Dietary Fiber NA
Saturated Fat 1g	**Protein** 0g	Sugars NA

Annie's, Organic Papaya Poppy Seed Dressing

2 tbsp

Amount per serving	Amount per serving	Amount per serving
Calories 90	**Cholesterol** NA	**Total Carbohydrate** 5g
Total Fat 8g	**Sodium** 180mg	Dietary Fiber NA
Saturated Fat 1g	**Protein** 0g	Sugars 4g

Annie's, Organic Pomegranate Vinaigrette Dressing

2 tbsp

Amount per serving	Amount per serving	Amount per serving
Calories 70	**Cholesterol** NA	**Total Carbohydrate** 2g
Total Fat 7g	**Sodium** 220mg	Dietary Fiber NA
Saturated Fat 0.5g	**Protein** 0g	Sugars 1g

Annie's, Organic Red Wine & Olive Oil Vinaigrette

2 tbsp

Amount per serving	Amount per serving	Amount per serving
Calories 130	**Cholesterol** NA	**Total Carbohydrate** 0g
Total Fat 14g	**Sodium** 190mg	Dietary Fiber NA
Saturated Fat 2g	**Protein** 0g	Sugars NA

Annie's, Organic Roasted Garlic Vinaigrette

2 tbsp

Amount per serving	Amount per serving	Amount per serving
Calories 110	**Cholesterol** NA	**Total Carbohydrate** 3g
Total Fat 11g	**Sodium** 220mg	Dietary Fiber NA
Saturated Fat 1g	**Protein** 0g	Sugars 2g

Annie's, Organic Sesame Ginger Vinaigrette

2 tbsp

Amount per serving	Amount per serving	Amount per serving
Calories 90	**Cholesterol** NA	**Total Carbohydrate** 4g
Total Fat 8g	**Sodium** 250mg	Dietary Fiber NA
Saturated Fat 1g	**Protein** 1g	Sugars 3g

Annie's, Organic Thousand Island Dressing

2 tbsp

Amount per serving	Amount per serving	Amount per serving
Calories 90	**Cholesterol** NA	**Total Carbohydrate** 5g
Total Fat 8g	**Sodium** 360mg	Dietary Fiber NA
Saturated Fat 1g	**Protein** 0g	Sugars 5g

Bragg, Organic Salad Dressings, Braggberry Organic Dressing & Marinade

2 tbsp (32g)

Amount per serving	Amount per serving	Amount per serving
Calories 20	**Cholesterol** 0mg	**Total Carbohydrate** 5g
Total Fat 0g	**Sodium** 0mg	Dietary Fiber 0g
Saturated Fat 0g	**Protein** 0g	Sugars 3g

Bragg, Organic Salad Dressings, Ginger & Sesame Dressing

2 tbsp (30g)

Amount per serving	Amount per serving	Amount per serving
Calories 90	**Cholesterol** 0mg	**Total Carbohydrate** 3g
Total Fat 9g	**Sodium** 170mg	Dietary Fiber 0g
Saturated Fat 1.5g	**Protein** 0g	Sugars 2g

Bragg, Organic Salad Dressings, Healthy Made with Organic Vinaigrette Dressing

2 tbsp (30g)

Amount per serving	Amount per serving	Amount per serving
Calories 90	**Cholesterol** 0mg	**Total Carbohydrate** 3g
Total Fat 9g	**Sodium** 60mg	Dietary Fiber 0g
Saturated Fat 1.5g	**Protein** 0g	Sugars 2g

Bragg, Organic Salad Dressings, Healthy Organic, Fat Free Vinaigrette Dressing

2 tbsp (30 ml)

Amount per serving	Amount per serving	Amount per serving
Calories 15	Cholesterol 0mg	Total Carbohydrate 4g
Total Fat 0g	Sodium 0mg	Dietary Fiber 0g
Saturated Fat 0g	Protein 0g	Sugars 3g

Bragg, Organic Salad Dressings, Organic Hawaiian Dressing & Marinade

2 tbsp (32g)

Amount per serving	Amount per serving	Amount per serving
Calories 20	Cholesterol 0mg	Total Carbohydrate 5g
Total Fat 0g	Sodium 0mg	Dietary Fiber 0g
Saturated Fat 0g	Protein 0g	Sugars 4g

Bragg, Organic Salad Dressings, Pomegranate Vinaigrette

2 tbsp (30 ml)

Amount per serving	Amount per serving	Amount per serving
Calories 15	Cholesterol 0mg	Total Carbohydrate 3g
Total Fat 0g	Sodium 10mg	Dietary Fiber 0g
Saturated Fat 0g	Protein 0g	Sugars 3g

Earth Balance, Organic Dressing

1 tbsp

Amount per serving	Amount per serving	Amount per serving
Calories 90	Cholesterol 0mg	Total Carbohydrate 0g
Total Fat 9g	Sodium 65mg	Dietary Fiber NA
Saturated Fat 0.5g	Protein 0g	Sugars NA

Marzetti®, Organic Balsamic Vinaigrette

2 tbsp

Amount per serving	Amount per serving	Amount per serving
Calories 100	Cholesterol 0mg	Total Carbohydrate 3g
Total Fat 9g	Sodium 360mg	Dietary Fiber 0g
Saturated Fat 2g	Protein 0g	Sugars 3g

Marzetti®, Organic Blue Cheese

2 tbsp

Amount per serving	Amount per serving	Amount per serving
Calories 130	Cholesterol 10mg	Total Carbohydrate 1g
Total Fat 14g	Sodium 300mg	Dietary Fiber 0g
Saturated Fat 3g	Protein 1g	Sugars 1g

Marzetti®, Organic Caesar

2 tbsp

Amount per serving	Amount per serving	Amount per serving
Calories 140	Cholesterol 5mg	Total Carbohydrate 1g
Total Fat 15g	Sodium 250mg	Dietary Fiber 0g
Saturated Fat 3g	Protein 0g	Sugars 1g

Marzetti®, Organic Parmesan Ranch

2 tbsp

Amount per serving	Amount per serving	Amount per serving
Calories 130	Cholesterol 5mg	Total Carbohydrate 2g
Total Fat 14g	Sodium 300mg	Dietary Fiber 0g
Saturated Fat 2g	Protein 1g	Sugars 1g

Newman's Own, Organic Lite Balsamic Salad Dressing

2 tbsp

Amount per serving	Amount per serving	Amount per serving
Calories 45	Cholesterol 0mg	Total Carbohydrate 2g
Total Fat 4g	Sodium 450mg	Dietary Fiber 0g
Saturated Fat 0.5g	Protein 0g	Sugars 2g

Newman's Own, Organic Tuscan Italian Salad Dressing

2 tbsp

Amount per serving	Amount per serving	Amount per serving
Calories 100	Cholesterol 0mg	Total Carbohydrate 2g
Total Fat 11g	Sodium 380mg	Dietary Fiber 0g
Saturated Fat 1.5g	Protein 0g	Sugars 1g

OrganicVille®, Dijon Organic Vinaigrette

2 tbsp (30g)

Amount per serving	Amount per serving	Amount per serving
Calories 60	Cholesterol 0mg	Total Carbohydrate 2g
Total Fat 6g	Sodium 240mg	Dietary Fiber 0g
Saturated Fat 0.5g	Protein 0g	Sugars 2g

OrganicVille®, Miso Ginger Organic Vinaigrette

2 tbsp (30g)

Amount per serving	Amount per serving	Amount per serving
Calories 100	Cholesterol 0mg	Total Carbohydrate 1g
Total Fat 10g	Sodium 250mg	Dietary Fiber 0g
Saturated Fat 1.5g	Protein 0g	Sugars <1g

OrganicVille®, Non Dairy Coleslaw Organic Dressing

2 tbsp (30g)

Amount per serving	Amount per serving	Amount per serving
Calories 70	**Cholesterol** 0mg	**Total Carbohydrate** 6g
Total Fat 4.5g	**Sodium** 125mg	Dietary Fiber 0g
Saturated Fat 1g	**Protein** 0g	Sugars 6g

OrganicVille®, Non Dairy Olive Oil & Balsamic Organic Vinaigrette

2 tbsp (30g)

Amount per serving	Amount per serving	Amount per serving
Calories 100	**Cholesterol** 0mg	**Total Carbohydrate** <1g
Total Fat 11g	**Sodium** 240mg	Dietary Fiber 0g
Saturated Fat 1.5g	**Protein** 0g	Sugars <1g

OrganicVille®, Non Dairy Thousand Island Dressing

2 tbsp (30g)

Amount per serving	Amount per serving	Amount per serving
Calories 80	**Cholesterol** 0mg	**Total Carbohydrate** 4g
Total Fat 7g	**Sodium** 160mg	Dietary Fiber 0g
Saturated Fat 1g	**Protein** 0g	Sugars 3g

OrganicVille®, Pomegranate Organic Vinaigrette

2 tbsp (30g)

Amount per serving	Amount per serving	Amount per serving
Calories 100	**Cholesterol** 0mg	**Total Carbohydrate** 2g
Total Fat 10g	**Sodium** 55mg	Dietary Fiber 0g
Saturated Fat 1.5g	**Protein** 0g	Sugars 2g

OrganicVille®, Sun Dried Tomato & Garlic Organic Vinaigrette

2 tbsp (30g)

Amount per serving	Amount per serving	Amount per serving
Calories 70	**Cholesterol** 0mg	**Total Carbohydrate** <1g
Total Fat 12g	**Sodium** 250mg	Dietary Fiber 0g
Saturated Fat 1.5g	**Protein** 0g	Sugars 0g

Simply Organic Foods, Classic Caesar Dressing

3/4 tsp

Amount per serving	Amount per serving	Amount per serving
Calories 15	**Cholesterol** 0mg	**Total Carbohydrate** 3g
Total Fat 0g	**Sodium** 240mg	Dietary Fiber 0g
Saturated Fat 0g	**Protein** 0g	Sugars 1g

Simply Organic Foods, Garlic Vinaigrette Dressing
3/4 tsp

Amount per serving	Amount per serving	Amount per serving
Calories 10	**Cholesterol** 0mg	**Total Carbohydrate** 2g
Total Fat 0g	**Sodium** 230mg	Dietary Fiber 0g
Saturated Fat 0g	**Protein** 0g	Sugars 1g

Simply Organic Foods, Italian Dressing
3/4 tsp

Amount per serving	Amount per serving	Amount per serving
Calories 5	**Cholesterol** 0mg	**Total Carbohydrate** 2g
Total Fat 0g	**Sodium** 150mg	Dietary Fiber 0g
Saturated Fat 0g	**Protein** 0g	Sugars 1g

Simply Organic Foods, Orange Ginger Vinaigrette
1 tsp

Amount per serving	Amount per serving	Amount per serving
Calories 5	**Cholesterol** 0mg	**Total Carbohydrate** 2g
Total Fat 0g	**Sodium** 170mg	Dietary Fiber 0g
Saturated Fat 0g	**Protein** 0g	Sugars 0g

Simply Organic Foods, Pineapple Cilantro Vinaigrette
1 tsp

Amount per serving	Amount per serving	Amount per serving
Calories 10	**Cholesterol** 0mg	**Total Carbohydrate** 2g
Total Fat 0g	**Sodium** 150mg	Dietary Fiber 0g
Saturated Fat 0g	**Protein** 0g	Sugars 0g

Simply Organic Foods, Ranch Dressing
1 tsp

Amount per serving	Amount per serving	Amount per serving
Calories 10	**Cholesterol** 0mg	**Total Carbohydrate** 1g
Total Fat 0g	**Sodium** 140mg	Dietary Fiber 0g
Saturated Fat 0g	**Protein** 1g	Sugars 1g

Spectrum®, Apple Cider Vinegar, Organic, Filtered
1 tbsp (15g)

Amount per serving	Amount per serving	Amount per serving
Calories 5	**Cholesterol** NA	**Total Carbohydrate** 1g
Total Fat 0g	**Sodium** 0mg	Dietary Fiber NA
Saturated Fat NA	**Protein** 0g	Sugars 1g

Spectrum®, Apple Cider Vinegar, Organic, Unfiltered

1 tbsp (15g)

Amount per serving	Amount per serving	Amount per serving
Calories 5	**Cholesterol** NA	**Total Carbohydrate** 1g
Total Fat 0g	**Sodium** 0mg	Dietary Fiber NA
Saturated Fat NA	**Protein** 0g	Sugars 1g

Spectrum®, Balsamic Vinegar, Organic

1 tbsp (15 ml)

Amount per serving	Amount per serving	Amount per serving
Calories 15	**Cholesterol** NA	**Total Carbohydrate** 4g
Total Fat 0g	**Sodium** 5mg	Dietary Fiber NA
Saturated Fat NA	**Protein** 0g	Sugars 2g

Spectrum®, Golden Balsamic Vinegar, Organic

1 tbsp (15 ml)

Amount per serving	Amount per serving	Amount per serving
Calories 20	**Cholesterol** NA	**Total Carbohydrate** 5g
Total Fat 0g	**Sodium** 5mg	Dietary Fiber NA
Saturated Fat NA	**Protein** 0g	Sugars 3g

Spectrum®, Red Wine Vinegar, Organic

1 tbsp (15 ml)

Amount per serving	Amount per serving	Amount per serving
Calories 0	**Cholesterol** NA	**Total Carbohydrate** 1g
Total Fat 0g	**Sodium** 5mg	Dietary Fiber NA
Saturated Fat NA	**Protein** 0g	Sugars 0g

Spectrum®, White Vinegar, Organic, Distilled

1 tbsp (15g)

Amount per serving	Amount per serving	Amount per serving
Calories 0	**Cholesterol** NA	**Total Carbohydrate** 0g
Total Fat 0g	**Sodium** 0mg	Dietary Fiber NA
Saturated Fat NA	**Protein** 0g	Sugars NA

Spectrum®, White Wine Vinegar, Organic

1 tbsp (15 ml)

Amount per serving	Amount per serving	Amount per serving
Calories 0	**Cholesterol** NA	**Total Carbohydrate** 1g
Total Fat 0g	**Sodium** 5mg	Dietary Fiber NA
Saturated Fat NA	**Protein** 0g	Sugars 0g

Spreads

Wildwood Organic, Organic Aioli Spread

1 tbsp (15 ml)

Amount per serving	Amount per serving	Amount per serving
Calories 80	**Cholesterol** 0mg	**Total Carbohydrate** <1g
Total Fat 9g	**Sodium** 80mg	Dietary Fiber 0g
Saturated Fat 1g	**Protein** 0g	Sugars 0g

Nut Butters

Arrowhead Mills, Gluten-Free Nut Butters, Organic Peanut Butter, Creamy

2 tbsp

Amount per serving	Amount per serving	Amount per serving
Calories 190	**Cholesterol** 0mg	**Total Carbohydrate** 6g
Total Fat 17g	**Sodium** 0mg	Dietary Fiber 2g
Saturated Fat 2.5g	**Protein** 8g	Sugars 1g

Arrowhead Mills, Gluten-Free Nut Butters, Organic Peanut Butter, Crunchy

2 tbsp

Amount per serving	Amount per serving	Amount per serving
Calories 190	**Cholesterol** 0mg	**Total Carbohydrate** 6g
Total Fat 17g	**Sodium** 0mg	Dietary Fiber 2g
Saturated Fat 2.5g	**Protein** 8g	Sugars 1g

Arrowhead Mills, Gluten-Free Nut Butters, Sesame Tahini, Organic

2 tbsp

Amount per serving	Amount per serving	Amount per serving
Calories 190	**Cholesterol** 0mg	**Total Carbohydrate** 3g
Total Fat 18g	**Sodium** 10mg	Dietary Fiber <1g
Saturated Fat 2.5g	**Protein** 8g	Sugars 1g

Manna Organics, Manna Butter Amaretto Almond

2 tbsp (28g)

Amount per serving	Amount per serving	Amount per serving
Calories 160	**Cholesterol** 0mg	**Total Carbohydrate** 6g
Total Fat 14g	**Sodium** 0mg	Dietary Fiber 3g
Saturated Fat 1g	**Protein** 6g	Sugars 1g

Manna Organics, Manna Butter Cashew Bliss

2 tbsp (28g/1 oz)

Amount per serving	Amount per serving	Amount per serving
Calories 160	**Cholesterol** 0mg	**Total Carbohydrate** 9g
Total Fat 12g	**Sodium** 0mg	Dietary Fiber 1g
Saturated Fat 2.5g	**Protein** 5g	Sugars 2g

Manna Organics, Manna Butter Cinnamon Chili

2 tbsp (28g)

Amount per serving	Amount per serving	Amount per serving
Calories 160	**Cholesterol** 0mg	**Total Carbohydrate** 9g
Total Fat 14g	**Sodium** 50mg	Dietary Fiber 2g
Saturated Fat 1.5g	**Protein** 3g	Sugars 4g

Manna Organics, Manna Butter Cinnamon Date

2 tbsp (28g)

Amount per serving	Amount per serving	Amount per serving
Calories 160	**Cholesterol** 0mg	**Total Carbohydrate** 8g
Total Fat 13g	**Sodium** 100mg	Dietary Fiber 3g
Saturated Fat 1g	**Protein** 4g	Sugars 4g

Manna Organics, Manna Butter Coconut Cashew

2 tbsp (28g)

Amount per serving	Amount per serving	Amount per serving
Calories 160	**Cholesterol** 0mg	**Total Carbohydrate** 9g
Total Fat 13g	**Sodium** 30mg	Dietary Fiber 1g
Saturated Fat 4.5g	**Protein** 4g	Sugars 3g

Manna Organics, Manna Butter Dark Chocolate Pecan

2 tbsp (28g)

Amount per serving	Amount per serving	Amount per serving
Calories 150	**Cholesterol** 0mg	**Total Carbohydrate** 12g
Total Fat 10g	**Sodium** 75mg	Dietary Fiber 1g
Saturated Fat 1.5g	**Protein** 3g	Sugars 8g

Manna Organics, Manna Butter Fig and Nut

2 tbsp (28g)

Amount per serving	Amount per serving	Amount per serving
Calories 140	**Cholesterol** 0mg	**Total Carbohydrate** 10g
Total Fat 11g	**Sodium** 0mg	Dietary Fiber 2g
Saturated Fat 1g	**Protein** 4g	Sugars 5g

Manna Organics, Manna Butter Nut Medley

2 tbsp (28g)

Amount per serving	Amount per serving	Amount per serving
Calories 170	**Cholesterol** 0mg	**Total Carbohydrate** 6g
Total Fat 15g	**Sodium** 95mg	Dietary Fiber 2g
Saturated Fat 1.5g	**Protein** 5g	Sugars 1g

Manna Organics, Manna Butter Tahini

2 tbsp (28g)

Amount per serving	Amount per serving	Amount per serving
Calories 160	**Cholesterol** 0mg	**Total Carbohydrate** 7g
Total Fat 14g	**Sodium** 0mg	Dietary Fiber 3g
Saturated Fat 2g	**Protein** 5g	Sugars 0g

MaraNatha Nut Butters, Organic Almond Butter, No Salt Added, Creamy

2 tbsp

Amount per serving	Amount per serving	Amount per serving
Calories 190	**Cholesterol** 0mg	**Total Carbohydrate** 6g
Total Fat 16g	**Sodium** 0mg	Dietary Fiber 4g
Saturated Fat 1.5g	**Protein** 7g	Sugars 2g

MaraNatha Nut Butters, Organic Almond Butter, No Salt Added, Crunchy

2 tbsp

Amount per serving	Amount per serving	Amount per serving
Calories 190	**Cholesterol** 0mg	**Total Carbohydrate** 6g
Total Fat 16g	**Sodium** 0mg	Dietary Fiber 4g
Saturated Fat 1.5g	**Protein** 7g	Sugars 2g

MaraNatha Nut Butters, Organic Peanut Butter, with Hint of Sea Salt, Creamy

2 tbsp

Amount per serving	Amount per serving	Amount per serving
Calories 190	**Cholesterol** 0mg	**Total Carbohydrate** 7g
Total Fat 16g	**Sodium** 80mg	Dietary Fiber 3g
Saturated Fat 2g	**Protein** 8g	Sugars 1g

MaraNatha Nut Butters, Organic Peanut Butter, with Hint of Sea Salt, Crunchy

2 tbsp

Amount per serving	Amount per serving	Amount per serving
Calories 190	**Cholesterol** 0mg	**Total Carbohydrate** 7g
Total Fat 16g	**Sodium** 80mg	Dietary Fiber 3g
Saturated Fat 2g	**Protein** 8g	Sugars 1g

MaraNatha Nut Butters, Organic Raw Almond Butter, No Salt, Creamy

2 tbsp

Amount per serving	Amount per serving	Amount per serving
Calories 190	**Cholesterol** 0mg	**Total Carbohydrate** 6g
Total Fat 17g	**Sodium** 0mg	Dietary Fiber 4g
Saturated Fat 1.5g	**Protein** 7g	Sugars 2g

MaraNatha Nut Butters, Organic Raw Almond Butter, No Salt, Crunchy

2 tbsp

Amount per serving	Amount per serving	Amount per serving
Calories 190	**Cholesterol** 0mg	**Total Carbohydrate** 6g
Total Fat 17g	**Sodium** 0mg	Dietary Fiber 4g
Saturated Fat 1.5g	**Protein** 7g	Sugars 2g

Once Again, 6-Pack Organic Almond Butter Lightly Toasted Creamy

30g

Amount per serving	Amount per serving	Amount per serving
Calories 190	**Cholesterol** 0mg	**Total Carbohydrate** 6g
Total Fat 17g	**Sodium** 0mg	Dietary Fiber 3g
Saturated Fat 1.5g	**Protein** 6g	Sugars 2g

Once Again, Organic Almond Butter Creamy

30g

Amount per serving	Amount per serving	Amount per serving
Calories 190	**Cholesterol** 0mg	**Total Carbohydrate** 6g
Total Fat 18g	**Sodium** 0mg	Dietary Fiber 1g
Saturated Fat 1.5g	**Protein** 5g	Sugars 2g

Once Again, Organic Almond Butter Lightly Toasted Creamy

30g

Amount per serving	Amount per serving	Amount per serving
Calories 190	**Cholesterol** 0mg	**Total Carbohydrate** 6g
Total Fat 17g	**Sodium** 0mg	Dietary Fiber 3g
Saturated Fat 1.5g	**Protein** 6g	Sugars 2g

Once Again, Organic Almond Butter Lightly Toasted Crunchy

30g

Amount per serving	Amount per serving	Amount per serving
Calories 190	**Cholesterol** 0mg	**Total Carbohydrate** 6g
Total Fat 17g	**Sodium** 0mg	Dietary Fiber 3g
Saturated Fat 1.5g	**Protein** 6g	Sugars 2g

Santa Cruz Organic, Creamy Dark Roasted Peanut Butter

2 tbsp (32g)

Amount per serving	Amount per serving	Amount per serving
Calories 210	**Cholesterol** 0mg	**Total Carbohydrate** 6g
Total Fat 17g	**Sodium** 50mg	Dietary Fiber 2g
Saturated Fat 2.5g	**Protein** 7g	Sugars 1g

Santa Cruz Organic, Creamy Light Roasted Peanut Butter

2 tbsp (32g)

Amount per serving	Amount per serving	Amount per serving
Calories 210	**Cholesterol** 0mg	**Total Carbohydrate** 6g
Total Fat 17g	**Sodium** 50mg	Dietary Fiber 2g
Saturated Fat 2.5g	**Protein** 7g	Sugars 1g

Santa Cruz Organic, Crunchy Dark Roasted Peanut Butter

2 tbsp (32g)

Amount per serving	Amount per serving	Amount per serving
Calories 210	**Cholesterol** 0mg	**Total Carbohydrate** 6g
Total Fat 17g	**Sodium** 45mg	Dietary Fiber 2g
Saturated Fat 2.5g	**Protein** 7g	Sugars 1g

Santa Cruz Organic, Crunchy Light Roasted Peanut Butter

2 tbsp (32g)

Amount per serving	Amount per serving	Amount per serving
Calories 210	**Cholesterol** 0mg	**Total Carbohydrate** 6g
Total Fat 17g	**Sodium** 45mg	Dietary Fiber 2g
Saturated Fat 2.5g	**Protein** 7g	Sugars 1g

SunButter, Organic Unsweetened

2 tbsp

Amount per serving	Amount per serving	Amount per serving
Calories 220	**Cholesterol** 0mg	**Total Carbohydrate** 5g
Total Fat 20g	**Sodium** 30mg	Dietary Fiber 2g
Saturated Fat 2g	**Protein** 6g	Sugars 1g

Nuts

Eden Foods, Pistachios, Shelled, Dry Roasted, Organic

3 tbsp

Amount per serving	Amount per serving	Amount per serving
Calories 160	**Cholesterol** 0mg	**Total Carbohydrate** 7g
Total Fat 12g	**Sodium** 60mg	Dietary Fiber 3g
Saturated Fat 1.5g	**Protein** 6g	Sugars 1g

Eden Foods, Tamari Roasted Almonds, Organic

3 tbsp

Amount per serving	Amount per serving	Amount per serving
Calories 160	**Cholesterol** 0mg	**Total Carbohydrate** 8g
Total Fat 11g	**Sodium** 65mg	Dietary Fiber 4g
Saturated Fat 1g	**Protein** 8g	Sugars <1g

Manna Organics, Organic Almonds

1 oz (28g)

Amount per serving	Amount per serving	Amount per serving
Calories 160	**Cholesterol** 0mg	**Total Carbohydrate** 6g
Total Fat 14g	**Sodium** 0mg	Dietary Fiber 3g
Saturated Fat 1g	**Protein** 6g	Sugars 1g

Manna Organics, Organic Cashews

1 oz (28g)

Amount per serving	Amount per serving	Amount per serving
Calories 160	**Cholesterol** 0mg	**Total Carbohydrate** 9g
Total Fat 12g	**Sodium** 0mg	Dietary Fiber 1g
Saturated Fat 2.5g	**Protein** 5g	Sugars 2g

Manna Organics, Organic Hazelnuts

1 oz (28g)

Amount per serving	Amount per serving	Amount per serving
Calories 180	**Cholesterol** 0mg	**Total Carbohydrate** 5g
Total Fat 17g	**Sodium** 0mg	Dietary Fiber 3g
Saturated Fat 1.5g	**Protein** 4g	Sugars 1g

Manna Organics, Organic Walnuts

1 oz (28g)

Amount per serving	Amount per serving	Amount per serving
Calories 190	**Cholesterol** 0mg	**Total Carbohydrate** 4g
Total Fat 18g	**Sodium** 0mg	Dietary Fiber 2g
Saturated Fat 1.5g	**Protein** 4g	Sugars 1g

Seeds

Arrowhead Mills, Organic Flax Seed Meal

2 tbsp

Amount per serving	Amount per serving	Amount per serving
Calories 80	**Cholesterol** 0mg	**Total Carbohydrate** 5g
Total Fat 4.5g	**Sodium** 0mg	Dietary Fiber 4g
Saturated Fat 0.5g	**Protein** 3g	Sugars 0g

Arrowhead Mills, Organic Golden Flax Seeds

3 tbsp

Amount per serving	Amount per serving	Amount per serving
Calories 160	**Cholesterol** 0mg	**Total Carbohydrate** 10g
Total Fat 10g	**Sodium** 10mg	Dietary Fiber 9g
Saturated Fat 1g	**Protein** 8g	Sugars 0g

Bob's Red Mill, Organic Brown Flaxseed Meal

2 tbsp

Amount per serving	Amount per serving	Amount per serving
Calories 60	**Cholesterol** 0mg	**Total Carbohydrate** 4g
Total Fat 4.5g	**Sodium** 0mg	Dietary Fiber 4g
Saturated Fat 0g	**Protein** 3g	Sugars 0g

Bob's Red Mill, Organic Brown Flaxseeds

2 tbsp

Amount per serving	Amount per serving	Amount per serving
Calories 90	**Cholesterol** 0mg	**Total Carbohydrate** 7g
Total Fat 8g	**Sodium** 5mg	Dietary Fiber 6g
Saturated Fat 0.5g	**Protein** 4g	Sugars 0g

Eden Foods, Pumpkin Seeds, Dry Roasted & Sea Salted, Organic

1/4 cup

Amount per serving	Amount per serving	Amount per serving
Calories 200	**Cholesterol** 0mg	**Total Carbohydrate** 5g
Total Fat 16g	**Sodium** 100mg	Dietary Fiber 5g
Saturated Fat 3g	**Protein** 10g	Sugars 0g

Eden Foods, Spicy Pumpkin Seeds, Tamari Dry Roasted, Organic

1/4 cup

Amount per serving	Amount per serving	Amount per serving
Calories 200	**Cholesterol** 0mg	**Total Carbohydrate** 5g
Total Fat 16g	**Sodium** 75mg	Dietary Fiber 5g
Saturated Fat 3g	**Protein** 10g	Sugars 0g

Eden Foods, Tamari Roasted Spicy Pumpkin Seeds, Organic

1/4 cup

Amount per serving	Amount per serving	Amount per serving
Calories 200	**Cholesterol** 0mg	**Total Carbohydrate** 5g
Total Fat 16g	**Sodium** 75mg	Dietary Fiber 5g
Saturated Fat 3g	**Protein** 10g	Sugars 1g

Hodgson Mill, Organic Golden Milled Flax Seed

2 tbsp

Amount per serving	Amount per serving	Amount per serving
Calories 65	**Cholesterol** 0mg	**Total Carbohydrate** 4g
Total Fat 4g	**Sodium** 0mg	Dietary Fiber 4g
Saturated Fat 0g	**Protein** 3g	Sugars 0g

Hodgson Mill, Organic Golden Milled Flax Seed "Travel Flax"

1 packet

Amount per serving	Amount per serving	Amount per serving
Calories 30	**Cholesterol** 0mg	**Total Carbohydrate** 2g
Total Fat 2g	**Sodium** 0mg	Dietary Fiber 2g
Saturated Fat 0g	**Protein** 1g	Sugars 0g

Manna Organics, Organic Brown Flax Seeds

2 tbsp (21g)

Amount per serving	Amount per serving	Amount per serving
Calories 90	**Cholesterol** 0mg	**Total Carbohydrate** 7g
Total Fat 8g	**Sodium** 5mg	Dietary Fiber 6g
Saturated Fat 0.5g	**Protein** 4g	Sugars 0g

Manna Organics, Organic Chia Seeds

28g (1 oz)

Amount per serving	Amount per serving	Amount per serving
Calories 140	**Cholesterol** 0mg	**Total Carbohydrate** 12g
Total Fat 9g	**Sodium** 5mg	Dietary Fiber 11g
Saturated Fat 1g	**Protein** 4g	Sugars 0g

Manna Organics, Organic Millet

45g (1.6 oz)

Amount per serving	Amount per serving	Amount per serving
Calories 170	**Cholesterol** 0mg	**Total Carbohydrate** 33g
Total Fat 2g	**Sodium** 0mg	Dietary Fiber 4g
Saturated Fat 0g	**Protein** 5g	Sugars 0g

Manna Organics, Organic Sesame Seeds

45g (1.6 oz)

Amount per serving	Amount per serving	Amount per serving
Calories 260	**Cholesterol** 0mg	**Total Carbohydrate** 11g
Total Fat 22g	**Sodium** 0mg	Dietary Fiber 5g
Saturated Fat 3g	**Protein** 8g	Sugars 0g

Manna Organics, Organic Sunflower Seeds

1 oz (28g/1 oz)

Amount per serving	Amount per serving	Amount per serving
Calories 180	**Cholesterol** 0mg	**Total Carbohydrate** 6g
Total Fat 16g	**Sodium** 0mg	Dietary Fiber 3g
Saturated Fat 1.5g	**Protein** 5g	Sugars 0g

Snacks

Why Eat Snacks?

Snacks help to keep you energized throughout the day and can tide you over until your next meal. In the book *Food Rules: An Eater's Manual* (2009), author Michael Pollan advises limiting snacks to unprocessed plant food—fruits, vegetables, nuts, and seeds. Even if you can't always limit your snacks to fresh, unprocessed foods, a wide variety of healthy, organic snack foods are readily available. Although nutrition bars made with whole grains, fruit, and nuts may be high in calories, they are healthier choices than snack foods that contain empty calories.

Carbohydrates Versus Sugar

On the snack's ingredients label, pay particular attention to the amount of total carbohydrates compared to the portion of that total separately labeled "sugars." The total carbohydrate count can include soluble and insoluble fiber, natural food components that can provide satisfying bulk but digest slowly, without taxing the body's production of insulin. Look for snacks where the amount of sugar is relatively small compared to the total carbohydrate count.

Some quality organic snacks are even considered "functional foods" because they contain natural ingredients with specific potential health benefits. While some snacks are fortified with synthetic vitamins and minerals, organic snacks are more likely to be made with naturally vitamin- and mineral-rich ingredients like organic vegetables, and seeds like flax and chia.

Various plant fibers also help the beneficial bacteria that live in the intestinal tract, where they assist in digestion and support the immune system. Look for snacks that contain *inulin*, a naturally sweet, soluble fiber from chicory root (not to be confused with insulin, a substance your body produces to process sugar), which also is sold as a prebiotic supplement to help healthful bacteria thrive in the gut.

Sugar by Any Other Name

Avoid products with added sugars—ripe fresh fruits and vegetables naturally contain plenty of sweetness. Sugars can also be listed under other names like corn syrup, dextrose, fructose, or sucrose (which is simply the name for table sugar). Other sweeteners like maple syrup, honey, and molasses may sound and actually be more natural—especially if they're organic—but they're still simple sugars that quickly enter the bloodstream and stress the body to produce more insulin.

Polyols, also known as sugar alcohols (don't worry—they are not the kind of alcohols that make you tipsy), are sweet compounds that aren't recognized by the body as sugars. A polyol called xylitol—which can be made from birch trees—tastes like sugar, has about 40% fewer calories and stimulates very little insulin demand. And because yeast and bacteria can't feed on it, xylitol won't promote tooth decay. Research suggests that xylitol can actually be good for the microbial ecosystem in our mouths. That's why some toothpastes, gum, and hard candies are sweetened with it.

The only downside of xylitol is that its metabolic products are cleared through the gut and large quantities can cause intestinal upset. Usually, starting with smaller quantities and building up over time can help a person develop a tolerance to this side effect. Another, similar polyol called maltitol isn't quite as sweet as xylitol, but it doesn't cause intestinal problems. You can find chocolates, ice cream, and pastries sweetened with maltitol.

Another sweetener that may be a good choice for healthful snacking is stevia—processed from the incredibly sweet leaves of a plant called Stevia *rebaudiana*. The whole leaf has a somewhat bitter taste, but a compound extracted from the leaf—which is hundreds of times sweeter than sugar—doesn't have this aftertaste.

Why Choose Organic Snacks?

Organic snacks are made with organic ingredients—meat, fish, dairy, eggs, grains, and produce raised or grown without the use of synthetic fertilizers, pesticides, or herbicides. Organic prepared foods contain no artificial ingredients, such as synthetic food coloring, additives, or preservatives.

Daily Goal

Plan ahead so you have a variety of healthy snacks at hand. That way, you won't be tempted by the limited choices in the vending machine or the candy jar on your coworker's desk.

Shopping Suggestions

Nuts	Popcorn	Fruits	Whole-grain cereal
Seeds	Dried fruit	Vegetables	Whole-grain crackers

Candy

Newman's Own Organics, Black Licorice Candy

5 pieces

Amount per serving	Amount per serving	Amount per serving
Calories 130	**Cholesterol** 0mg	**Total Carbohydrate** 31g
Total Fat 1g	**Sodium** 20mg	Dietary Fiber 2g
Saturated Fat NA	**Protein** 2g	Sugars 14g

Newman's Own Organics, Cinnamon Mints (in Tin)

2 pieces (2.0g)

Amount per serving	Amount per serving	Amount per serving
Calories 10	**Cholesterol** NA	**Total Carbohydrate** 2g
Total Fat 0g	**Sodium** 0mg	Dietary Fiber NA
Saturated Fat NA	**Protein** 0g	Sugars 2g

Newman's Own Organics, Cinnamon Mints (Rolls)

3 pieces (2.0g)

Amount per serving	Amount per serving	Amount per serving
Calories 10	**Cholesterol** NA	**Total Carbohydrate** 2g
Total Fat 0g	**Sodium** 0mg	Dietary Fiber NA
Saturated Fat NA	**Protein** 0g	Sugars 2g

Newman's Own Organics, Ginger Mints (in Tin)

2 pieces (2.0g)

Amount per serving	Amount per serving	Amount per serving
Calories 10	**Cholesterol** NA	**Total Carbohydrate** 2g
Total Fat 0g	**Sodium** 0mg	Dietary Fiber NA
Saturated Fat NA	**Protein** 0g	Sugars 2g

Newman's Own Organics, Ginger Mints (Rolls)

3 pieces (2.0g)

Amount per serving	Amount per serving	Amount per serving
Calories 10	**Cholesterol** NA	**Total Carbohydrate** 2g
Total Fat 0g	**Sodium** 0mg	Dietary Fiber NA
Saturated Fat NA	**Protein** 0g	Sugars 2g

Newman's Own Organics, Peppermint Mints (in Tin)

2 pieces (2.0g)

Amount per serving	Amount per serving	Amount per serving
Calories 10	**Cholesterol** NA	**Total Carbohydrate** 2g
Total Fat 0g	**Sodium** 0mg	Dietary Fiber NA
Saturated Fat NA	**Protein** 0g	Sugars 2g

Newman's Own Organics, Peppermint Mints (Rolls)

3 pieces (2.0g)

Amount per serving	Amount per serving	Amount per serving
Calories 10	**Cholesterol** NA	**Total Carbohydrate** 2g
Total Fat 0g	**Sodium** 0mg	Dietary Fiber NA
Saturated Fat NA	**Protein** 0g	Sugars 2g

Newman's Own Organics, Pomegranate Licorice Candy

5 pieces

Amount per serving	Amount per serving	Amount per serving
Calories 130	**Cholesterol** 0mg	**Total Carbohydrate** 32g
Total Fat 0.5g	**Sodium** 5mg	Dietary Fiber 2g
Saturated Fat NA	**Protein** 2g	Sugars 10g

Newman's Own Organics, Sour Apple Licorice Candy Twists

4 pieces

Amount per serving	Amount per serving	Amount per serving
Calories 120	**Cholesterol** 0mg	**Total Carbohydrate** 0g
Total Fat 0.5g	**Sodium** 0mg	Dietary Fiber 0g
Saturated Fat NA	**Protein** 1g	Sugars 13g

Newman's Own Organics, Sour Cherry Licorice Candy Twists

4 pieces

Amount per serving	Amount per serving	Amount per serving
Calories 130	**Cholesterol** 0mg	**Total Carbohydrate** 29g
Total Fat 0.5g	**Sodium** 0mg	Dietary Fiber 0g
Saturated Fat NA	**Protein** 1g	Sugars 13g

Newman's Own Organics, Sour Mango Licorice Candy Twists

4 pieces

Amount per serving	Amount per serving	Amount per serving
Calories 120	**Cholesterol** 0mg	**Total Carbohydrate** 28g
Total Fat 0.5g	**Sodium** 0mg	Dietary Fiber 0g
Saturated Fat NA	**Protein** 1g	Sugars 13g

Newman's Own Organics, Sour Strawberry Licorice Candy Twists

4 pieces

Amount per serving	Amount per serving	Amount per serving
Calories 130	**Cholesterol** 0mg	**Total Carbohydrate** 29g
Total Fat 0.5g	**Sodium** 0mg	Dietary Fiber 0g
Saturated Fat NA	**Protein** 1g	Sugars 14g

Newman's Own Organics, Strawberry Licorice Candy

5 pieces

Amount per serving	Amount per serving	Amount per serving
Calories 130	**Cholesterol** 0mg	**Total Carbohydrate** 32g
Total Fat 0.5g	**Sodium** 5mg	Dietary Fiber 2g
Saturated Fat NA	**Protein** 2g	Sugars 10g

Newman's Own Organics, Wintergreen Mints (in Tin)

2 pieces (2.0g)

Amount per serving	Amount per serving	Amount per serving
Calories 10	**Cholesterol** NA	**Total Carbohydrate** 2g
Total Fat 0g	**Sodium** 0mg	Dietary Fiber NA
Saturated Fat NA	**Protein** 0g	Sugars 2g

Newman's Own Organics, Wintergreen Mints (Rolls)

3 pieces (2.0g)

Amount per serving	Amount per serving	Amount per serving
Calories 10	**Cholesterol** NA	**Total Carbohydrate** 2g
Total Fat 0g	**Sodium** 0mg	Dietary Fiber NA
Saturated Fat NA	**Protein** 0g	Sugars 2g

Tru Joy Sweets, Organic Candy Canes

1 cane (15g)

Amount per serving	Amount per serving	Amount per serving
Calories 60	**Cholesterol** 0mg	**Total Carbohydrate** 15g
Total Fat 0g	**Sodium** 5mg	Dietary Fiber 0g
Saturated Fat 0g	**Protein** 0g	Sugars 10g

Chocolate

Newman's Own Organics, Dark Chocolate Bar

1 2.25 oz bar (64g)

Amount per serving	Amount per serving	Amount per serving
Calories 330	**Cholesterol** 0mg	**Total Carbohydrate** 37g
Total Fat 22g	**Sodium** 5mg	Dietary Fiber 4g
Saturated Fat 13g	**Protein** 3g	Sugars 28g

Newman's Own Organics, Dark Chocolate Caramel Cup

1 package (34g)

Amount per serving	Amount per serving	Amount per serving
Calories 160	**Cholesterol** 0mg	**Total Carbohydrate** 20g
Total Fat 9g	**Sodium** 30mg	Dietary Fiber 2g
Saturated Fat 5g	**Protein** 1g	Sugars 14g

Newman's Own Organics, Dark Chocolate Peanut Butter Cup

1 package (34g)

Amount per serving	Amount per serving	Amount per serving
Calories 180	**Cholesterol** 0mg	**Total Carbohydrate** 16g
Total Fat 13g	**Sodium** 0mg	Dietary Fiber 2g
Saturated Fat 7g	**Protein** 3g	Sugars 12g

Newman's Own Organics, Dark Chocolate Peppermint Cup

1 package (34g)

Amount per serving	Amount per serving	Amount per serving
Calories 190	**Cholesterol** 5mg	**Total Carbohydrate** 18g
Total Fat 11g	**Sodium** 0mg	Dietary Fiber 1g
Saturated Fat 7g	**Protein** 2g	Sugars 15g

Newman's Own Organics, Espresso Dark Chocolate Bar

1 2.25 oz bar (64g)

Amount per serving	Amount per serving	Amount per serving
Calories 320	**Cholesterol** 0mg	**Total Carbohydrate** 237g
Total Fat 22g	**Sodium** 5mg	Dietary Fiber 4g
Saturated Fat 13g	**Protein** 3g	Sugars 28g

Newman's Own Organics, Milk Chocolate Bar

1 2.25 oz bar (64g)

Amount per serving	Amount per serving	Amount per serving
Calories 340	**Cholesterol** 5mg	**Total Carbohydrate** 38g
Total Fat 21g	**Sodium** 35mg	Dietary Fiber 1g
Saturated Fat 12g	**Protein** 3g	Sugars 33g

Newman's Own Organics, Milk Chocolate Caramel Cup

1 package (34g)

Amount per serving	Amount per serving	Amount per serving
Calories 160	**Cholesterol** 5mg	**Total Carbohydrate** 21g
Total Fat 8g	**Sodium** 40mg	Dietary Fiber 0g
Saturated Fat 5g	**Protein** 2g	Sugars 16g

Newman's Own Organics, Milk Chocolate Peanut Butter Cup

1 package (34g)

Amount per serving	Amount per serving	Amount per serving
Calories 180	**Cholesterol** 5mg	**Total Carbohydrate** 17g
Total Fat 12g	**Sodium** 10mg	Dietary Fiber 1g
Saturated Fat 6g	**Protein** 4g	Sugars 14g

Newman's Own Organics, Mocha Milk Chocolate Bar

1 2.25 oz bar (64g)

Amount per serving	Amount per serving	Amount per serving
Calories 340	**Cholesterol** 5mg	**Total Carbohydrate** 37g
Total Fat 23g	**Sodium** 30mg	Dietary Fiber 1g
Saturated Fat 12g	**Protein** 3g	Sugars 33g

Newman's Own Organics, Orange Dark Chocolate Bar

1 2.25 oz bar (64g)

Amount per serving	Amount per serving	Amount per serving
Calories 320	**Cholesterol** 0mg	**Total Carbohydrate** 36g
Total Fat 22g	**Sodium** 5mg	Dietary Fiber 2g
Saturated Fat 13g	**Protein** 3g	Sugars 28g

Newman's Own Organics, Super Dark Chocolate Bar

1 2.25 oz bar (64g)

Amount per serving	Amount per serving	Amount per serving
Calories 330	**Cholesterol** 0mg	**Total Carbohydrate** 30g
Total Fat 28g	**Sodium** 0mg	Dietary Fiber 6g
Saturated Fat 16g	**Protein** 5g	Sugars 16g

Sunspire, Organic Fair Trade 100% Cacao Unsweetened Baking Bar

1 section (14g)

Amount per serving	Amount per serving	Amount per serving
Calories 90	**Cholesterol** 0mg	**Total Carbohydrate** 4g
Total Fat 7.5g	**Sodium** 0mg	Dietary Fiber 2g
Saturated Fat 4.5g	**Protein** 2g	Sugars 0g

Sunspire, Organic Fair Trade 42% Cacao Semi-Sweet Baking Chips

2 tbsp (15g)

Amount per serving	Amount per serving	Amount per serving
Calories 70	**Cholesterol** 0mg	**Total Carbohydrate** 10g
Total Fat 4g	**Sodium** 0mg	Dietary Fiber 1g
Saturated Fat 2.5g	**Protein** 1g	Sugars 8g

Sunspire, Organic Fair Trade 65% Cacao Bittersweet Baking Chips

2 tbsp (15g)

Amount per serving	Amount per serving	Amount per serving
Calories 80	**Cholesterol** 0mg	**Total Carbohydrate** 8g
Total Fat 5g	**Sodium** 0mg	Dietary Fiber 2g
Saturated Fat 3g	**Protein** 1g	Sugars 5g

Sunspire, Organic Fair Trade 65% Cacao Semi-Sweet Baking Bar

1 section (14g)

Amount per serving	Amount per serving	Amount per serving
Calories 80	**Cholesterol** 0mg	**Total Carbohydrate** 7g
Total Fat 5g	**Sodium** 0mg	Dietary Fiber 2g
Saturated Fat 3g	**Protein** 1g	Sugars 5g

Tru Joy Sweets, Organic Choco Chews

7 pieces (42g)

Amount per serving	Amount per serving	Amount per serving
Calories 160	**Cholesterol** 0mg	**Total Carbohydrate** 16g
Total Fat 4.5g	**Sodium** 0mg	Dietary Fiber 1g
Saturated Fat 3.5g	**Protein** 1g	Sugars 15g

Cookies

Back to Nature, Organic Shortbread Cookies

2 cookies

Amount per serving	Amount per serving	Amount per serving
Calories 150	**Cholesterol** 20mg	**Total Carbohydrate** 17g
Total Fat 8g	**Sodium** 100mg	Dietary Fiber 0g
Saturated Fat 5g	**Protein** 1g	Sugars 5g

Country Choice Organic, Ginger Snaps

5 cookies

Amount per serving	Amount per serving	Amount per serving
Calories 140	**Cholesterol** 0mg	**Total Carbohydrate** 22g
Total Fat 5g	**Sodium** 85mg	Dietary Fiber 0g
Saturated Fat 0g	**Protein** 1g	Sugars 0g

Country Choice Organic, Iced Oatmeal Cookies

4 cookies

Amount per serving	Amount per serving	Amount per serving
Calories 120	**Cholesterol** 0mg	**Total Carbohydrate** 21g
Total Fat 4g	**Sodium** 120mg	Dietary Fiber <1g
Saturated Fat 0g	**Protein** 1g	Sugars 12g

Country Choice Organic, Sandwich Cookies, Chocolate

2 cookies

Amount per serving	Amount per serving	Amount per serving
Calories 130	**Cholesterol** 0mg	**Total Carbohydrate** 19g
Total Fat 5g	**Sodium** 100mg	Dietary Fiber <1g
Saturated Fat 0.5g	**Protein** 1g	Sugars 11g

Country Choice Organic, Sandwich Cookies, Duplex

2 cookies

Amount per serving	Amount per serving	Amount per serving
Calories 130	**Cholesterol** 0mg	**Total Carbohydrate** 19g
Total Fat 5g	**Sodium** 110mg	Dietary Fiber <1g
Saturated Fat 0.5g	**Protein** 1g	Sugars 11g

Country Choice Organic, Sandwich Cookies, Ginger Lemon

2 cookies

Amount per serving	Amount per serving	Amount per serving
Calories 130	**Cholesterol** 0mg	**Total Carbohydrate** 19g
Total Fat 5g	**Sodium** 120mg	Dietary Fiber <1g
Saturated Fat 0.5g	**Protein** 1g	Sugars 11g

Country Choice Organic, Sandwich Cookies, Vanilla

2 cookies

Amount per serving	Amount per serving	Amount per serving
Calories 130	**Cholesterol** 0mg	**Total Carbohydrate** 19g
Total Fat 5g	**Sodium** 120mg	Dietary Fiber 0g
Saturated Fat 0.5g	**Protein** 1g	Sugars 11g

Country Choice Organic, Vanilla Wafers

7 cookies

Amount per serving	Amount per serving	Amount per serving
Calories 140	**Cholesterol** 5mg	**Total Carbohydrate** 22g
Total Fat 5g	**Sodium** 100mg	Dietary Fiber 0g
Saturated Fat 0g	**Protein** 1g	Sugars 8g

Go Raw, 100% Organic Carrot Cake Super Cookies

about 20 pieces (28g) 1 oz

Amount per serving	Amount per serving	Amount per serving
Calories 150	**Cholesterol** 0mg	**Total Carbohydrate** 22g
Total Fat 7g	**Sodium** 20mg	Dietary Fiber 4g
Saturated Fat 5g	**Protein** 1g	Sugars 14g

Go Raw, 100% Organic Chocolate Super Cookies

about 18 pieces (28g) 1 oz

Amount per serving	Amount per serving	Amount per serving
Calories 160	**Cholesterol** 0mg	**Total Carbohydrate** 17g
Total Fat 9g	**Sodium** 10mg	Dietary Fiber 4g
Saturated Fat 5g	**Protein** 2g	Sugars 11g

Go Raw, 100% Organic Ginger Snaps Super Cookies

about 18 pieces (28g) 1 oz

Amount per serving	Amount per serving	Amount per serving
Calories 160	**Cholesterol** 0mg	**Total Carbohydrate** 18g
Total Fat 9g	**Sodium** 10mg	Dietary Fiber 4g
Saturated Fat 5g	**Protein** 2g	Sugars 11g

Go Raw, 100% Organic Lemon Super Cookies

about 18 pieces (28g) 1 oz

Amount per serving	Amount per serving	Amount per serving
Calories 160	**Cholesterol** 0mg	**Total Carbohydrate** 21g
Total Fat 8g	**Sodium** 5mg	Dietary Fiber 4g
Saturated Fat 4g	**Protein** 2g	Sugars 16g

Go Raw, 100% Organic Masala Chai Super Cookies

about 18 pieces (28g) 1 oz

Amount per serving	Amount per serving	Amount per serving
Calories 160	**Cholesterol** 0mg	**Total Carbohydrate** 22g
Total Fat 8g	**Sodium** 5mg	Dietary Fiber 4g
Saturated Fat 4g	**Protein** 2g	Sugars 16g

Go Raw, 100% Organic Original Super Cookies

about 18 pieces (28g) 1 oz

Amount per serving	Amount per serving	Amount per serving
Calories 160	**Cholesterol** 0mg	**Total Carbohydrate** 18g
Total Fat 9g	**Sodium** 10mg	Dietary Fiber 4g
Saturated Fat 5g	**Protein** 2g	Sugars 11g

Jovial Foods, Jovial Checkerboard Einkorn Cookies

2 cookies (25g)

Amount per serving	Amount per serving	Amount per serving
Calories 120	**Cholesterol** 20mg	**Total Carbohydrate** 15g
Total Fat 5.5g	**Sodium** 70mg	Dietary Fiber 1g
Saturated Fat 2.5g	**Protein** 3g	Sugars 6g

Jovial Foods, Jovial Crispy Cocoa Einkorn Cookies

3 cookies (28g)

Amount per serving	Amount per serving	Amount per serving
Calories 140	**Cholesterol** 0mg	**Total Carbohydrate** 18g
Total Fat 6g	**Sodium** 80mg	Dietary Fiber 1g
Saturated Fat 2.5g	**Protein** 3g	Sugars 6g

Jovial Foods, Jovial Ginger Spice Einkorn Cookies

2 cookies (32g)

Amount per serving	Amount per serving	Amount per serving
Calories 150	**Cholesterol** 25mg	**Total Carbohydrate** 21g
Total Fat 6g	**Sodium** 70mg	Dietary Fiber 1g
Saturated Fat 2.5g	**Protein** 3g	Sugars 7g

Jovial Foods, Jovial Gluten Free Chocolate Cream Chocolate Cookies

2 cookies (33g)

Amount per serving	Amount per serving	Amount per serving
Calories 160	**Cholesterol** 15mg	**Total Carbohydrate** 20g
Total Fat 7g	**Sodium** 75mg	Dietary Fiber 1g
Saturated Fat 2.5g	**Protein** 2g	Sugars 9g

Jovial Foods, Jovial Gluten Free Fig Fruit Filled Cookies

2 cookies (33g)

Amount per serving	Amount per serving	Amount per serving
Calories 130	**Cholesterol** 5mg	**Total Carbohydrate** 23g
Total Fat 4g	**Sodium** 65mg	Dietary Fiber 1g
Saturated Fat 1.5g	**Protein** 1g	Sugars 12g

Jovial Foods, Jovial Gluten Free Vanilla Cream Chocolate Cookies

2 cookies (33g)

Amount per serving	Amount per serving	Amount per serving
Calories 160	**Cholesterol** 15mg	**Total Carbohydrate** 21g
Total Fat 7g	**Sodium** 75mg	Dietary Fiber 1g
Saturated Fat 2.5g	**Protein** 2g	Sugars 10g

Mary's Gone Crackers, "N" Oatmeal Raisin Cookies

2 cookies

Amount per serving	Amount per serving	Amount per serving
Calories 120	**Cholesterol** 0mg	**Total Carbohydrate** 20g
Total Fat 4g	**Sodium** 110mg	Dietary Fiber 1.5g
Saturated Fat 23g	**Protein** 1g	Sugars 9g

Mary's Gone Crackers, Chocolate Chip Cookies

2 cookies

Amount per serving	Amount per serving	Amount per serving
Calories 130	**Cholesterol** 0mg	**Total Carbohydrate** 19g
Total Fat 6g	**Sodium** 95mg	Dietary Fiber 1.5g
Saturated Fat 3g	**Protein** 1g	Sugars 9g

Mary's Gone Crackers, Double Chocolate Cookies

2 cookies

Amount per serving	Amount per serving	Amount per serving
Calories 130	**Cholesterol** 0mg	**Total Carbohydrate** 19g
Total Fat 6g	**Sodium** 100mg	Dietary Fiber 1.5g
Saturated Fat 3g	**Protein** 1g	Sugars 9g

Mary's Gone Crackers, Ginger Snaps Cookies

3 cookies

Amount per serving	Amount per serving	Amount per serving
Calories 140	**Cholesterol** 0mg	**Total Carbohydrate** 23g
Total Fat 5g	**Sodium** 120mg	Dietary Fiber 1g
Saturated Fat 3g	**Protein** 1g	Sugars 9g

Newman's Own Organics, Alphabet Cookies, Chocolate

7 oz bag

Amount per serving	Amount per serving	Amount per serving
Calories 120	**Cholesterol** 0mg	**Total Carbohydrate** 21g
Total Fat 3g	**Sodium** 140mg	Dietary Fiber 1g
Saturated Fat 1.5g	**Protein** 2g	Sugars 9g

Newman's Own Organics, Alphabet Cookies, Cinnamon Graham

7 oz bag

Amount per serving	Amount per serving	Amount per serving
Calories 120	**Cholesterol** 0mg	**Total Carbohydrate** 21g
Total Fat 3g	**Sodium** 90mg	Dietary Fiber <1g
Saturated Fat 1.5g	**Protein** 2g	Sugars 8g

Newman's Own Organics, Alphabet Cookies, Vanilla

7 oz bag

Amount per serving	Amount per serving	Amount per serving
Calories 120	**Cholesterol** 0mg	**Total Carbohydrate** 21g
Total Fat 3g	**Sodium** 135mg	Dietary Fiber <1g
Saturated Fat 1.5g	**Protein** 2g	Sugars 7g

Newman's Own Organics, Family Recipe Cookies, Chocolate Chip

5 cookies (33g)

Amount per serving	Amount per serving	Amount per serving
Calories 150	**Cholesterol** 0mg	**Total Carbohydrate** 22g
Total Fat 7g	**Sodium** 100mg	Dietary Fiber <1g
Saturated Fat 3.5g	**Protein** 2g	Sugars 11g

Newman's Own Organics, Family Recipe Cookies, Double Chocolate Chip

5 cookies (33g)

Amount per serving	Amount per serving	Amount per serving
Calories 150	**Cholesterol** 0mg	**Total Carbohydrate** 22g
Total Fat 8g	**Sodium** 70mg	Dietary Fiber 1g
Saturated Fat 4g	**Protein** 2g	Sugars 11g

Newman's Own Organics, Family Recipe Cookies, Ginger Snaps

5 cookies (30g)

Amount per serving	Amount per serving	Amount per serving
Calories 130	**Cholesterol** 0mg	**Total Carbohydrate** 24g
Total Fat 3.5g	**Sodium** 180mg	Dietary Fiber 0g
Saturated Fat 1.5g	**Protein** 2g	Sugars 11g

Newman's Own Organics, Family Recipe Cookies, Oatmeal Chocolate Chip

5 cookies (33g)

Amount per serving	Amount per serving	Amount per serving
Calories 140	**Cholesterol** 0mg	**Total Carbohydrate** 23g
Total Fat 6g	**Sodium** 70mg	Dietary Fiber 1g
Saturated Fat 3g	**Protein** 2g	Sugars 12g

Newman's Own Organics, Family Recipe Cookies, Orange Chocolate Chip

5 cookies (33g)

Amount per serving	Amount per serving	Amount per serving
Calories 160	**Cholesterol** 0mg	**Total Carbohydrate** 22g
Total Fat 7g	**Sodium** 110mg	Dietary Fiber 1g
Saturated Fat 4g	**Protein** 2g	Sugars 11g

Newman's Own Organics, Family Recipe Cookies, Spelt Ginger Snaps

5 cookies (30g)

Amount per serving	Amount per serving	Amount per serving
Calories 140	**Cholesterol** 0mg	**Total Carbohydrate** 25g
Total Fat 4g	**Sodium** 200mg	Dietary Fiber 2g
Saturated Fat 2g	**Protein** 2g	Sugars 12g

Newman's Own Organics, Fat Free, Fig Newman's

2 bars (32g)

Amount per serving	Amount per serving	Amount per serving
Calories 100	**Cholesterol** 0mg	**Total Carbohydrate** 24g
Total Fat 0g	**Sodium** 150mg	Dietary Fiber <1g
Saturated Fat NA	**Protein** 2g	Sugars 13g

Newman's Own Organics, Hermits, Cinnamon

1 cookie (22g)

Amount per serving	Amount per serving	Amount per serving
Calories 80	**Cholesterol** 0mg	**Total Carbohydrate** 17g
Total Fat 1.5g	**Sodium** 60mg	Dietary Fiber <1g
Saturated Fat 1g	**Protein** 1g	Sugars 10g

Newman's Own Organics, Hermits, Ginger

1 cookie (22g)

Amount per serving	Amount per serving	Amount per serving
Calories 80	**Cholesterol** 0mg	**Total Carbohydrate** 16g
Total Fat 1.5g	**Sodium** 65mg	Dietary Fiber <1g
Saturated Fat 1g	**Protein** 1g	Sugars 10g

Newman's Own Organics, Hermits, Original

1 cookie (22g)

Amount per serving	Amount per serving	Amount per serving
Calories 80	**Cholesterol** 0mg	**Total Carbohydrate** 16g
Total Fat 1.5g	**Sodium** 65mg	Dietary Fiber <1g
Saturated Fat 1g	**Protein** 1g	Sugars 10g

Newman's Own Organics, Low Fat, Fig Newman's

2 bars (32g)

Amount per serving	Amount per serving	Amount per serving
Calories 110	**Cholesterol** 0mg	**Total Carbohydrate** 23g
Total Fat 1.5g	**Sodium** 135mg	Dietary Fiber <1g
Saturated Fat 0.5g	**Protein** 2g	Sugars 12g

Newman's Own Organics, Newman-O's Cream Filled Chocolate Cookies

2 cookies (27g)

Amount per serving	Amount per serving	Amount per serving
Calories 130	**Cholesterol** 0mg	**Total Carbohydrate** 18g
Total Fat 5g	**Sodium** 90mg	Dietary Fiber 0g
Saturated Fat 2g	**Protein** 1g	Sugars 10g

Newman's Own Organics, Newman-O's Cream Filled Chocolate Cookies, Chocolate Crème

2 cookies (27g)

Amount per serving	Amount per serving	Amount per serving
Calories 120	**Cholesterol** 0mg	**Total Carbohydrate** 19g
Total Fat 5g	**Sodium** 85mg	Dietary Fiber <1g
Saturated Fat 1.5g	**Protein** 2g	Sugars 10g

Newman's Own Organics, Newman-O's Cream Filled Chocolate Cookies, Ginger-O's

2 cookies (27g)

Amount per serving	Amount per serving	Amount per serving
Calories 130	**Cholesterol** 0mg	**Total Carbohydrate** 20g
Total Fat 4.5g	**Sodium** 85mg	Dietary Fiber 0g
Saturated Fat 2g	**Protein** 1g	Sugars 10g

Newman's Own Organics, Newman-O's Cream Filled Chocolate Cookies, Mint Crème

2 cookies (27g)

Amount per serving	Amount per serving	Amount per serving
Calories 130	**Cholesterol** 0mg	**Total Carbohydrate** 19g
Total Fat 5g	**Sodium** 85mg	Dietary Fiber <1g
Saturated Fat 1.5g	**Protein** 2g	Sugars 11g

Newman's Own Organics, Newman-O's Cream Filled Chocolate Cookies, Original

2 cookies (27g)

Amount per serving	Amount per serving	Amount per serving
Calories 130	**Cholesterol** 0mg	**Total Carbohydrate** 19g
Total Fat 5g	**Sodium** 85mg	Dietary Fiber <1g
Saturated Fat 1.5g	**Protein** 2g	Sugars 11g

Newman's Own Organics, Newman-O's Cream Filled Chocolate Cookies, Peanut Butter

2 cookies (27g)

Amount per serving	Amount per serving	Amount per serving
Calories 130	**Cholesterol** 0mg	**Total Carbohydrate** 18g
Total Fat 5g	**Sodium** 135mg	Dietary Fiber <1g
Saturated Fat 1.5g	**Protein** 3g	Sugars 9g

Newman's Own Organics, Wheat Free-Dairy Free, Fig Newman's

2 bars (38g)

Amount per serving	Amount per serving	Amount per serving
Calories 120	**Cholesterol** 0mg	**Total Carbohydrate** 26g
Total Fat 1.5g	**Sodium** 170mg	Dietary Fiber 1g
Saturated Fat 0g	**Protein** 2g	Sugars 12g

Crackers

Annie's, Organic Buttery Rich Classic Crackers

7 crackers (15g)

Amount per serving	Amount per serving	Amount per serving
Calories 70	**Cholesterol** 0mg	**Total Carbohydrate** 10g
Total Fat 2.5g	**Sodium** 100mg	Dietary Fiber 0g
Saturated Fat 0g	**Protein** 1g	Sugars 0g

Annie's, Organic Cheddar Bunnies

51 crackers (30g)

Amount per serving	Amount per serving	Amount per serving
Calories 150	**Cholesterol** 0mg	**Total Carbohydrate** 19g
Total Fat 7g	**Sodium** 250mg	Dietary Fiber 0g
Saturated Fat 1g	**Protein** 3g	Sugars 0g

Annie's, Organic Cheddar Classic Crackers

7 crackers (15g)

Amount per serving	Amount per serving	Amount per serving
Calories 70	**Cholesterol** 0mg	**Total Carbohydrate** 10g
Total Fat 2.5g	**Sodium** 100mg	Dietary Fiber 0g
Saturated Fat 0g	**Protein** 1g	Sugars 0g

Annie's, Organic Cinnamon Graham Crackers

2 full cracker sheets (31g)

Amount per serving	Amount per serving	Amount per serving
Calories 130	**Cholesterol** 0mg	**Total Carbohydrate** 25g
Total Fat 3g	**Sodium** 160mg	Dietary Fiber 2g
Saturated Fat 0g	**Protein** 2g	Sugars 9g

Annie's, Organic Honey Graham Crackers

2 full cracker sheets (31g)

Amount per serving	Amount per serving	Amount per serving
Calories 130	**Cholesterol** 0mg	**Total Carbohydrate** 25g
Total Fat 3g	**Sodium** 160mg	Dietary Fiber 2g
Saturated Fat 0g	**Protein** 2g	Sugars 8g

Annie's, Organic Saltine Classic Crackers

7 crackers (15g)

Amount per serving	Amount per serving	Amount per serving
Calories 70	**Cholesterol** 0mg	**Total Carbohydrate** 10g
Total Fat 2.5g	**Sodium** 100mg	Dietary Fiber 0g
Saturated Fat 0g	**Protein** 1g	Sugars 0g

Back to Nature, Organic Saltines

5 crackers

Amount per serving	Amount per serving	Amount per serving
Calories 60	**Cholesterol** 0mg	**Total Carbohydrate** 12g
Total Fat 1.5g	**Sodium** 150mg	Dietary Fiber 0g
Saturated Fat 0g	**Protein** 1g	Sugars 0g

Back to Nature, Organic Stoneground Wheat Crackers

10 crackers

Amount per serving	Amount per serving	Amount per serving
Calories 70	**Cholesterol** 0mg	**Total Carbohydrate** 11g
Total Fat 2.5g	**Sodium** 125mg	Dietary Fiber 1g
Saturated Fat 0g	**Protein** 1g	Sugars 1g

Edward & Sons, Brown Rice Snaps, Black Sesame Crackers, with Organic Brown Rice

8 crackers

Amount per serving	Amount per serving	Amount per serving
Calories 60	**Cholesterol** 0mg	**Total Carbohydrate** 11g
Total Fat 2g	**Sodium** 70mg	Dietary Fiber 1g
Saturated Fat 0g	**Protein** 2g	Sugars 0g

Edward & Sons, Brown Rice Snaps, Onion Garlic Crackers

9 crackers

Amount per serving	Amount per serving	Amount per serving
Calories 50	**Cholesterol** 0mg	**Total Carbohydrate** 10g
Total Fat 1g	**Sodium** 50mg	Dietary Fiber <1g
Saturated Fat 0.5g	**Protein** 1g	Sugars 0g

Edward & Sons, Brown Rice Snaps, Tamari Seaweed Crackers

9 crackers

Amount per serving	Amount per serving	Amount per serving
Calories 60	**Cholesterol** 0mg	**Total Carbohydrate** 12g
Total Fat 0g	**Sodium** 120mg	Dietary Fiber <1g
Saturated Fat 0g	**Protein** 1g	Sugars 0g

Edward & Sons, Brown Rice Snaps, Tamari Sesame Crackers

9 crackers

Amount per serving	Amount per serving	Amount per serving
Calories 60	**Cholesterol** 0mg	**Total Carbohydrate** 13g
Total Fat 0.5g	**Sodium** 120mg	Dietary Fiber <1g
Saturated Fat 0g	**Protein** 1g	Sugars 0g

Edward & Sons, Brown Rice Snaps, Toasted Onion Crackers, with Organic Brown Rice

8 crackers

Amount per serving	Amount per serving	Amount per serving
Calories 60	**Cholesterol** 0mg	**Total Carbohydrate** 12g
Total Fat 1g	**Sodium** 30mg	Dietary Fiber <1g
Saturated Fat 0g	**Protein** 1g	Sugars <1g

Edward & Sons, Brown Rice Snaps, Unsalted Plain Crackers, with Organic Brown Rice

8 crackers

Amount per serving	Amount per serving	Amount per serving
Calories 60	**Cholesterol** 0mg	**Total Carbohydrate** 12g
Total Fat 1g	**Sodium** 0mg	Dietary Fiber <1g
Saturated Fat 0g	**Protein** 1g	Sugars <1g

Edward & Sons, Brown Rice Snaps, Unsalted Sesame Crackers

9 crackers

Amount per serving	Amount per serving	Amount per serving
Calories 60	**Cholesterol** 0mg	**Total Carbohydrate** 12g
Total Fat 1g	**Sodium** 0mg	Dietary Fiber <1g
Saturated Fat 0g	**Protein** 1g	Sugars 0g

Erewhon, Cinnamon Grahams

2 full cracker sheets

Amount per serving	Amount per serving	Amount per serving
Calories 130	**Cholesterol** 0mg	**Total Carbohydrate** 24g
Total Fat 2.5g	**Sodium** 120mg	Dietary Fiber 1g
Saturated Fat 0g	**Protein** 2g	Sugars 8g

Erewhon, Honey Grahams

2 full cracker sheets

Amount per serving	Amount per serving	Amount per serving
Calories 130	**Cholesterol** 0mg	**Total Carbohydrate** 23g
Total Fat 2.5g	**Sodium** 125mg	Dietary Fiber 1g
Saturated Fat 0g	**Protein** 2g	Sugars 7g

Mary's Gone Crackers, Black Pepper Crackers

13 crackers

Amount per serving	Amount per serving	Amount per serving
Calories 140	**Cholesterol** 0mg	**Total Carbohydrate** 21g
Total Fat 5g	**Sodium** 180mg	Dietary Fiber 3g
Saturated Fat 0.5g	**Protein** 3g	Sugars 0g

Mary's Gone Crackers, Caraway Crackers

13 crackers

Amount per serving	Amount per serving	Amount per serving
Calories 140	**Cholesterol** 0mg	**Total Carbohydrate** 21g
Total Fat 5g	**Sodium** 190mg	Dietary Fiber 3g
Saturated Fat 0.5g	**Protein** 3g	Sugars 0g

Mary's Gone Crackers, Herb Crackers

13 crackers

Amount per serving | Amount per serving | Amount per serving

Calories 140
Total Fat 5g
  Saturated Fat 0.5g

Cholesterol 0mg
Sodium 180mg
Protein 3g

Total Carbohydrate 21g
  Dietary Fiber 3g
  Sugars 0g

Mary's Gone Crackers, Onion Crackers

13 crackers

Amount per serving | Amount per serving | Amount per serving

Calories 140
Total Fat 5g
  Saturated Fat 0.5g

Cholesterol 0mg
Sodium 190mg
Protein 3g

Total Carbohydrate 21g
  Dietary Fiber 3g
  Sugars 0g

Mary's Gone Crackers, Original Seed Crackers

13 crackers

Amount per serving | Amount per serving | Amount per serving

Calories 140
Total Fat 5g
  Saturated Fat 0.5g

Cholesterol 0mg
Sodium 190mg
Protein 3g

Total Carbohydrate 21g
  Dietary Fiber 3g
  Sugars 0g

Fruit Snacks

Annie's, Organic Berry Patch Fruit Snacks

1 pouch

Amount per serving | Amount per serving | Amount per serving

Calories 70
Total Fat 0g
  Saturated Fat NA

Cholesterol 0mg
Sodium 45mg
Protein 0g

Total Carbohydrate 18g
  Dietary Fiber NA
  Sugars 10g

Annie's, Organic Grapes Galore Fruit Snacks

1 pouch

Amount per serving | Amount per serving | Amount per serving

Calories 70
Total Fat 0g
  Saturated Fat NA

Cholesterol 0mg
Sodium 45mg
Protein 0g

Total Carbohydrate 18g
  Dietary Fiber NA
  Sugars 10g

Annie's, Organic Orchard Apple Fruit Bites

1 pouch

Amount per serving | Amount per serving | Amount per serving

Calories 60
Total Fat 0g
  Saturated Fat NA

Cholesterol 0mg
Sodium 5mg
Protein 0g

Total Carbohydrate 15g
  Dietary Fiber 1g
  Sugars 12g

Annie's, Organic Orchard Cherry Fruit Bites

1 pouch

Amount per serving	Amount per serving	Amount per serving
Calories 60	**Cholesterol** 0mg	**Total Carbohydrate** 15g
Total Fat 0g	**Sodium** 5mg	Dietary Fiber 1g
Saturated Fat NA	**Protein** 0g	Sugars 12g

Annie's, Organic Orchard Grape Fruit Bites

1 pouch

Amount per serving	Amount per serving	Amount per serving
Calories 60	**Cholesterol** 0mg	**Total Carbohydrate** 15g
Total Fat 0g	**Sodium** 5mg	Dietary Fiber 1g
Saturated Fat NA	**Protein** 0g	Sugars 12g

Annie's, Organic Orchard Strawberry Fruit Bites

1 pouch

Amount per serving	Amount per serving	Amount per serving
Calories 60	**Cholesterol** 0mg	**Total Carbohydrate** 15g
Total Fat 0g	**Sodium** 5mg	Dietary Fiber 1g
Saturated Fat NA	**Protein** 0g	Sugars 12g

Annie's, Organic Pink Lemonade Bunny Fruit Snacks

1 pouch

Amount per serving	Amount per serving	Amount per serving
Calories 70	**Cholesterol** 0mg	**Total Carbohydrate** 18g
Total Fat 0g	**Sodium** 45mg	Dietary Fiber NA
Saturated Fat NA	**Protein** 0g	Sugars 10g

Annie's, Organic Summer Strawberry Fruit Snacks

1 pouch

Amount per serving	Amount per serving	Amount per serving
Calories 70	**Cholesterol** 0mg	**Total Carbohydrate** 18g
Total Fat 0g	**Sodium** 45mg	Dietary Fiber NA
Saturated Fat NA	**Protein** 0g	Sugars 10g

Annie's, Organic Sunny Citrus Fruit Snacks

1 pouch

Amount per serving	Amount per serving	Amount per serving
Calories 70	**Cholesterol** 0mg	**Total Carbohydrate** 18g
Total Fat 0g	**Sodium** 45mg	Dietary Fiber NA
Saturated Fat NA	**Protein** 0g	Sugars 10g

Annie's, Organic Tropical Treat Bunny Fruit Snacks

1 pouch

Amount per serving	Amount per serving	Amount per serving
Calories 70	**Cholesterol** 0mg	**Total Carbohydrate** 18g
Total Fat 0g	**Sodium** 45mg	Dietary Fiber NA
Saturated Fat NA	**Protein** 0g	Sugars 10g

Columbia Gorge Organic, Almond Banana CoGo Organic Gluten-Free Food Bar

1 bar (50g)

Amount per serving	Amount per serving	Amount per serving
Calories 180	**Cholesterol** 0mg	**Total Carbohydrate** 29g
Total Fat 5g	**Sodium** 100mg	Dietary Fiber 3g
Saturated Fat 1g	**Protein** 5g	Sugars 10g

Columbia Gorge Organic, Double Chocolate Organic Gluten-Free Food Bar

1 bar (50g)

Amount per serving	Amount per serving	Amount per serving
Calories 170	**Cholesterol** 0mg	**Total Carbohydrate** 33g
Total Fat 3g	**Sodium** 115mg	Dietary Fiber 2g
Saturated Fat 1.5g	**Protein** 3g	Sugars 16g

Columbia Gorge Organic, Hemp Apricot Organic Gluten-Free Food Bar

1 bar (50g)

Amount per serving	Amount per serving	Amount per serving
Calories 170	**Cholesterol** 0mg	**Total Carbohydrate** 30g
Total Fat 4.5g	**Sodium** 115mg	Dietary Fiber 2g
Saturated Fat 1g	**Protein** 4g	Sugars 13g

Columbia Gorge Organic, Peanut Chocolate Chip Organic Gluten-Free Food Bar

1 bar (50g)

Amount per serving	Amount per serving	Amount per serving
Calories 190	**Cholesterol** 0mg	**Total Carbohydrate** 30g
Total Fat 7g	**Sodium** 170mg	Dietary Fiber 2g
Saturated Fat 1.5g	**Protein** 4g	Sugars 14g

Columbia Gorge Organic, Superberry CoGo Organic Gluten-Free Food Bar

1 bar (50g)

Amount per serving	Amount per serving	Amount per serving
Calories 160	**Cholesterol** 0mg	**Total Carbohydrate** 34g
Total Fat 3g	**Sodium** 85mg	Dietary Fiber 2g
Saturated Fat 1g	**Protein** 2g	Sugars 16g

Let's Do...Organic, Organic Super Sour Gummi Bears

1 packet

Amount per serving	Amount per serving	Amount per serving
Calories 100	**Cholesterol** 0mg	**Total Carbohydrate** 23g
Total Fat 0g	**Sodium** 15mg	Dietary Fiber 0g
Saturated Fat 0g	**Protein** 0g	Sugars 19g

Tru Joy Sweets, Organic Original Fruit Chews

8 pieces (40g)

Amount per serving	Amount per serving	Amount per serving
Calories 160	**Cholesterol** 0mg	**Total Carbohydrate** 34g
Total Fat 3g	**Sodium** 0mg	Dietary Fiber 0g
Saturated Fat 2g	**Protein** 0g	Sugars 21g

Yum Earth® Organics, YumEarth Naturals Sour Jelly Beans

1 snack pack (20g)

Amount per serving	Amount per serving	Amount per serving
Calories 69	**Cholesterol** 0mg	**Total Carbohydrate** 18g
Total Fat 0g	**Sodium** 7mg	Dietary Fiber 0g
Saturated Fat 0g	**Protein** 0g	Sugars 15g

Yum Earth® Organics, YumEarth Organic Fruit Snacks

1 snack pack (20g)

Amount per serving	Amount per serving	Amount per serving
Calories 70	**Cholesterol** 0mg	**Total Carbohydrate** 16g
Total Fat 0g	**Sodium** 0mg	Dietary Fiber 0g
Saturated Fat 0g	**Protein** 0g	Sugars 11g

Yum Earth® Organics, YumEarth Organic Gummy Bears

1 snack pack (20g)

Amount per serving	Amount per serving	Amount per serving
Calories 69	**Cholesterol** 0mg	**Total Carbohydrate** 18g
Total Fat 0g	**Sodium** 7mg	Dietary Fiber 0g
Saturated Fat 0g	**Protein** 0g	Sugars 15g

Yum Earth® Organics, YumEarth Organic Lollipops

17g (approx 3 pops)

Amount per serving	Amount per serving	Amount per serving
Calories 70	**Cholesterol** 0mg	**Total Carbohydrate** 17g
Total Fat 0g	**Sodium** 0mg	Dietary Fiber 0g
Saturated Fat 0g	**Protein** 0g	Sugars 17g

Nut Candies

Justin's, Dark Chocolate Peanut Butter Cup

2 cups

Amount per serving	Amount per serving	Amount per serving
Calories 200	**Cholesterol** 0mg	**Total Carbohydrate** 20g
Total Fat 16g	**Sodium** 120mg	Dietary Fiber 2g
Saturated Fat 7g	**Protein** 4g	Sugars 14g

Justin's, Milk Chocolate Peanut Butter Cup

2 cups

Amount per serving	Amount per serving	Amount per serving
Calories 200	**Cholesterol** 0mg	**Total Carbohydrate** 18g
Total Fat 14g	**Sodium** 120mg	Dietary Fiber 2g
Saturated Fat 6g	**Protein** 4g	Sugars 14g

Rice Cakes / Chips

Barbara's Bakery, Barbara's Organic Brown Rice Crisps

1 cup (30g)

Amount per serving	Amount per serving	Amount per serving
Calories 120	**Cholesterol** 0mg	**Total Carbohydrate** 25g
Total Fat 1g	**Sodium** 95mg	Dietary Fiber <1g
Saturated Fat 0g	**Protein** 0g	Sugars 1g

Eden Foods, Popcorn, 100% Whole Grain, Organic

2 tbsp

Amount per serving	Amount per serving	Amount per serving
Calories 80	**Cholesterol** NA	**Total Carbohydrate** 20g
Total Fat 1g	**Sodium** 0mg	Dietary Fiber 5g
Saturated Fat 0g	**Protein** 2g	Sugars 0g

Garden of Eatin', Baked Blue Chips, Tortilla Chips

28g/about 19 chips

Amount per serving	Amount per serving	Amount per serving
Calories 120	**Cholesterol** 0mg	**Total Carbohydrate** 20g
Total Fat 3g	**Sodium** 120mg	Dietary Fiber 3g
Saturated Fat 1g	**Protein** 3g	Sugars 0g

Garden of Eatin', Baked Cheddar Puffs

28g/about 35 chips

Amount per serving	Amount per serving	Amount per serving
Calories 140	**Cholesterol** <5mg	**Total Carbohydrate** 18g
Total Fat 7g	**Sodium** 310mg	Dietary Fiber 1g
Saturated Fat 1g	**Protein** 2g	Sugars 1g

Garden of Eatin', Baked Crunchitos

28g/about 35 chips

Amount per serving	Amount per serving	Amount per serving
Calories 140	**Cholesterol** <5mg	**Total Carbohydrate** 18g
Total Fat 7g	**Sodium** 310mg	Dietary Fiber 1g
Saturated Fat 1g	**Protein** 2g	Sugars 1g

Garden of Eatin', Baked Yellow Tortilla Chips

28g/about 19 chips

Amount per serving	Amount per serving	Amount per serving
Calories 120	**Cholesterol** 0mg	**Total Carbohydrate** 21g
Total Fat 2g	**Sodium** 120mg	Dietary Fiber 3g
Saturated Fat 0g	**Protein** 3g	Sugars 0g

Garden of Eatin', Black Bean Chili, All Natural Tortilla Chips with Jalapeno

28g/about 13 chips

Amount per serving	Amount per serving	Amount per serving
Calories 140	**Cholesterol** 0mg	**Total Carbohydrate** 17g
Total Fat 7g	**Sodium** 130mg	Dietary Fiber 4g
Saturated Fat 0.5g	**Protein** 3g	Sugars 0g

Garden of Eatin', Black Bean, All Natural Tortilla Chips with Black Beans

28g/about 13 chips

Amount per serving	Amount per serving	Amount per serving
Calories 140	**Cholesterol** 0mg	**Total Carbohydrate** 18g
Total Fat 7g	**Sodium** 70mg	Dietary Fiber 1g
Saturated Fat 0.5g	**Protein** 2g	Sugars 0g

Garden of Eatin', Blue Chips, All Natural Tortilla Chips, No Salt Added

28g/about 16 chips

Amount per serving	Amount per serving	Amount per serving
Calories 140	**Cholesterol** 0mg	**Total Carbohydrate** 18g
Total Fat 7g	**Sodium** 10mg	Dietary Fiber 2g
Saturated Fat 0.5g	**Protein** 2g	Sugars 0g

Garden of Eatin', Blue Chips, Blue Corn Tortilla Chips

28g/about 16 chips

Amount per serving	Amount per serving	Amount per serving
Calories 140	**Cholesterol** 0mg	**Total Carbohydrate** 18g
Total Fat 7g	**Sodium** 10mg	Dietary Fiber 2g
Saturated Fat 0.5g	**Protein** 2g	Sugars 0g

Garden of Eatin', Chili & Lime, All Natural Cantina Chips

28g/about 10 chips

Amount per serving	Amount per serving	Amount per serving
Calories 140	**Cholesterol** 0mg	**Total Carbohydrate** 18g
Total Fat 7g	**Sodium** 125mg	Dietary Fiber 2g
Saturated Fat 1g	**Protein** 2g	Sugars 1g

Garden of Eatin', Guac-A-Mole, All Natural Tortilla Chips

28g/about 9 chips

Amount per serving	Amount per serving	Amount per serving
Calories 140	**Cholesterol** 0mg	**Total Carbohydrate** 19g
Total Fat 6g	**Sodium** 170mg	Dietary Fiber 2g
Saturated Fat 0.5g	**Protein** 2g	Sugars <1g

Garden of Eatin', Key Lime Jalapeno, All Natural Tortilla Chips, Bold Flavor

28g/about 15 chips

Amount per serving	Amount per serving	Amount per serving
Calories 140	**Cholesterol** 0mg	**Total Carbohydrate** 18g
Total Fat 7g	**Sodium** 80mg	Dietary Fiber 3g
Saturated Fat 1g	**Protein** 2g	Sugars 0g

Garden of Eatin', Little Soy Blues, All Natural Tortilla Chips with Soybeans

28g/about 13 chips

Amount per serving	Amount per serving	Amount per serving
Calories 140	**Cholesterol** 0mg	**Total Carbohydrate** 17g
Total Fat 7g	**Sodium** 70mg	Dietary Fiber 2g
Saturated Fat 0.5g	**Protein** 3g	Sugars 0g

Garden of Eatin', Maui Style Onion, All Natural Tortilla Chips, Bold Flavor

28g/about 15 chips

Amount per serving	Amount per serving	Amount per serving
Calories 140	**Cholesterol** 0mg	**Total Carbohydrate** 19g
Total Fat 6g	**Sodium** 80mg	Dietary Fiber 1g
Saturated Fat 0.5g	**Protein** 2g	Sugars 0g

Garden of Eatin', Mini White Rounds, All Natural Bite-Size Tortilla Chips

28g/about 18 chips

Amount per serving	Amount per serving	Amount per serving
Calories 140	**Cholesterol** 0mg	**Total Carbohydrate** 19g
Total Fat 6g	**Sodium** 60mg	Dietary Fiber 2g
Saturated Fat 0.5g	**Protein** 2g	Sugars 0g

Garden of Eatin', Mini White Strips, All Natural Bite-Size Tortilla Chips

28g/about 18 chips

Amount per serving	Amount per serving	Amount per serving
Calories 140	**Cholesterol** 0mg	**Total Carbohydrate** 19g
Total Fat 6g	**Sodium** 60mg	Dietary Fiber 2g
Saturated Fat 0.5g	**Protein** 2g	Sugars 0g

Garden of Eatin', Mini Yellow rounds, All Natural Bite-Size Tortilla Chips

28g/about 19 chips

Amount per serving	Amount per serving	Amount per serving
Calories 140	**Cholesterol** 0mg	**Total Carbohydrate** 18g
Total Fat 7g	**Sodium** 60mg	Dietary Fiber 2g
Saturated Fat 0.5g	**Protein** 2g	Sugars 0g

Garden of Eatin', Multigrain Blues, Sea Salt, All Natural Tortilla Chips

28g/about 14 chips

Amount per serving	Amount per serving	Amount per serving
Calories 130	**Cholesterol** 0mg	**Total Carbohydrate** 16g
Total Fat 7g	**Sodium** 110mg	Dietary Fiber 2g
Saturated Fat 0.5g	**Protein** 2g	Sugars 1g

Garden of Eatin', Multigrain Tortilla Chips, Everything

28g/about 16 chips

Amount per serving	Amount per serving	Amount per serving
Calories 140	**Cholesterol** 0mg	**Total Carbohydrate** 19g
Total Fat 7g	**Sodium** 140mg	Dietary Fiber 3g
Saturated Fat 1g	**Protein** 2g	Sugars 1g

Garden of Eatin', Multigrain Tortilla Chips, Sea Salt with Flax Seeds

28g/about 16 chips

Amount per serving	Amount per serving	Amount per serving
Calories 140	**Cholesterol** 0mg	**Total Carbohydrate** 19g
Total Fat 7g	**Sodium** 140mg	Dietary Fiber 3g
Saturated Fat 1g	**Protein** 2g	Sugars 1g

Garden of Eatin', Nacho Cheese, All Natural Tortilla Chips

28g/about 9 chips

Amount per serving	Amount per serving	Amount per serving
Calories 140	**Cholesterol** 0mg	**Total Carbohydrate** 18g
Total Fat 6g	**Sodium** 140mg	Dietary Fiber 2g
Saturated Fat 0.5g	**Protein** 2g	Sugars <1g

Garden of Eatin', Pico De Gallo, All Natural Tortilla Chips

28g/about 7 chips

Amount per serving	Amount per serving	Amount per serving
Calories 140	**Cholesterol** 0mg	**Total Carbohydrate** 18g
Total Fat 7g	**Sodium** 150mg	Dietary Fiber 3g
Saturated Fat 0.5g	**Protein** 2g	Sugars 0g

Garden of Eatin', Pita Chips with Whole Grain, Greek Isle

28g/about 9 chips

Amount per serving	Amount per serving	Amount per serving
Calories 120	**Cholesterol** 0mg	**Total Carbohydrate** 20g
Total Fat 3g	**Sodium** 190mg	Dietary Fiber 2g
Saturated Fat 0g	**Protein** 3g	Sugars 2g

Garden of Eatin', Pita Chips with Whole Grain, Sea Salt

28g/about 9 chips

Amount per serving	Amount per serving	Amount per serving
Calories 120	**Cholesterol** 0mg	**Total Carbohydrate** 21g
Total Fat 3g	**Sodium** 260mg	Dietary Fiber 2g
Saturated Fat 0g	**Protein** 3g	Sugars 1g

Garden of Eatin', Popped Blues, Multigrain—Sea Salt, All Natural Tortilla Chips

28g/about 20 chips

Amount per serving	Amount per serving	Amount per serving
Calories 120	**Cholesterol** 0mg	**Total Carbohydrate** 20g
Total Fat 3g	**Sodium** 280mg	Dietary Fiber 3g
Saturated Fat 0g	**Protein** 2g	Sugars 1g

Garden of Eatin', Popped Tortillas, All Natural Tortilla Chips

28g/about 20 chips

Amount per serving	Amount per serving	Amount per serving
Calories 110	**Cholesterol** 0mg	**Total Carbohydrate** 19g
Total Fat 3g	**Sodium** 280mg	Dietary Fiber 3g
Saturated Fat 0g	**Protein** 2g	Sugars 1g

Garden of Eatin', Red Chips, All Natural Tortilla Chips

28g/about 15 chips

Amount per serving	Amount per serving	Amount per serving
Calories 140	**Cholesterol** 0mg	**Total Carbohydrate** 18g
Total Fat 7g	**Sodium** 70mg	Dietary Fiber 1g
Saturated Fat 1g	**Protein** 2g	Sugars 0g

Garden of Eatin', Red Hot Blues, Spicy All Natural Tortilla Chips

28g/about 15 chips

Amount per serving	Amount per serving	Amount per serving
Calories 140	**Cholesterol** 0mg	**Total Carbohydrate** 18g
Total Fat 7g	**Sodium** 150mg	Dietary Fiber 2g
Saturated Fat 0.5g	**Protein** 2g	Sugars 0g

Garden of Eatin', Salsa Reds, Zesty All Natural Tortilla Chips

28g/about 15 chips

Amount per serving	Amount per serving	Amount per serving
Calories 140	**Cholesterol** 0mg	**Total Carbohydrate** 18g
Total Fat 7g	**Sodium** 170mg	Dietary Fiber 3g
Saturated Fat 1g	**Protein** 2g	Sugars 0g

Garden of Eatin', Sesame Blues, All Natural Tortilla Chips with Sesame Seeds

28g/about 9 chips

Amount per serving	Amount per serving	Amount per serving
Calories 150	**Cholesterol** 0mg	**Total Carbohydrate** 16g
Total Fat 8g	**Sodium** 90mg	Dietary Fiber 2g
Saturated Fat 1g	**Protein** 3g	Sugars 0g

Garden of Eatin', Sunny Blues, All Natural Tortilla Chips with Sunflower Seeds

28g/about 9 chips

Amount per serving	Amount per serving	Amount per serving
Calories 150	**Cholesterol** 0mg	**Total Carbohydrate** 17g
Total Fat 8g	**Sodium** 70mg	Dietary Fiber 2g
Saturated Fat 0.5g	**Protein** 2g	Sugars 0g

Garden of Eatin', Tamari Chips, All Natural Tortilla Chips

28g/about 8 chips

Amount per serving	Amount per serving	Amount per serving
Calories 140	**Cholesterol** 0mg	**Total Carbohydrate** 18g
Total Fat 7g	**Sodium** 160mg	Dietary Fiber 3g
Saturated Fat 1g	**Protein** 2g	Sugars 0g

Garden of Eatin', Three Pepper, All Natural Tortilla Chips, Bold Flavor

28g/about 15 chips

Amount per serving	Amount per serving	Amount per serving
Calories 140	**Cholesterol** 0mg	**Total Carbohydrate** 18g
Total Fat 7g	**Sodium** 125mg	Dietary Fiber 2g
Saturated Fat 0.5g	**Protein** 2g	Sugars 0g

Garden of Eatin', Veggie Chips, Beet & Garlic All Natural Tortilla Chips

28g/about 17 chips

Amount per serving	Amount per serving	Amount per serving
Calories 140	Cholesterol 0mg	Total Carbohydrate 19g
Total Fat 6g	Sodium 120mg	Dietary Fiber 2g
Saturated Fat 1g	Protein 2g	Sugars 1g

Garden of Eatin', Veggie Chips, Vegetable Medley, All Natural Tortilla Chips

28g/about 17 chips

Amount per serving	Amount per serving	Amount per serving
Calories 140	Cholesterol 0mg	Total Carbohydrate 19g
Total Fat 6g	Sodium 120mg	Dietary Fiber 2g
Saturated Fat 1g	Protein 2g	Sugars 1g

Garden of Eatin', White Chips, All Natural Cantina Chips

28g/about 10 chips

Amount per serving	Amount per serving	Amount per serving
Calories 140	Cholesterol 0mg	Total Carbohydrate 19g
Total Fat 6g	Sodium 70mg	Dietary Fiber 2g
Saturated Fat 0.5g	Protein 2g	Sugars 0g

Garden of Eatin', Yellow Chips, All Natural Tortilla Chips

28g/about 13 chips

Amount per serving	Amount per serving	Amount per serving
Calories 140	Cholesterol 0mg	Total Carbohydrate 18g
Total Fat 7g	Sodium 70mg	Dietary Fiber 2g
Saturated Fat 0.5g	Protein 2g	Sugars 0g

Go Raw, Pumpkin Super Chips

About 20 pieces (28g)

Amount per serving	Amount per serving	Amount per serving
Calories 190	Cholesterol 0mg	Total Carbohydrate 12g
Total Fat 13g	Sodium 120mg	Dietary Fiber 3g
Saturated Fat 2g	Protein 6g	Sugars 8g

Go Raw, Spirulina Super Chips

About 22 pieces (28g)

Amount per serving	Amount per serving	Amount per serving
Calories 160	Cholesterol 0mg	Total Carbohydrate 20g
Total Fat 8g	Sodium 20mg	Dietary Fiber 4g
Saturated Fat 1g	Protein 3g	Sugars 12g

KOYO, Organic Buckwheat Rice Cakes Lightly Salted - 6 oz

1 cake (10g)

Amount per serving	Amount per serving	Amount per serving
Calories 40	**Cholesterol** 0mg	**Total Carbohydrate** 8g
Total Fat 0g	**Sodium** 80mg	Dietary Fiber 0g
Saturated Fat 0g	**Protein** <1g	Sugars 0g

KOYO, Organic Dulse Rice Cakes No Salt - 6 oz

1 cake (10g)

Amount per serving	Amount per serving	Amount per serving
Calories 40	**Cholesterol** 0mg	**Total Carbohydrate** 8g
Total Fat 0g	**Sodium** 0mg	Dietary Fiber 0g
Saturated Fat 0g	**Protein** <1g	Sugars 0g

KOYO, Organic Millet Rice Cakes Lightly Salted - 6 oz

1 cake (10g)

Amount per serving	Amount per serving	Amount per serving
Calories 40	**Cholesterol** 0mg	**Total Carbohydrate** 8g
Total Fat 0g	**Sodium** 80mg	Dietary Fiber 0g
Saturated Fat 0g	**Protein** <1g	Sugars 0g

KOYO, Organic Mixed Grain Rice Cakes Lightly Salted - 6 oz

1 cake (10g)

Amount per serving	Amount per serving	Amount per serving
Calories 40	**Cholesterol** 0mg	**Total Carbohydrate** 8g
Total Fat 0g	**Sodium** 80mg	Dietary Fiber 0g
Saturated Fat 0g	**Protein** <1g	Sugars 0g

KOYO, Organic Mixed Grain Rice Cakes No Salt - 6 oz

1 cake (10g)

Amount per serving	Amount per serving	Amount per serving
Calories 35	**Cholesterol** 0mg	**Total Carbohydrate** 8g
Total Fat 0g	**Sodium** 0mg	Dietary Fiber 0g
Saturated Fat 0g	**Protein** <1g	Sugars 0g

KOYO, Organic Nori Rice Cakes No Salt - 6 oz

1 cake (10g)

Amount per serving	Amount per serving	Amount per serving
Calories 40	**Cholesterol** 0mg	**Total Carbohydrate** 8g
Total Fat 0g	**Sodium** 0mg	Dietary Fiber 0g
Saturated Fat 0g	**Protein** <1g	Sugars 0g

KOYO, Organic Plain Rice Cakes Lightly Salted - 6 oz

1 cake (10g)

Amount per serving	Amount per serving	Amount per serving
Calories 35	Cholesterol 0mg	Total Carbohydrate 8g
Total Fat 0g	Sodium 80mg	Dietary Fiber 0g
Saturated Fat 0g	Protein <1g	Sugars 0g

KOYO, Organic Plain Rice Cakes No Salt - 6 oz

1 cake (10g)

Amount per serving	Amount per serving	Amount per serving
Calories 40	Cholesterol 0mg	Total Carbohydrate 8g
Total Fat 0g	Sodium 0mg	Dietary Fiber 0g
Saturated Fat 0g	Protein <1g	Sugars 0g

Lundberg Family Farms, Organic Brown Rice Cake—Lightly Salted

1 cake

Amount per serving	Amount per serving	Amount per serving
Calories 60	Cholesterol 0mg	Total Carbohydrate 14g
Total Fat 0.5g	Sodium 35mg	Dietary Fiber 1g
Saturated Fat 0g	Protein 1g	Sugars 0g

Lundberg Family Farms, Organic Brown Rice Cake—Salt Free

1 cake

Amount per serving	Amount per serving	Amount per serving
Calories 60	Cholesterol 0mg	Total Carbohydrate 14g
Total Fat 0.5g	Sodium 0mg	Dietary Fiber 1g
Saturated Fat 0g	Protein 1g	Sugars 0g

Lundberg Family Farms, Organic Caramel Corn Rice Cake

1 cake

Amount per serving	Amount per serving	Amount per serving
Calories 80	Cholesterol 0mg	Total Carbohydrate 18g
Total Fat 0.5g	Sodium 40mg	Dietary Fiber 1g
Saturated Fat 0g	Protein 1g	Sugars 2g

Lundberg Family Farms, Organic Cinnamon Toast Rice Cake

1 cake

Amount per serving	Amount per serving	Amount per serving
Calories 80	Cholesterol 0mg	Total Carbohydrate 18g
Total Fat 0.5g	Sodium 0mg	Dietary Fiber 1g
Saturated Fat 0g	Protein 1g	Sugars 3g

Lundberg Family Farms, Organic Cracked Black Pepper Rice Chips

About 9 chips (28g)

Amount per serving	Amount per serving	Amount per serving
Calories 140	**Cholesterol** 0mg	**Total Carbohydrate** 19g
Total Fat 6g	**Sodium** 110mg	Dietary Fiber 1g
Saturated Fat 0.5g	**Protein** 2g	Sugars 0g

Lundberg Family Farms, Organic Flax with Tamari Rice Cake

1 cake

Amount per serving	Amount per serving	Amount per serving
Calories 60	**Cholesterol** 0mg	**Total Carbohydrate** 13g
Total Fat 0g	**Sodium** 75mg	Dietary Fiber 1g
Saturated Fat 0g	**Protein** 1g	Sugars 0g

Lundberg Family Farms, Organic Hemp-A-Licious Rice Cake

1 cake (21g)

Amount per serving	Amount per serving	Amount per serving
Calories 80	**Cholesterol** 0mg	**Total Carbohydrate** 16g
Total Fat 1g	**Sodium** 60mg	Dietary Fiber 1g
Saturated Fat 0g	**Protein** 2g	Sugars 1g

Lundberg Family Farms, Organic Kettle Corn Rice Cake

1 cake (22g)

Amount per serving	Amount per serving	Amount per serving
Calories 80	**Cholesterol** 0mg	**Total Carbohydrate** 18g
Total Fat 0.5g	**Sodium** 70mg	Dietary Fiber 1g
Saturated Fat 0g	**Protein** 1g	Sugars 3g

Lundberg Family Farms, Organic Koku Seaweed Rice Cake

1 cake

Amount per serving	Amount per serving	Amount per serving
Calories 60	**Cholesterol** 0mg	**Total Carbohydrate** 14g
Total Fat 0.5g	**Sodium** 75mg	Dietary Fiber 1g
Saturated Fat 0g	**Protein** 1g	Sugars 1g

Lundberg Family Farms, Organic Mochi Sweet Rice Cake

1 cake

Amount per serving	Amount per serving	Amount per serving
Calories 60	**Cholesterol** 0mg	**Total Carbohydrate** 14g
Total Fat 0.5g	**Sodium** 35mg	Dietary Fiber 1g
Saturated Fat 0g	**Protein** 1g	Sugars 0g

Lundberg Family Farms, Organic Popcorn Rice Cake

1 cake

Amount per serving	Amount per serving	Amount per serving
Calories 60	**Cholesterol** 0mg	**Total Carbohydrate** 14g
Total Fat 0.5g	**Sodium** 35mg	Dietary Fiber 1g
Saturated Fat 0g	**Protein** 1g	Sugars 0g

Lundberg Family Farms, Organic Sesame Tamari Rice Cake

1 cake (20g)

Amount per serving	Amount per serving	Amount per serving
Calories 60	**Cholesterol** 0mg	**Total Carbohydrate** 14g
Total Fat 1g	**Sodium** 75mg	Dietary Fiber 1g
Saturated Fat 0g	**Protein** 1g	Sugars 0g

Lundberg Family Farms, Organic Spicy Black Bean Rice Chips

About 9 chips (28g)

Amount per serving	Amount per serving	Amount per serving
Calories 140	**Cholesterol** 0mg	**Total Carbohydrate** 18g
Total Fat 6g	**Sodium** 170mg	Dietary Fiber 1g
Saturated Fat 0.5g	**Protein** 2g	Sugars 1g

Lundberg Family Farms, Organic Sweet Chili Rice Cake

1 cake (21g)

Amount per serving	Amount per serving	Amount per serving
Calories 70	**Cholesterol** 0mg	**Total Carbohydrate** 16g
Total Fat 0.5g	**Sodium** 75mg	Dietary Fiber 1g
Saturated Fat 0g	**Protein** 1g	Sugars 2g

Lundberg Family Farms, Organic Wild Rice Lightly Salted Rice Cake

1 cake

Amount per serving	Amount per serving	Amount per serving
Calories 60	**Cholesterol** 0mg	**Total Carbohydrate** 14g
Total Fat 0.5g	**Sodium** 35mg	Dietary Fiber 1g
Saturated Fat 0g	**Protein** 1g	Sugars 0g

Manna Organics, Manna Munchies Kale Chips Café Mocha

1 oz (28g)

Amount per serving	Amount per serving	Amount per serving
Calories 100	**Cholesterol** 0mg	**Total Carbohydrate** 12g
Total Fat 4.5g	**Sodium** 40mg	Dietary Fiber 2g
Saturated Fat 1g	**Protein** 3g	Sugars 6g

Manna Organics, Manna Munchies Kale Chips Curry Bliss

1 oz (28g)

Amount per serving	Amount per serving	Amount per serving
Calories 120	**Cholesterol** 0mg	**Total Carbohydrate** 11g
Total Fat 7g	**Sodium** 200mg	Dietary Fiber 2g
Saturated Fat 1.5g	**Protein** 5g	Sugars 4g

Manna Organics, Manna Munchies Kale Chips Pizza Margherita

1 oz (28g)

Amount per serving	Amount per serving	Amount per serving
Calories 110	**Cholesterol** 0mg	**Total Carbohydrate** 13g
Total Fat 6g	**Sodium** 200mg	Dietary Fiber 2g
Saturated Fat 1g	**Protein** 5g	Sugars 4g

Manna Organics, Manna Munchies Kale Chips Say Cheese

1 oz (28g)

Amount per serving	Amount per serving	Amount per serving
Calories 130	**Cholesterol** 0mg	**Total Carbohydrate** 11g
Total Fat 9g	**Sodium** 170mg	Dietary Fiber 2g
Saturated Fat 1.5g	**Protein** 5g	Sugars 1g

Utz, Organic 7 Grain Pretzel Sticks

1 oz (28g/about 7 pretzels)

Amount per serving	Amount per serving	Amount per serving
Calories 120	**Cholesterol** 0mg	**Total Carbohydrate** 22g
Total Fat 2g	**Sodium** 200mg	Dietary Fiber 3g
Saturated Fat 0g	**Protein** 3g	Sugars 1g

Utz, Organic Blue Corn Tortillas

1 oz (28g/about 12 chips)

Amount per serving	Amount per serving	Amount per serving
Calories 140	**Cholesterol** 0mg	**Total Carbohydrate** 19g
Total Fat 6g	**Sodium** 100mg	Dietary Fiber 1g
Saturated Fat 0.5g	**Protein** 2g	Sugars 0g

Utz, Organic White Corn Tortillas

1 oz (28g/about 12 chips)

Amount per serving	Amount per serving	Amount per serving
Calories 140	**Cholesterol** 0mg	**Total Carbohydrate** 19g
Total Fat 6g	**Sodium** 100mg	Dietary Fiber 2g
Saturated Fat 0.5g	**Protein** 2g	Sugars 0g

YogaVive, Apple Chips - Caramel

10g

Amount per serving	Amount per serving	Amount per serving
Calories 35	**Cholesterol** 0mg	**Total Carbohydrate** 9g
Total Fat 0g	**Sodium** 0mg	Dietary Fiber <1g
Saturated Fat 0g	**Protein** 0g	Sugars 7g

YogaVive, Apple Chips - Chocolate

10g

Amount per serving	Amount per serving	Amount per serving
Calories 35	**Cholesterol** 0mg	**Total Carbohydrate** 9g
Total Fat 0g	**Sodium** 0mg	Dietary Fiber <1g
Saturated Fat 0g	**Protein** 0g	Sugars 7g

YogaVive, Apple Chips - Cinnamon

10g

Amount per serving	Amount per serving	Amount per serving
Calories 35	**Cholesterol** 0mg	**Total Carbohydrate** 9g
Total Fat 0g	**Sodium** 0mg	Dietary Fiber <1g
Saturated Fat 0g	**Protein** 0g	Sugars 7g

YogaVive, Apple Chips - Ginger

10g

Amount per serving	Amount per serving	Amount per serving
Calories 35	**Cholesterol** 0mg	**Total Carbohydrate** 9g
Total Fat 0g	**Sodium** 0mg	Dietary Fiber <1g
Saturated Fat 0g	**Protein** 0g	Sugars 7g

YogaVive, Apple Chips - Original

10g

Amount per serving	Amount per serving	Amount per serving
Calories 35	**Cholesterol** 0mg	**Total Carbohydrate** 9g
Total Fat 0g	**Sodium** 0mg	Dietary Fiber <1g
Saturated Fat 0g	**Protein** 0g	Sugars 7g

YogaVive, Apple Chips - Peach

10g

Amount per serving	Amount per serving	Amount per serving
Calories 35	**Cholesterol** 0mg	**Total Carbohydrate** 9g
Total Fat 0g	**Sodium** 0mg	Dietary Fiber <1g
Saturated Fat 0g	**Protein** 0g	Sugars 7g

YogaVive, Apple Chips - Strawberry

10g

Amount per serving	Amount per serving	Amount per serving
Calories 35	**Cholesterol** 0mg	**Total Carbohydrate** 9g
Total Fat 0g	**Sodium** 0mg	Dietary Fiber <1g
Saturated Fat 0g	**Protein** 0g	Sugars 7g

YogaVive, Mango Chips - Chili

10g

Amount per serving	Amount per serving	Amount per serving
Calories 40	**Cholesterol** 0mg	**Total Carbohydrate** 9g
Total Fat 0g	**Sodium** 0mg	Dietary Fiber <1g
Saturated Fat 0g	**Protein** 1g	Sugars 8g

YogaVive, Mango Chips - Original

10g

Amount per serving	Amount per serving	Amount per serving
Calories 40	**Cholesterol** 0mg	**Total Carbohydrate** 9g
Total Fat 0g	**Sodium** 0mg	Dietary Fiber <1g
Saturated Fat 0g	**Protein** 1g	Sugars 8g

YogaVive, Mango Chips - Sea Salt

10g

Amount per serving	Amount per serving	Amount per serving
Calories 40	**Cholesterol** 0mg	**Total Carbohydrate** 9g
Total Fat 0g	**Sodium** 0.1mg	Dietary Fiber <1g
Saturated Fat 0g	**Protein** 1g	Sugars 8g

Snacks

Annie's, Organic Cheddar Snack Mix

1 oz (28g/about 1/2 cup)

Amount per serving	Amount per serving	Amount per serving
Calories 140	**Cholesterol** 0mg	**Total Carbohydrate** 19g
Total Fat 5g	**Sodium** 270mg	Dietary Fiber 0g
Saturated Fat 0.5g	**Protein** 3g	Sugars 1g

Annie's, Organic Honey Wheat Pretzel Bunnies

1 oz (28g/about 32 pieces)

Amount per serving	Amount per serving	Amount per serving
Calories 100	**Cholesterol** 0mg	**Total Carbohydrate** 20g
Total Fat 1g	**Sodium** 360mg	Dietary Fiber 1g
Saturated Fat 0g	**Protein** 3g	Sugars 3g

Annie's, Organic Pizza Snack Mix

1 oz (28g/about 1/2 cup)

Amount per serving	Amount per serving	Amount per serving
Calories 140	**Cholesterol** 0mg	**Total Carbohydrate** 19g
Total Fat 5g	**Sodium** 250mg	Dietary Fiber 0g
Saturated Fat 0.5g	**Protein** 3g	Sugars 1g

Annie's, Organic Pretzel Bunnies

1 oz (28g/about 32 pieces)

Amount per serving	Amount per serving	Amount per serving
Calories 110	**Cholesterol** 0mg	**Total Carbohydrate** 22g
Total Fat 0g	**Sodium** 360mg	Dietary Fiber 1g
Saturated Fat 0g	**Protein** 3g	Sugars 1g

Annie's, Organic Traditional Party Mix

1 oz (28g/about 1/2 cup)

Amount per serving	Amount per serving	Amount per serving
Calories 130	**Cholesterol** 0mg	**Total Carbohydrate** 19g
Total Fat 5g	**Sodium** 260mg	Dietary Fiber 1g
Saturated Fat 0.5g	**Protein** 3g	Sugars 1g

Go Raw, Pizza Flax Snax

About 22 pieces (28g)

Amount per serving	Amount per serving	Amount per serving
Calories 180	**Cholesterol** 0mg	**Total Carbohydrate** 10g
Total Fat 13g	**Sodium** 290mg	Dietary Fiber 5g
Saturated Fat 1g	**Protein** 5g	Sugars 1g

Go Raw, Simple Flax Snax

About 22 pieces (28g)

Amount per serving	Amount per serving	Amount per serving
Calories 180	**Cholesterol** 0mg	**Total Carbohydrate** 10g
Total Fat 13g	**Sodium** 20mg	Dietary Fiber 8g
Saturated Fat 1g	**Protein** 6g	Sugars 1g

Go Raw, Spicy Flax Snax

About 22 pieces (28g)

Amount per serving	Amount per serving	Amount per serving
Calories 180	**Cholesterol** 0mg	**Total Carbohydrate** 10g
Total Fat 13g	**Sodium** 290mg	Dietary Fiber 5g
Saturated Fat 1g	**Protein** 5g	Sugars 1g

Go Raw, Sunflower Flax Snax

About 22 pieces (28g)

Amount per serving	Amount per serving	Amount per serving
Calories 180	**Cholesterol** 0mg	**Total Carbohydrate** 10g
Total Fat 13g	**Sodium** 240mg	Dietary Fiber 5g
Saturated Fat 1g	**Protein** 5g	Sugars 1g

Manna Munchies™, Snack Crunchies Banana Coconut

1 1/4 oz (35g)

Amount per serving	Amount per serving	Amount per serving
Calories 190	**Cholesterol** 0mg	**Total Carbohydrate** 12g
Total Fat 14g	**Sodium** 30mg	Dietary Fiber 3g
Saturated Fat 2.5g	**Protein** 5g	Sugars 6g

Manna Munchies™, Snack Crunchies Ginger Fig Date

1 1/4 oz (35g)

Amount per serving	Amount per serving	Amount per serving
Calories 170	**Cholesterol** 0mg	**Total Carbohydrate** 14g
Total Fat 13g	**Sodium** 30mg	Dietary Fiber 3g
Saturated Fat 1.5g	**Protein** 5g	Sugars 8g

Newman's Own Organics, High Protein Pretzels

About 22 pretzels (30g)

Amount per serving	Amount per serving	Amount per serving
Calories 120	**Cholesterol** 0mg	**Total Carbohydrate** 22g
Total Fat 1.5g	**Sodium** 230mg	Dietary Fiber 4g
Saturated Fat 0g	**Protein** 5g	Sugars 1g

Newman's Own Organics, Honey Wheat Pretzels

About 20 pretzels (30g)

Amount per serving	Amount per serving	Amount per serving
Calories 110	**Cholesterol** 0mg	**Total Carbohydrate** 22g
Total Fat 1g	**Sodium** 180mg	Dietary Fiber 3g
Saturated Fat 0g	**Protein** 2g	Sugars 2g

Newman's Own Organics, Mighty Mini Pretzels

About 20 pretzels (30g)

Amount per serving	Amount per serving	Amount per serving
Calories 110	**Cholesterol** 0mg	**Total Carbohydrate** 22g
Total Fat 1g	**Sodium** 180mg	Dietary Fiber 4g
Saturated Fat 0g	**Protein** 3g	Sugars 0g

Newman's Own Organics, Pop's Corn, Butter

About 3 cups (28g)

Amount per serving	Amount per serving	Amount per serving
Calories 42	**Cholesterol** 0mg	**Total Carbohydrate** 17g
Total Fat 5g	**Sodium** 187mg	Dietary Fiber 4g
Saturated Fat 2g	**Protein** 3g	Sugars 1g

Newman's Own Organics, Pop's Corn, Light Butter

About 3 cups (28g)

Amount per serving	Amount per serving	Amount per serving
Calories 112	**Cholesterol** 0mg	**Total Carbohydrate** 19g
Total Fat 3g	**Sodium** NA	Dietary Fiber 3.5g
Saturated Fat 2g	**Protein** 3g	Sugars 1g

Newman's Own Organics, Pop's Corn, Unsalted

About 3 cups (28g)

Amount per serving	Amount per serving	Amount per serving
Calories 100	**Cholesterol** 0mg	**Total Carbohydrate** 20g
Total Fat 1.5g	**Sodium** 0mg	Dietary Fiber 3g
Saturated Fat 0g	**Protein** 3g	Sugars 0g

Newman's Own Organics, Pretzel Rods

4 rods (30g)

Amount per serving	Amount per serving	Amount per serving
Calories 120	**Cholesterol** 0mg	**Total Carbohydrate** 25g
Total Fat 1.5g	**Sodium** 330mg	Dietary Fiber 2g
Saturated Fat 0g	**Protein** 3g	Sugars 1g

Newman's Own Organics, Pretzel Spelt

20 pretzels (30g)

Amount per serving	Amount per serving	Amount per serving
Calories 120	**Cholesterol** 0mg	**Total Carbohydrate** 23g
Total Fat 1g	**Sodium** 240mg	Dietary Fiber 4g
Saturated Fat 0g	**Protein** 4g	Sugars 0g

Newman's Own Organics, Salted Pretzel Rounds

8 rounds (30g)

Amount per serving	Amount per serving	Amount per serving
Calories 110	**Cholesterol** 0mg	**Total Carbohydrate** 24g
Total Fat 1g	**Sodium** 400mg	Dietary Fiber <1g
Saturated Fat 0g	**Protein** 2g	Sugars 1g

Newman's Own Organics, Salted Pretzel Sticks

About 13 sticks (30g)

Amount per serving	Amount per serving	Amount per serving
Calories 110	**Cholesterol** 0mg	**Total Carbohydrate** 24g
Total Fat 1g	**Sodium** 350mg	Dietary Fiber 1g
Saturated Fat 0g	**Protein** 2g	Sugars 1g

Newman's Own Organics, Salted Pretzel Thins

About 10 pretzels (30g)

Amount per serving	Amount per serving	Amount per serving
Calories 110	**Cholesterol** 0mg	**Total Carbohydrate** 24g
Total Fat 1g	**Sodium** 400mg	Dietary Fiber <1g
Saturated Fat 0g	**Protein** 2g	Sugars 1g

Newman's Own Organics, Thin Pretzel Sticks

About 22 pretzels (30g)

Amount per serving	Amount per serving	Amount per serving
Calories 110	**Cholesterol** 0mg	**Total Carbohydrate** 22g
Total Fat 1.5g	**Sodium** 180mg	Dietary Fiber 4g
Saturated Fat 0g	**Protein** 3g	Sugars 0g

Newman's Own Organics, Unsalted Pretzel Rounds

About 8 pretzels (30g)

Amount per serving	Amount per serving	Amount per serving
Calories 30	**Cholesterol** 0mg	**Total Carbohydrate** 24g
Total Fat 1g	**Sodium** 105mg	Dietary Fiber <1g
Saturated Fat 0g	**Protein** 2g	Sugars 1g

Rudi's Organic Bakery, Soft Pretzels, Multigrain Organic Soft Pretzels

1 pretzel (64g)

Amount per serving	Amount per serving	Amount per serving
Calories 170	**Cholesterol** 0mg	**Total Carbohydrate** 32g
Total Fat 3g	**Sodium** 360mg	Dietary Fiber 2g
Saturated Fat 0g	**Protein** 5g	Sugars 4g

Rudi's Organic Bakery, Soft Pretzels, Organic Soft Pretzels

1 pretzel (64g)

Amount per serving	Amount per serving	Amount per serving
Calories 170	**Cholesterol** 0mg	**Total Carbohydrate** 35g
Total Fat 0g	**Sodium** 45mg	Dietary Fiber 1g
Saturated Fat 0g	**Protein** 6g	Sugars 2g

Toppings

Let's Do Organic..., Confetti Sprinkelz

1 tsp

Amount per serving	Amount per serving	Amount per serving
Calories 25	**Cholesterol** 0mg	**Total Carbohydrate** 7g
Total Fat 0g	**Sodium** 0mg	Dietary Fiber 0g
Saturated Fat 0g	**Protein** 0g	Sugars 6g

Sugar Alternatives

Pyure, Premium Organic Stevia Sweetener

1 packet (1g)

Amount per serving	Amount per serving	Amount per serving
Calories 0	**Cholesterol** NA	**Total Carbohydrate** 1g
Total Fat 0g	**Sodium** 0mg	Dietary Fiber 1g
Saturated Fat NA	**Protein** 0g	Sugars 0g

Wholesome Sweeteners, Fair Trade Certified Organic Sucanat

1 tsp

Amount per serving	Amount per serving	Amount per serving
Calories 15	**Cholesterol** 0mg	**Total Carbohydrate** 4g
Total Fat 0g	**Sodium** 0mg	Dietary Fiber 0g
Saturated Fat 0g	**Protein** 0g	Sugars 4g

Wholesome Sweeteners, Organic Coconut Palm Sugar

1 tsp

Amount per serving	Amount per serving	Amount per serving
Calories 16	**Cholesterol** 0mg	**Total Carbohydrate** 4g
Total Fat 0g	**Sodium** 0mg	Dietary Fiber 0g
Saturated Fat 0g	**Protein** NA	Sugars 4g

Wholesome Sweeteners, Organic Stevia

1 packet

Amount per serving	Amount per serving	Amount per serving
Calories 0	**Cholesterol** 0mg	**Total Carbohydrate** 1g
Total Fat 0g	**Sodium** 0mg	Dietary Fiber 0.6g
Saturated Fat 0g	**Protein** 0g	Sugars 0g

Sugars

Hain Pure Foods, Organic Light Brown Sugar

1 tsp

Amount per serving	Amount per serving	Amount per serving
Calories 15	**Cholesterol** NA	**Total Carbohydrate** 4g
Total Fat 0g	**Sodium** 0mg	Dietary Fiber NA
Saturated Fat NA	**Protein** 0g	Sugars 4g

Hain Pure Foods, Organic Powdered Sugar

1/4 cup

Amount per serving	Amount per serving	Amount per serving
Calories 140	**Cholesterol** NA	**Total Carbohydrate** 37g
Total Fat 0g	**Sodium** 0mg	Dietary Fiber NA
Saturated Fat NA	**Protein** 0g	Sugars 34g

Hain Pure Foods, Organic Sugar

1 tsp

Amount per serving	Amount per serving	Amount per serving
Calories 10	**Cholesterol** NA	**Total Carbohydrate** 3g
Total Fat 0g	**Sodium** 0mg	Dietary Fiber NA
Saturated Fat NA	**Protein** 0g	Sugars 3g

Wholesome Sweeteners, Fair Trade Certified Organic Dark Brown Sugar

1 tsp

Amount per serving	Amount per serving	Amount per serving
Calories 15	**Cholesterol** 0mg	**Total Carbohydrate** 4g
Total Fat 0g	**Sodium** 0mg	Dietary Fiber 0g
Saturated Fat 0g	**Protein** 0g	Sugars 4g

Wholesome Sweeteners, Fair Trade Certified Organic Powdered Sugar

1/4 cup

Amount per serving	Amount per serving	Amount per serving
Calories 120	**Cholesterol** 0mg	**Total Carbohydrate** 30g
Total Fat 0g	**Sodium** 0mg	Dietary Fiber 0g
Saturated Fat 0g	**Protein** 0g	Sugars 30g

Wholesome Sweeteners, Fair Trade Certified Organic Sugar

1 tsp

Amount per serving	Amount per serving	Amount per serving
Calories 15	**Cholesterol** 0mg	**Total Carbohydrate** 4g
Total Fat 0g	**Sodium** 0mg	Dietary Fiber 0g
Saturated Fat 0g	**Protein** 0g	Sugars 4g

Wholesome Sweeteners, Organic Turbinado Sugar

1 tsp

Amount per serving	Amount per serving	Amount per serving
Calories 15	**Cholesterol** 0mg	**Total Carbohydrate** 4g
Total Fat 0g	**Sodium** 0mg	Dietary Fiber 0g
Saturated Fat 0g	**Protein** 0g	Sugars 4g

Syrups

Lundberg Family Farms, Organic Sweet Dreams Brown Rice Syrup

2 tbsp (30 ml)

Amount per serving

Calories 150
Total Fat 0g
  Saturated Fat 0g

Amount per serving

Cholesterol 0mg
Sodium 70mg
Protein 0g

Amount per serving

Total Carbohydrate 36g
  Dietary Fiber 0g
  Sugars 22g

Maple Grove Farms, Organic Dark Amber Maple Syrup

1/4 cup

Amount per serving

Calories 200
Total Fat 0g
  Saturated Fat NA

Amount per serving

Cholesterol NA
Sodium 5mg
Protein 0g

Amount per serving

Total Carbohydrate 53g
  Dietary Fiber NA
  Sugars 53g

Santa Cruz Organic, Chocolate Flavored Syrup

2 tbsp (40g)

Amount per serving

Calories 110
Total Fat 0g
  Saturated Fat NA

Amount per serving

Cholesterol NA
Sodium 15mg
Protein 1g

Amount per serving

Total Carbohydrate 26g
  Dietary Fiber 1g
  Sugars 24g

Santa Cruz Organic, Mint Chocolate Flavored Syrup

2 tbsp (40g)

Amount per serving

Calories 110
Total Fat 0g
  Saturated Fat NA

Amount per serving

Cholesterol NA
Sodium 10mg
Protein 1g

Amount per serving

Total Carbohydrate 26g
  Dietary Fiber 1g
  Sugars 25g

Wholesome Sweeteners, Fair Trade Certified Organic Amber Honey

1 tbsp

Amount per serving

Calories 60
Total Fat 0g
  Saturated Fat 0g

Amount per serving

Cholesterol 0mg
Sodium 0mg
Protein 0g

Amount per serving

Total Carbohydrate 17g
  Dietary Fiber 0g
  Sugars 16g

Wholesome Sweeteners, Fair Trade Certified Organic Blackstrap Molasses

1 tbsp

Amount per serving

Calories 60
Total Fat 0g
  Saturated Fat 0g

Amount per serving

Cholesterol 0mg
Sodium 0mg
Protein 0g

Amount per serving

Total Carbohydrate 14g
  Dietary Fiber 0g
  Sugars 10g

Wholesome Sweeteners, Fair Trade Certified Organic Raw Honey

1 tbsp

Amount per serving	Amount per serving	Amount per serving
Calories 60	**Cholesterol** 0mg	**Total Carbohydrate** 17g
Total Fat 0g	**Sodium** 0mg	Dietary Fiber 0g
Saturated Fat 0g	**Protein** 0g	Sugars 16g

Wholesome Sweeteners, Organic Blue Agave

1 tbsp

Amount per serving	Amount per serving	Amount per serving
Calories 60	**Cholesterol** 0mg	**Total Carbohydrate** 16g
Total Fat 0g	**Sodium** 0mg	Dietary Fiber 0g
Saturated Fat 0g	**Protein** 0g	Sugars 16g

Wholesome Sweeteners, Organic Cinnamon Flavored Blue Agave Syrup

2 tbsp

Amount per serving	Amount per serving	Amount per serving
Calories 120	**Cholesterol** 0mg	**Total Carbohydrate** 32g
Total Fat 0g	**Sodium** 0mg	Dietary Fiber 0g
Saturated Fat 0g	**Protein** 0g	Sugars 32g

Wholesome Sweeteners, Organic Maple Flavored Blue Agave Syrup

2 tbsp

Amount per serving	Amount per serving	Amount per serving
Calories 120	**Cholesterol** 0mg	**Total Carbohydrate** 32g
Total Fat 0g	**Sodium** 0mg	Dietary Fiber 0g
Saturated Fat 0g	**Protein** 0g	Sugars 32g

Wholesome Sweeteners, Organic Raw Blue Agave

1 tbsp

Amount per serving	Amount per serving	Amount per serving
Calories 60	**Cholesterol** 0mg	**Total Carbohydrate** 16g
Total Fat 0g	**Sodium** 0mg	Dietary Fiber 0g
Saturated Fat 0g	**Protein** 0g	Sugars 16g

Wholesome Sweeteners, Organic Strawberry Flavored Blue Agave Syrup

2 tbsp

Amount per serving	Amount per serving	Amount per serving
Calories 120	**Cholesterol** 0mg	**Total Carbohydrate** 32g
Total Fat 0g	**Sodium** 0mg	Dietary Fiber 0g
Saturated Fat 0g	**Protein** 0g	Sugars 32g

Wholesome Sweeteners, Organic Vanilla Blue Agave

2 tbsp

Amount per serving	Amount per serving	Amount per serving
Calories 120	**Cholesterol** 0mg	**Total Carbohydrate** 32g
Total Fat 0g	**Sodium** 0mg	Dietary Fiber 0g
Saturated Fat 0g	**Protein** 0g	Sugars 32g

Beverages

Water is the ideal beverage for quenching your thirst and restoring fluids lost through breathing, sweating, and elimination. It's essential for proper digestion, kidney function, and brain function and is used by every cell of the body. Plus it's clean, refreshing, sugar-free, and contains no calories. Drink water throughout the day to rehydrate and even more when exercising—especially in hot, humid weather.

All beverages count toward meeting daily fluid requirements—fruit and vegetable juices, flavored water, tea, coffee, dairy milk and milk alternatives, and even soft drinks.

Find milk and milk alternatives in the Dairy Foods section and juice in the Fruit section.

Why Choose Organic Beverages?

Organic beverages are distinguished from their non-organic counterparts by the fact that they do not contain artificial ingredients—no artificial colors, flavors, preservatives, or synthetic sweeteners. Fruit and other produce used in organic beverages are grown without the use of synthetic pesticides or herbicides.

The USDA criteria for 100% organic beverages are the same as the criteria for organic food products—all ingredients and processing aids must be organic. In addition, organic beverages must be produced without using genetically engineered ingredients, ionizing radiation, or sewage sludge and must not contain any of the prohibited substances on the National List of Allowed and Prohibited Substances (National List). Certification also requires oversight by a USDA National Organic Program certifying agent to ensure adherence to all USDA organic regulations.

Beverages certified as "organic," as opposed to "100% organic," may contain up to 5% of non-organic content excluding salt and water. To claim that a beverage is "made with" organic ingredients, at least 70% of it, excluding salt and water, must be certified organic ingredients.

Look for the USDA organic seal on cows' milk, as well as almond milk, rice milk, coconut milk, soy milk, flax milk, and hemp milk. There is also an expanding array of organic water and flavored water as well as coffees, teas, fruit juices, energy drinks, and soft drinks.

There are even organic wines and malt beverages. Many consumers seek out organic wines because grapes are among the most frequently chemically treated fruits—they are often sprayed with synthetic insecticides and herbicides. In addition to meeting the USDA organic requirements, alcoholic beverages must meet the Alcohol and Tobacco Tax and Trade Bureau (TTB) regulations, including labeling requirements for sulfites. Sulfites are naturally occurring chemical compounds that are produced during fermentation. They preserve wine's distinctive flavor and color. Sulfites may be added during the fermentation stage to prevent the wine from fermenting to vinegar. Wine with added sulfites cannot bear the USDA organic seal and is only eligible for the "made with" organic ingredients label. In addition, in order to be considered organic, only wine made from organic grapes may contain added sulfites. Sulfites may not be added to wine made with other organic fruit.

Daily Goal or Target

The Institute of Medicine (IOM) suggests that healthy adults can let their thirst guide their fluid intake and encourages men to aim for total fluid consumption of about 125 ounces (15 cups) per day and women 91 ounces (about 11 cups). It's important to remember that about 20% of required fluid comes from foods like fruits and vegetables that contain water. To obtain that balance—the remaining 80%—the IOM guidelines recommend that men consume 12.5 cups of fluid per day and women 9 cups.

Coffee

Newman's Own Organics Coffee (All Varieties)

1 tbsp

Amount per serving	Amount per serving	Amount per serving
Calories 0	**Cholesterol** 0mg	**Total Carbohydrate** 0g
Total Fat 0g	**Sodium** 0mg	Dietary Fiber 0g
Saturated Fat 0g	**Protein** 0g	Sugars 0g

Juice

Amazing Grass, Chocolate Green SuperFood

1 scoop/8g

Amount per serving	Amount per serving	Amount per serving
Calories 30	**Cholesterol** 4mg	**Total Carbohydrate** 2g
Total Fat 1g	**Sodium** 65mg	Dietary Fiber 0g
Saturated Fat NA	**Protein** 8g	Sugars 2g

Blue Print Juice, Cold Pressed, Beet Apple Carrot Lemon Ginger

16 fl oz (473 ml)

Amount per serving	Amount per serving	Amount per serving
Calories 190	**Cholesterol** 0mg	**Total Carbohydrate** 44g
Total Fat 0g	**Sodium** 85mg	Dietary Fiber 0g
Saturated Fat 0g	**Protein** 2g	Sugars 37g

Blue Print Juice, Cold Pressed, C.A.B.

16 fl oz (473 ml)

Amount per serving	Amount per serving	Amount per serving
Calories 190	**Cholesterol** 0mg	**Total Carbohydrate** 44g
Total Fat 0g	**Sodium** 85mg	Dietary Fiber 0g
Saturated Fat 0g	**Protein** 2g	Sugars 37g

Blue Print Juice, Cold Pressed, Cashew Milk

16 fl oz (473 ml)

Amount per serving	Amount per serving	Amount per serving
Calories 300	**Cholesterol** 0mg	**Total Carbohydrate** 26g
Total Fat 19g	**Sodium** 45mg	Dietary Fiber 5g
Saturated Fat 3g	**Protein** 7g	Sugars 21g

Blue Print Juice, Cold Pressed, Cashew Vanilla Cinnamon Agave

16 fl oz (473 ml)

Amount per serving	Amount per serving	Amount per serving
Calories 300	**Cholesterol** 0mg	**Total Carbohydrate** 45g
Total Fat 19g	**Sodium** 45mg	Dietary Fiber 26g
Saturated Fat 3g	**Protein** 7g	Sugars 21g

Blue Print Juice, Cold Pressed, Kale Apple Ginger Romaine Spinach

16 fl oz (473 ml)

Amount per serving	Amount per serving	Amount per serving
Calories 110	**Cholesterol** 0mg	**Total Carbohydrate** 24g
Total Fat 0g	**Sodium** 90mg	Dietary Fiber 0g
Saturated Fat 0g	**Protein** 3g	Sugars 24g

Blue Print Juice, Cold Pressed, Lime Ginger Lemon Agave

16 fl oz (473 ml)

Amount per serving	Amount per serving	Amount per serving
Calories 170	**Cholesterol** 0mg	**Total Carbohydrate** 42g
Total Fat 0g	**Sodium** 10mg	Dietary Fiber 0g
Saturated Fat 0g	**Protein** 0g	Sugars 38g

Blue Print Juice, Cold Pressed, Pineapple Apple Mint

16 fl oz (473 ml)

Amount per serving	Amount per serving	Amount per serving
Calories 210	**Cholesterol** 0mg	**Total Carbohydrate** 49g
Total Fat 0g	**Sodium** 55mg	Dietary Fiber 0g
Saturated Fat 0g	**Protein** 1g	Sugars 45g

Blue Print Juice, Cold Pressed, Spicy Lemonade

16 fl oz (473 ml)

Amount per serving	Amount per serving	Amount per serving
Calories 120	**Cholesterol** 0mg	**Total Carbohydrate** 30g
Total Fat 0g	**Sodium** 10mg	Dietary Fiber 0g
Saturated Fat 0g	**Protein** 0g	Sugars 29g

Bragg, Organic Apple Cider Vinegar Drinks, Apple-Cinnamon

8 fl oz (240 ml)

Amount per serving	Amount per serving	Amount per serving
Calories 16	**Cholesterol** NA	**Total Carbohydrate** 4g
Total Fat 0g	**Sodium** 0mg	Dietary Fiber NA
Saturated Fat NA	**Protein** 0g	Sugars 4g

Bragg, Organic Apple Cider Vinegar Drinks, Concord Grape-Acai

8 fl oz (240 ml)

Amount per serving	Amount per serving	Amount per serving
Calories 20	**Cholesterol** NA	**Total Carbohydrate** 5g
Total Fat 0g	**Sodium** 0mg	Dietary Fiber NA
Saturated Fat NA	**Protein** 0g	Sugars 5g

Bragg, Organic Apple Cider Vinegar Drinks, Ginger Spice

8 fl oz (240 ml)

Amount per serving	Amount per serving	Amount per serving
Calories 0	**Cholesterol** NA	**Total Carbohydrate** 0g
Total Fat 0g	**Sodium** 0mg	Dietary Fiber NA
Saturated Fat NA	**Protein** 0g	Sugars NA

Bragg, Organic Apple Cider Vinegar Drinks, Honey

8 fl oz (240 ml)

Amount per serving	Amount per serving	Amount per serving
Calories 60	**Cholesterol** 0mg	**Total Carbohydrate** 14g
Total Fat 0g	**Sodium** 0mg	Dietary Fiber 0g
Saturated Fat 0g	**Protein** 0g	Sugars 13g

Bragg, Organic Apple Cider Vinegar Drinks, Limeaid

8 fl oz (240 ml)

Amount per serving	Amount per serving	Amount per serving
Calories 0	**Cholesterol** NA	**Total Carbohydrate** 0g
Total Fat 0g	**Sodium** 0mg	Dietary Fiber NA
Saturated Fat NA	**Protein** 0g	Sugars NA

Bragg, Organic Apple Cider Vinegar Drinks, Stevia

8 fl oz (240 ml)

Amount per serving	Amount per serving	Amount per serving
Calories 0	**Cholesterol** NA	**Total Carbohydrate** 0g
Total Fat 0g	**Sodium** 0mg	Dietary Fiber NA
Saturated Fat NA	**Protein** 0g	Sugars NA

Chia Star, Blackberry Lime Refresh

1 bottle (236 ml)

Amount per serving	Amount per serving	Amount per serving
Calories 60	**Cholesterol** NA	**Total Carbohydrate** 8g
Total Fat 3g	**Sodium** 0mg	Dietary Fiber 4g
Saturated Fat NA	**Protein** 2g	Sugars 3g

Chia Star, Lemonberry Splash

1 bottle (236 ml)

Amount per serving	Amount per serving	Amount per serving
Calories 47	**Cholesterol** NA	**Total Carbohydrate** 5g
Total Fat 3g	**Sodium** 0mg	Dietary Fiber 4g
Saturated Fat NA	**Protein** 2g	Sugars 0g

Chia Star, Peach Green Tea Fusion

1 bottle (236 ml)

Amount per serving	Amount per serving	Amount per serving
Calories 60	**Cholesterol** NA	**Total Carbohydrate** 8g
Total Fat 3g	**Sodium** 0mg	Dietary Fiber 4g
Saturated Fat NA	**Protein** 2g	Sugars 3g

Chia Star, Pineapple Honey Love

1 bottle (236 ml)

Amount per serving	Amount per serving	Amount per serving
Calories 49	**Cholesterol** NA	**Total Carbohydrate** 5g
Total Fat 3g	**Sodium** 0mg	Dietary Fiber 4g
Saturated Fat NA	**Protein** 2g	Sugars 2g

Chia Star, Pomegranate Apple Power

1 bottle (236 ml)

Amount per serving	Amount per serving	Amount per serving
Calories 90	**Cholesterol** NA	**Total Carbohydrate** 13g
Total Fat 3g	**Sodium** 1mg	Dietary Fiber 4g
Saturated Fat NA	**Protein** 2g	Sugars 8g

Coco Libre, Pure Coconut Water

1 bottle (330 ml)

Amount per serving	Amount per serving	Amount per serving
Calories 60	**Cholesterol** 0mg	**Total Carbohydrate** 14g
Total Fat 0g	**Sodium** 120mg	Dietary Fiber NA
Saturated Fat NA	**Protein** 0g	Sugars 13g

Coco Libre, Pure Coconut Water with Pineapple

1 bottle (330 ml)

Amount per serving	Amount per serving	Amount per serving
Calories 75	**Cholesterol** 0mg	**Total Carbohydrate** 18g
Total Fat 0g	**Sodium** 100mg	Dietary Fiber NA
Saturated Fat NA	**Protein** 0g	Sugars 17g

Columbia Gorge Organic Farm to Bottle, Pure Juices, Blood Orange Juice

(227g)

Amount per serving	Amount per serving	Amount per serving
Calories 100	**Cholesterol** 0mg	**Total Carbohydrate** 24g
Total Fat 0g	**Sodium** 30mg	Dietary Fiber 4g
Saturated Fat 0g	**Protein** 2g	Sugars 21g

Columbia Gorge Organic Farm to Bottle, Pure Juices, Ginger Juice

227g

Amount per serving	Amount per serving	Amount per serving
Calories 180	**Cholesterol** 0mg	**Total Carbohydrate** 40g
Total Fat 1.5g	**Sodium** 30mg	Dietary Fiber 5g
Saturated Fat 0g	**Protein** 4g	Sugars 4g

Columbia Gorge Organic Farm to Bottle, Pure Juices, Lemon Juice

227g

Amount per serving	Amount per serving	Amount per serving
Calories 60	**Cholesterol** 0mg	**Total Carbohydrate** 20g
Total Fat 0g	**Sodium** 0mg	Dietary Fiber 1g
Saturated Fat 0g	**Protein** 1g	Sugars 5g

Columbia Gorge Organic Farm to Bottle, Pure Juices, Lime Juice

227g

Amount per serving	Amount per serving	Amount per serving
Calories 60	**Cholesterol** 0mg	**Total Carbohydrate** 19g
Total Fat 0g	**Sodium** 0mg	Dietary Fiber 1g
Saturated Fat 0g	**Protein** 1g	Sugars 4g

Columbia Gorge Organic Farm to Bottle, Pure Juices, Meyer Lemon Juice

227g

Amount per serving	Amount per serving	Amount per serving
Calories 60	**Cholesterol** 0mg	**Total Carbohydrate** 20g
Total Fat 0g	**Sodium** 0mg	Dietary Fiber 1g
Saturated Fat 0g	**Protein** 1g	Sugars 5g

Columbia Gorge Organic Farm to Bottle, Pure Juices, Pomegranate Juice

227g

Amount per serving	Amount per serving	Amount per serving
Calories 150	**Cholesterol** 0mg	**Total Carbohydrate** 38g
Total Fat 0g	**Sodium** 30mg	Dietary Fiber 0g
Saturated Fat 0g	**Protein** 0g	Sugars 39g

Columbia Gorge Organic Farm to Bottle, Pure Originals, 100% Organic Apple Cider

8 fl oz (236 ml)

Amount per serving	Amount per serving	Amount per serving
Calories 110	**Cholesterol** 0mg	**Total Carbohydrate** 27g
Total Fat 0g	**Sodium** 20mg	Dietary Fiber 0g
Saturated Fat 0g	**Protein** 0g	Sugars 22g

Columbia Gorge Organic Farm to Bottle, Pure Originals, 100% Organic Carrot Juice

8 fl oz (236 ml)

Amount per serving	Amount per serving	Amount per serving
Calories 70	**Cholesterol** 0mg	**Total Carbohydrate** 17g
Total Fat 0g	**Sodium** 95mg	Dietary Fiber 0g
Saturated Fat 0g	**Protein** 1g	Sugars 14g

Columbia Gorge Organic Farm to Bottle, Smoothies, Mango CoGo™ Smoothie

8 fl oz (236 ml)

Amount per serving	Amount per serving	Amount per serving
Calories 150	**Cholesterol** 0mg	**Total Carbohydrate** 28g
Total Fat 4.5g	**Sodium** 30mg	Dietary Fiber 1g
Saturated Fat 4g	**Protein** 1g	Sugars 23g

Columbia Gorge Organic Farm to Bottle, Smoothies, Orange Carrot Banana Smoothie

8 fl oz (236 ml)

Amount per serving	Amount per serving	Amount per serving
Calories 120	**Cholesterol** 0mg	**Total Carbohydrate** 29g
Total Fat 0g	**Sodium** 35mg	Dietary Fiber 2g
Saturated Fat 0g	**Protein** 1g	Sugars 25g

Columbia Gorge Organic Farm to Bottle, Smoothies, Raspberry Peach Smoothie

8 fl oz (236 ml)

Amount per serving	Amount per serving	Amount per serving
Calories 120	**Cholesterol** 0mg	**Total Carbohydrate** 30g
Total Fat 0g	**Sodium** 15mg	Dietary Fiber 2g
Saturated Fat 0g	**Protein** 1g	Sugars 24g

Columbia Gorge Organic Farm to Bottle, Smoothies, Strawberry Banana Smoothie

8 fl oz (236 ml)

Amount per serving	Amount per serving	Amount per serving
Calories 130	**Cholesterol** 0mg	**Total Carbohydrate** 31g
Total Fat 1g	**Sodium** 20mg	Dietary Fiber 2g
Saturated Fat 0g	**Protein** 1g	Sugars 25g

Columbia Gorge Organic Farm to Bottle, Smoothies, Wild Blackberry Smoothie

8 fl oz (236 ml)

Amount per serving	Amount per serving	Amount per serving
Calories 130	**Cholesterol** 0mg	**Total Carbohydrate** 31g
Total Fat 0g	**Sodium** 15mg	Dietary Fiber 2g
Saturated Fat 0g	**Protein** 2g	Sugars 25g

Columbia Gorge Organic Farm to Bottle, Vitatrition™, Blueberry B'Mega™

8 fl oz (236 ml)

Amount per serving	Amount per serving	Amount per serving
Calories 140	**Cholesterol** 0mg	**Total Carbohydrate** 32g
Total Fat 1.5g	**Sodium** 15mg	Dietary Fiber 3g
Saturated Fat 0g	**Protein** 1g	Sugars 21g

Columbia Gorge Organic Farm to Bottle, Vitatrition™, Pomegranate Blueberry Cherry

8 fl oz (236 ml)

Amount per serving	Amount per serving	Amount per serving
Calories 120	**Cholesterol** 0mg	**Total Carbohydrate** 30g
Total Fat 0g	**Sodium** 20mg	Dietary Fiber 0g
Saturated Fat 0g	**Protein** 1g	Sugars 23g

Columbia Gorge Organic Farm to Bottle, Vitatrition™, Strawberry Super C™

8 fl oz (236 ml)

Amount per serving	Amount per serving	Amount per serving
Calories 110	**Cholesterol** 0mg	**Total Carbohydrate** 25g
Total Fat 0g	**Sodium** 30mg	Dietary Fiber 1g
Saturated Fat 0g	**Protein** 1g	Sugars 21g

Columbia Gorge Organic Farm to Bottle, Vitatrition™, Super C™

8 fl oz (236 ml)

Amount per serving	Amount per serving	Amount per serving
Calories 160	**Cholesterol** 0mg	**Total Carbohydrate** 39g
Total Fat 0g	**Sodium** 30mg	Dietary Fiber 2g
Saturated Fat 0g	**Protein** 1g	Sugars 34g

Columbia Gorge Organic Farm to Bottle, Vitatrition™, Vita Sea™ Superfoods

8 fl oz (236 ml)

Amount per serving	Amount per serving	Amount per serving
Calories 140	**Cholesterol** 0mg	**Total Carbohydrate** 33g
Total Fat 0.5g	**Sodium** 20mg	Dietary Fiber 1g
Saturated Fat 0g	**Protein** 2g	Sugars 27g

Columbia Gorge Organic, Pure Originals, 100% Organic Amazing Ginger Apple Cider

8 fl oz (236 ml)

Amount per serving	Amount per serving	Amount per serving
Calories 110	**Cholesterol** 0mg	**Total Carbohydrate** 27g
Total Fat 0g	**Sodium** 20mg	Dietary Fiber 0g
Saturated Fat 0g	**Protein** 0g	Sugars 22g

Columbia Gorge Organic, Pure Originals, 100% Organic Apple Pear Cider

8 fl oz (236 ml)

Amount per serving	Amount per serving	Amount per serving
Calories 100	**Cholesterol** 0mg	**Total Carbohydrate** 25g
Total Fat 0g	**Sodium** 25mg	Dietary Fiber 1g
Saturated Fat 0g	**Protein** 0g	Sugars 18g

Columbia Gorge Organic, Pure Originals, 100% Organic Grapefruit Juice

8 fl oz (236 ml)

Amount per serving	Amount per serving	Amount per serving
Calories 90	**Cholesterol** 0mg	**Total Carbohydrate** 21g
Total Fat 0g	**Sodium** 0mg	Dietary Fiber 0g
Saturated Fat 0g	**Protein** 1g	Sugars 16g

Columbia Gorge Organic, Pure Originals, 100% Organic Orange Juice

8 fl oz (236 ml)

Amount per serving	Amount per serving	Amount per serving
Calories 100	**Cholesterol** 0mg	**Total Carbohydrate** 24g
Total Fat 0g	**Sodium** 30mg	Dietary Fiber 4g
Saturated Fat 0g	**Protein** 2g	Sugars 21g

Columbia Gorge Organic, Pure Originals, 100% Organic Tangerine Juice

8 fl oz (236 ml)

Amount per serving	Amount per serving	Amount per serving
Calories 100	**Cholesterol** 0mg	**Total Carbohydrate** 23g
Total Fat 0g	**Sodium** 0mg	Dietary Fiber 0g
Saturated Fat 0g	**Protein** 1g	Sugars 22g

Columbia Gorge Organic, Satisfiers, 100% Organic Lemonade with Organic Agave

8 fl oz (236 ml)

Amount per serving	Amount per serving	Amount per serving
Calories 90	**Cholesterol** 0mg	**Total Carbohydrate** 23g
Total Fat 0g	**Sodium** 0mg	Dietary Fiber 0g
Saturated Fat 0g	**Protein** 0g	Sugars 21g

Columbia Gorge Organic, Satisfiers, 100% Organic Limeade with Organic Agave

8 fl oz (236 ml)

Amount per serving	Amount per serving	Amount per serving
Calories 80	**Cholesterol** 0mg	**Total Carbohydrate** 21g
Total Fat 0g	**Sodium** 0mg	Dietary Fiber 0g
Saturated Fat 0g	**Protein** 0g	Sugars 19g

Columbia Gorge Organic, Satisfiers, 100% Organic Meyer Ginger Lemonade

8 fl oz (236 ml)

Amount per serving	Amount per serving	Amount per serving
Calories 110	**Cholesterol** 0mg	**Total Carbohydrate** 29g
Total Fat 0g	**Sodium** 0mg	Dietary Fiber 0g
Saturated Fat 0g	**Protein** 0g	Sugars 25g

Columbia Gorge Organic, Satisfiers, 100% Organic Pomegranate Ginger Limeade

8 fl oz (236 ml)

Amount per serving	Amount per serving	Amount per serving
Calories 110	**Cholesterol** 0mg	**Total Carbohydrate** 28g
Total Fat 0g	**Sodium** 10mg	Dietary Fiber 0g
Saturated Fat 0g	**Protein** 0g	Sugars 25g

Columbia Gorge Organic, Satisfiers, 100% Organic Raspberry Cranberry

8 fl oz (236 ml)

Amount per serving	Amount per serving	Amount per serving
Calories 110	**Cholesterol** 0mg	**Total Carbohydrate** 28g
Total Fat 0g	**Sodium** 10mg	Dietary Fiber 1g
Saturated Fat 0g	**Protein** 1g	Sugars 25g

Columbia Gorge Organic, Satisfiers, 100% Organic Red Ginger Limeade

8 fl oz (236 ml)

Amount per serving	Amount per serving	Amount per serving
Calories 110	**Cholesterol** 0mg	**Total Carbohydrate** 28g
Total Fat 0g	**Sodium** 0mg	Dietary Fiber 0g
Saturated Fat 0g	**Protein** 0g	Sugars 25g

Columbia Gorge Organic, Satisfiers, 100% Organic Strawberry Honey Lemonade

8 fl oz (236 ml)

Amount per serving	Amount per serving	Amount per serving
Calories 90	**Cholesterol** 0mg	**Total Carbohydrate** 23g
Total Fat 0g	**Sodium** 0mg	Dietary Fiber 0g
Saturated Fat 0g	**Protein** 0g	Sugars 20g

Columbia Gorge Organic, Smoothies, Blue Green Spirulina with Coconut Water

8 fl oz (236 ml)

Amount per serving	Amount per serving	Amount per serving
Calories 130	**Cholesterol** 0mg	**Total Carbohydrate** 30g
Total Fat 0g	**Sodium** 45mg	Dietary Fiber 2g
Saturated Fat 0g	**Protein** 2g	Sugars 25g

Columbia Gorge Organic, Smoothies, Mango Mango™ with Coconut water Smoothie

8 fl oz (236 ml)

Amount per serving	Amount per serving	Amount per serving
Calories 110	Cholesterol 0mg	Total Carbohydrate 28g
Total Fat 0g	Sodium 70mg	Dietary Fiber 2g
Saturated Fat 0g	Protein 1g	Sugars 23g

Columbia Gorge Organic, Vegan Protein, Berry Almond Soy Hemp Milk Juice Blend

8 fl oz (236 ml)

Amount per serving	Amount per serving	Amount per serving
Calories 220	Cholesterol 0mg	Total Carbohydrate 35g
Total Fat 4.5g	Sodium 70mg	Dietary Fiber 3g
Saturated Fat 0.5g	Protein 11g	Sugars 29g

Columbia Gorge Organic, Vegan Protein, Chocolate Soymilk Protein Drink

8 fl oz (236 ml)

Amount per serving	Amount per serving	Amount per serving
Calories 190	Cholesterol 0mg	Total Carbohydrate 30g
Total Fat 3.5g	Sodium 60mg	Dietary Fiber 3g
Saturated Fat 1.5g	Protein 11g	Sugars 26g

Columbia Gorge Organic, Vegan Protein, Protein CoGo™ 20g Soy Protein Per Bottle

8 fl oz (236 ml)

Amount per serving	Amount per serving	Amount per serving
Calories 190	Cholesterol 0mg	Total Carbohydrate 29g
Total Fat 4g	Sodium 30mg	Dietary Fiber 4g
Saturated Fat 2.5g	Protein 11g	Sugars 23g

Columbia Gorge Organic, Veggie Blends, Carrot Beet Celery 100% Organic Veggies

8 fl oz (236 ml)

Amount per serving	Amount per serving	Amount per serving
Calories 70	Cholesterol 0mg	Total Carbohydrate 16g
Total Fat 0g	Sodium 135mg	Dietary Fiber 0g
Saturated Fat 0g	Protein 1g	Sugars 12g

Columbia Gorge Organic, Veggie Blends, Carrot Leafy Greens 100% Organic Veggies

8 fl oz (236 ml)

Amount per serving	Amount per serving	Amount per serving
Calories 60	Cholesterol 0mg	Total Carbohydrate 12g
Total Fat 0g	Sodium 85mg	Dietary Fiber 0g
Saturated Fat 0g	Protein 1g	Sugars 10g

Columbia Gorge Organic, Veggie Blends, Celery Kale with Coconut Water

8 fl oz (236 ml)

Amount per serving	Amount per serving	Amount per serving
Calories 40	Cholesterol 0mg	Total Carbohydrate 7g
Total Fat 0g	Sodium 250mg	Dietary Fiber 2g
Saturated Fat 0g	Protein 2g	Sugars 4g

Columbia Gorge Organic, Veggie Blends, Green Apple Greens™ Cold Pressed

8 fl oz (236 ml)

Amount per serving	Amount per serving	Amount per serving
Calories 70	Cholesterol 0mg	Total Carbohydrate 17g
Total Fat 0g	Sodium 100mg	Dietary Fiber 0g
Saturated Fat 0g	Protein 1g	Sugars 13g

Columbia Gorge Organic, Veggie Blends, Just Greens™ 100% Organic Veggies

8 fl oz (236 ml)

Amount per serving	Amount per serving	Amount per serving
Calories 25	Cholesterol 0mg	Total Carbohydrate 4g
Total Fat 0g	Sodium 210mg	Dietary Fiber 0g
Saturated Fat 0g	Protein 2g	Sugars 1g

Columbia Gorge Organic, Veggie Blends, Kale Apple Lemon Cold Pressed

8 fl oz (236 ml)

Amount per serving	Amount per serving	Amount per serving
Calories 100	Cholesterol 0mg	Total Carbohydrate 25g
Total Fat 0g	Sodium 25mg	Dietary Fiber 1g
Saturated Fat 0g	Protein 1g	Sugars 19g

Columbia Gorge Organic, Veggie Blends, Lemon Ginger Greens 100% Organic Veggies

8 fl oz (236 ml)

Amount per serving	Amount per serving	Amount per serving
Calories 60	Cholesterol 0mg	Total Carbohydrate 15g
Total Fat 0g	Sodium 105mg	Dietary Fiber 0g
Saturated Fat 0g	Protein 1g	Sugars 11g

Columbia Gorge Organic, Veggie Blends, Red Apple Greens™ 100% Organic Veggies

8 fl oz (236 ml)

Amount per serving	Amount per serving	Amount per serving
Calories 80	Cholesterol 0mg	Total Carbohydrate 19g
Total Fat 0g	Sodium 105mg	Dietary Fiber 0g
Saturated Fat 0g	Protein 1g	Sugars 13g

Columbia Gorge Organic, Vitatrition™, CoGo Beta™ Vitamins, A, C, & E

8 fl oz (236 ml)

Amount per serving	Amount per serving	Amount per serving
Calories 110	**Cholesterol** 0mg	**Total Carbohydrate** 26g
Total Fat 0g	**Sodium** 20mg	Dietary Fiber 2g
Saturated Fat 0g	**Protein** 1g	Sugars 23g

Columbia Gorge Organic, Vitatrition™, Radical Red™ Vitamins A, C, & E

8 fl oz (236 ml)

Amount per serving	Amount per serving	Amount per serving
Calories 110	**Cholesterol** 0mg	**Total Carbohydrate** 25g
Total Fat 1g	**Sodium** 30mg	Dietary Fiber 1g
Saturated Fat 0g	**Protein** 1g	Sugars 19g

GoodBelly, GoodBelly + Blueberry Acai

1 bottle (80 ml)

Amount per serving	Amount per serving	Amount per serving
Calories 50	**Cholesterol** 0mg	**Total Carbohydrate** 12g
Total Fat 0g	**Sodium** 5mg	Dietary Fiber <1g
Saturated Fat 0g	**Protein** <1g	Sugars 9g

GoodBelly, GoodBelly + Mango

1 bottle (80 ml)

Amount per serving	Amount per serving	Amount per serving
Calories 50	**Cholesterol** 0mg	**Total Carbohydrate** 13g
Total Fat 0g	**Sodium** 10mg	Dietary Fiber <1g
Saturated Fat 0g	**Protein** <1g	Sugars 9g

GoodBelly, GoodBelly + Pomegranate Blackberry

1 bottle (80 ml)

Amount per serving	Amount per serving	Amount per serving
Calories 50	**Cholesterol** 0mg	**Total Carbohydrate** 12g
Total Fat 0g	**Sodium** 5mg	Dietary Fiber <1g
Saturated Fat 0g	**Protein** <1g	Sugars 9g

GoodBelly, GoodBelly + Strawberry

1 bottle (80 ml)

Amount per serving	Amount per serving	Amount per serving
Calories 50	**Cholesterol** 0mg	**Total Carbohydrate** 12g
Total Fat 0g	**Sodium** 5mg	Dietary Fiber <1g
Saturated Fat 0g	**Protein** <1g	Sugars 9g

GoodBelly, GoodBelly BigShot, Lemon Ginger

1 bottle (80 ml)

Amount per serving	Amount per serving	Amount per serving
Calories 60	**Cholesterol** 0mg	**Total Carbohydrate** 11g
Total Fat 1g	**Sodium** 0mg	Dietary Fiber 1g
Saturated Fat 0g	**Protein** 2g	Sugars 5g

GoodBelly, GoodBelly BigShot, Vanilla Chamomile

1 bottle (80 ml)

Amount per serving	Amount per serving	Amount per serving
Calories 60	**Cholesterol** 0mg	**Total Carbohydrate** 11g
Total Fat 1g	**Sodium** 0mg	Dietary Fiber 1g
Saturated Fat 0g	**Protein** 2g	Sugars 5g

GoodBelly, GoodBelly Quarts, Blueberry Acai

8 oz (240 ml)

Amount per serving	Amount per serving	Amount per serving
Calories 120	**Cholesterol** 0mg	**Total Carbohydrate** 29g
Total Fat 0g	**Sodium** 20mg	Dietary Fiber 0g
Saturated Fat 0g	**Protein** <1g	Sugars 24g

GoodBelly, GoodBelly Quarts, Cranberry Watermelon

8 oz (240 ml)

Amount per serving	Amount per serving	Amount per serving
Calories 110	**Cholesterol** 0mg	**Total Carbohydrate** 28g
Total Fat 0g	**Sodium** 30mg	Dietary Fiber <1g
Saturated Fat 0g	**Protein** <1g	Sugars 26g

GoodBelly, GoodBelly Quarts, Gluten-Free Carrot Ginger

8 oz (240 ml)

Amount per serving	Amount per serving	Amount per serving
Calories 80	**Cholesterol** 0mg	**Total Carbohydrate** 19g
Total Fat 0g	**Sodium** 60mg	Dietary Fiber 0g
Saturated Fat 0g	**Protein** 1g	Sugars 17g

GoodBelly, GoodBelly Quarts, Gluten-Free GoodBelly Fermented Coconut Water

8 oz (240 ml)

Amount per serving	Amount per serving	Amount per serving
Calories 70	**Cholesterol** 0mg	**Total Carbohydrate** 14g
Total Fat 0g	**Sodium** 110mg	Dietary Fiber 0g
Saturated Fat 0g	**Protein** 1g	Sugars 13g

GoodBelly, GoodBelly Quarts, Gluten-Free GoodBelly Pink Grapefruit

8 oz (240 ml)

Amount per serving	Amount per serving	Amount per serving
Calories 120	**Cholesterol** 0mg	**Total Carbohydrate** 27g
Total Fat 0g	**Sodium** 10mg	Dietary Fiber 0g
Saturated Fat 0g	**Protein** 1g	Sugars 23g

GoodBelly, GoodBelly Quarts, Gluten-Free GoodBelly Tropical Orange

8 oz (240 ml)

Amount per serving	Amount per serving	Amount per serving
Calories 120	**Cholesterol** 0mg	**Total Carbohydrate** 28g
Total Fat 0g	**Sodium** 10mg	Dietary Fiber 0g
Saturated Fat 0g	**Protein** 1g	Sugars 26g

GoodBelly, GoodBelly Quarts, GoodBelly Tropical Green

8 oz (240 ml)

Amount per serving	Amount per serving	Amount per serving
Calories 110	**Cholesterol** 0mg	**Total Carbohydrate** 25g
Total Fat 0g	**Sodium** 20mg	Dietary Fiber 0g
Saturated Fat 0g	**Protein** 2g	Sugars 20g

GoodBelly, GoodBelly Quarts, Mango

8 oz (240 ml)

Amount per serving	Amount per serving	Amount per serving
Calories 110	**Cholesterol** 0mg	**Total Carbohydrate** 26g
Total Fat 0g	**Sodium** 10mg	Dietary Fiber 1g
Saturated Fat 0g	**Protein** <1g	Sugars 22g

GoodBelly, GoodBelly Quarts, Pomegranate Blackberry

8 oz (240 ml)

Amount per serving	Amount per serving	Amount per serving
Calories 110	**Cholesterol** 0mg	**Total Carbohydrate** 24g
Total Fat 0g	**Sodium** 20mg	Dietary Fiber 0g
Saturated Fat 0g	**Protein** <1g	Sugars 22g

GoodBelly, GoodBelly StraightShot

1 bottle (80 ml)

Amount per serving	Amount per serving	Amount per serving
Calories 30	**Cholesterol** 0mg	**Total Carbohydrate** 6g
Total Fat 0g	**Sodium** 0mg	Dietary Fiber 0g
Saturated Fat 0g	**Protein** 1g	Sugars 3g

Harmless Harvest®, 100% Raw Coconut Water

8 oz

Amount per serving	Amount per serving	Amount per serving
Calories 56	**Cholesterol** 0mg	**Total Carbohydrate** 14g
Total Fat 0g	**Sodium** 4mg	Dietary Fiber 1g
Saturated Fat 0g	**Protein** 0g	Sugars 12g

Harmless Harvest®, Namacha, Raw Honey & Lemon

10 fl oz

Amount per serving	Amount per serving	Amount per serving
Calories 60	**Cholesterol** NA	**Total Carbohydrate** 16g
Total Fat 0g	**Sodium** 0mg	Dietary Fiber NA
Saturated Fat NA	**Protein** 0g	Sugars 13g

Harmless Harvest®, Namacha, Raw Peppermint

10 fl oz

Amount per serving	Amount per serving	Amount per serving
Calories 30	**Cholesterol** NA	**Total Carbohydrate** 8g
Total Fat 0g	**Sodium** 0mg	Dietary Fiber NA
Saturated Fat NA	**Protein** 0g	Sugars 5g

Harmless Harvest®, Namacha, Unsweetened

10 fl oz

Amount per serving	Amount per serving	Amount per serving
Calories 0	**Cholesterol** NA	**Total Carbohydrate** 0g
Total Fat 0g	**Sodium** 0mg	Dietary Fiber NA
Saturated Fat NA	**Protein** 0g	Sugars NA

Honest Ade, Cranberry Lemonade

16.9 fl oz

Amount per serving	Amount per serving	Amount per serving
Calories 100	**Cholesterol** NA	**Total Carbohydrate** 25g
Total Fat 0g	**Sodium** 10mg	Dietary Fiber NA
Saturated Fat NA	**Protein** 0g	Sugars 24g

Honest Ade, Orange Mango

16.9 fl oz

Amount per serving	Amount per serving	Amount per serving
Calories 100	**Cholesterol** NA	**Total Carbohydrate** 25g
Total Fat 0g	**Sodium** 10mg	Dietary Fiber NA
Saturated Fat NA	**Protein** 0g	Sugars 25g

Honest Ade, Pomegranate Blue

16.9 fl oz

Amount per serving	Amount per serving	Amount per serving
Calories 100	**Cholesterol** NA	**Total Carbohydrate** 25g
Total Fat 0g	**Sodium** 10mg	Dietary Fiber NA
Saturated Fat NA	**Protein** 0g	Sugars 25g

Honest Kids, Appley Ever After, Organic Juice Drink

6.75 fl oz

Amount per serving	Amount per serving	Amount per serving
Calories 40	**Cholesterol** NA	**Total Carbohydrate** 10g
Total Fat 0g	**Sodium** 5mg	Dietary Fiber NA
Saturated Fat NA	**Protein** 0g	Sugars 9g

Honest Kids, Berry Berry Good Lemonade, Organic Juice Drink

6.75 fl oz

Amount per serving	Amount per serving	Amount per serving
Calories 40	**Cholesterol** NA	**Total Carbohydrate** 10g
Total Fat 0g	**Sodium** 10mg	Dietary Fiber NA
Saturated Fat NA	**Protein** 0g	Sugars 9g

Honest Kids, Goodness Grapeness, Organic Juice Drink

6.75 fl oz

Amount per serving	Amount per serving	Amount per serving
Calories 40	**Cholesterol** NA	**Total Carbohydrate** 10g
Total Fat 0g	**Sodium** 15mg	Dietary Fiber NA
Saturated Fat NA	**Protein** 0g	Sugars 9g

Honest Kids, Super Fruit Punch, Organic Juice Drink

6.75 fl oz

Amount per serving	Amount per serving	Amount per serving
Calories 40	**Cholesterol** NA	**Total Carbohydrate** 10g
Total Fat 0g	**Sodium** 10mg	Dietary Fiber NA
Saturated Fat NA	**Protein** 0g	Sugars 9g

Honest Kids, Tropical Tango Punch, Organic Juice Drink

6.75 fl oz

Amount per serving	Amount per serving	Amount per serving
Calories 40	**Cholesterol** NA	**Total Carbohydrate** 10g
Total Fat 0g	**Sodium** 10mg	Dietary Fiber NA
Saturated Fat NA	**Protein** 0g	Sugars 9g

Honest Splash, Goodness Grapeness

12 fl oz

Amount per serving	Amount per serving	Amount per serving
Calories 70	**Cholesterol** NA	**Total Carbohydrate** 17g
Total Fat 0g	**Sodium** 15mg	Dietary Fiber NA
Saturated Fat NA	**Protein** 0g	Sugars 17g

Honest Splash, Super Fruit Punch

12 fl oz

Amount per serving	Amount per serving	Amount per serving
Calories 70	**Cholesterol** NA	**Total Carbohydrate** 17g
Total Fat 0g	**Sodium** 15mg	Dietary Fiber NA
Saturated Fat NA	**Protein** 0g	Sugars 16g

Honest Zero, Zero Calorie Lemonade

8 fl oz

Amount per serving	Amount per serving	Amount per serving
Calories 0	**Cholesterol** NA	**Total Carbohydrate** 0g
Total Fat 0g	**Sodium** 5mg	Dietary Fiber NA
Saturated Fat 0g	**Protein** 0g	Sugars 0g

Old Orchard Organics, 100% Apple Juice

8 fl oz

Amount per serving	Amount per serving	Amount per serving
Calories 120	**Cholesterol** 0mg	**Total Carbohydrate** 29g
Total Fat 0g	**Sodium** 25mg	Dietary Fiber NA
Saturated Fat NA	**Protein** 0g	Sugars 27g

OrganicVille®, OrangeVille Carbonated Beverage

1 bottle 12 fl oz (355 ml)

Amount per serving	Amount per serving	Amount per serving
Calories 140	**Cholesterol** 0mg	**Total Carbohydrate** 35g
Total Fat 0g	**Sodium** 5mg	Dietary Fiber 0g
Saturated Fat 0g	**Protein** 0g	Sugars 34g

Santa Cruz Organic, Apple Juice

8 fl oz

Amount per serving	Amount per serving	Amount per serving
Calories 120	**Cholesterol** NA	**Total Carbohydrate** 30g
Total Fat 0g	**Sodium** 25mg	Dietary Fiber NA
Saturated Fat NA	**Protein** <1g	Sugars 30g

Santa Cruz Organic, Apricot Mango Juice

8 fl oz

Amount per serving	Amount per serving	Amount per serving
Calories 130	**Cholesterol** NA	**Total Carbohydrate** 31g
Total Fat 0g	**Sodium** 15mg	Dietary Fiber NA
Saturated Fat NA	**Protein** 0g	Sugars 25g

Santa Cruz Organic, Apricot Nectar Juice

8 fl oz (240 ml)

Amount per serving	Amount per serving	Amount per serving
Calories 120	**Cholesterol** 0mg	**Total Carbohydrate** 29g
Total Fat 0g	**Sodium** 15mg	Dietary Fiber <1g
Saturated Fat 0g	**Protein** 0g	Sugars 25g

Santa Cruz Organic, Berry Nectar Juice

8 fl oz (240 ml)

Amount per serving	Amount per serving	Amount per serving
Calories 120	**Cholesterol** NA	**Total Carbohydrate** 29g
Total Fat 0g	**Sodium** 15mg	Dietary Fiber 1g
Saturated Fat NA	**Protein** 0g	Sugars 25g

Santa Cruz Organic, Cherry Lemonade

8 fl oz (240 ml)

Amount per serving	Amount per serving	Amount per serving
Calories 100	**Cholesterol** NA	**Total Carbohydrate** 26g
Total Fat 0g	**Sodium** 5mg	Dietary Fiber NA
Saturated Fat NA	**Protein** 0g	Sugars 25g

Santa Cruz Organic, Concord Grape Juice

8 fl oz (240 ml)

Amount per serving	Amount per serving	Amount per serving
Calories 160	**Cholesterol** 0mg	**Total Carbohydrate** 39g
Total Fat 0g	**Sodium** 20mg	Dietary Fiber <1g
Saturated Fat 0g	**Protein** 1g	Sugars 38g

Santa Cruz Organic, Cranberry Nectar Juice

8 fl oz (240 ml)

Amount per serving	Amount per serving	Amount per serving
Calories 120	**Cholesterol** NA	**Total Carbohydrate** 29g
Total Fat 0g	**Sodium** 20mg	Dietary Fiber NA
Saturated Fat NA	**Protein** 0g	Sugars 27g

Santa Cruz Organic, Hibiscus Cooler Juice

8 fl oz (240 ml)

Amount per serving	Amount per serving	Amount per serving
Calories 100	**Cholesterol** NA	**Total Carbohydrate** 25g
Total Fat 0g	**Sodium** 15mg	Dietary Fiber NA
Saturated Fat NA	**Protein** 0g	Sugars 24g

Santa Cruz Organic, Lemon Lime Carbonated Beverage

1 can

Amount per serving	Amount per serving	Amount per serving
Calories 130	**Cholesterol** NA	**Total Carbohydrate** 32g
Total Fat 0g	**Sodium** 10mg	Dietary Fiber NA
Saturated Fat NA	**Protein** 0g	Sugars 32g

Santa Cruz Organic, Lemonade

8 fl oz (240 ml)

Amount per serving	Amount per serving	Amount per serving
Calories 100	**Cholesterol** NA	**Total Carbohydrate** 22g
Total Fat 0g	**Sodium** 5mg	Dietary Fiber NA
Saturated Fat NA	**Protein** 0g	Sugars 22g

Santa Cruz Organic, Limeade

8 fl oz (240 ml)

Amount per serving	Amount per serving	Amount per serving
Calories 100	**Cholesterol** NA	**Total Carbohydrate** 25g
Total Fat 0g	**Sodium** 10mg	Dietary Fiber NA
Saturated Fat NA	**Protein** 0g	Sugars 24g

Santa Cruz Organic, Mango Lemonade

8 fl oz (240 ml)

Amount per serving	Amount per serving	Amount per serving
Calories 90	**Cholesterol** NA	**Total Carbohydrate** 22g
Total Fat 0g	**Sodium** 10mg	Dietary Fiber NA
Saturated Fat NA	**Protein** 0g	Sugars 21g

Santa Cruz Organic, Mango Lemonade Carbonated Beverage

1 can

Amount per serving	Amount per serving	Amount per serving
Calories 110	**Cholesterol** NA	**Total Carbohydrate** 28g
Total Fat 0g	**Sodium** 10mg	Dietary Fiber NA
Saturated Fat NA	**Protein** 0g	Sugars 28g

Santa Cruz Organic, Orange Mango Carbonated Beverage

1 can

Amount per serving	Amount per serving	Amount per serving
Calories 120	**Cholesterol** NA	**Total Carbohydrate** 29g
Total Fat 0g	**Sodium** 10mg	Dietary Fiber NA
Saturated Fat NA	**Protein** 0g	Sugars 29g

Santa Cruz Organic, Orange Mango Juice

8 fl oz (240 ml)

Amount per serving	Amount per serving	Amount per serving
Calories 130	**Cholesterol** NA	**Total Carbohydrate** 32g
Total Fat 0g	**Sodium** 20mg	Dietary Fiber NA
Saturated Fat NA	**Protein** 1g	Sugars 31g

Santa Cruz Organic, Peach Lemonade

8 fl oz (240 ml)

Amount per serving	Amount per serving	Amount per serving
Calories 90	**Cholesterol** NA	**Total Carbohydrate** 22g
Total Fat 0g	**Sodium** 5mg	Dietary Fiber NA
Saturated Fat NA	**Protein** 0g	Sugars 22g

Santa Cruz Organic, Pear Nectar Juice

8 fl oz (240 ml)

Amount per serving	Amount per serving	Amount per serving
Calories 130	**Cholesterol** NA	**Total Carbohydrate** 33g
Total Fat 0g	**Sodium** 15mg	Dietary Fiber 1g
Saturated Fat NA	**Protein** 0g	Sugars 25g

Santa Cruz Organic, Pomegranate Limeade Carbonated Beverage

1 can

Amount per serving	Amount per serving	Amount per serving
Calories 140	**Cholesterol** NA	**Total Carbohydrate** 36g
Total Fat 0g	**Sodium** 10mg	Dietary Fiber NA
Saturated Fat NA	**Protein** 0g	Sugars 34g

Santa Cruz Organic, Pure Lemon Juice

1 tsp (5 ml)

Amount per serving	Amount per serving	Amount per serving
Calories 0	**Cholesterol** NA	**Total Carbohydrate** 0g
Total Fat 0g	**Sodium** 0mg	Dietary Fiber NA
Saturated Fat NA	**Protein** 0g	Sugars NA

Santa Cruz Organic, Pure Lime Juice

1 tsp (5 ml)

Amount per serving	Amount per serving	Amount per serving
Calories 0	**Cholesterol** NA	**Total Carbohydrate** 0g
Total Fat 0g	**Sodium** 0mg	Dietary Fiber NA
Saturated Fat NA	**Protein** 0g	Sugars NA

Santa Cruz Organic, Raspberry Lemonade

8 fl oz (240 ml)

Amount per serving	Amount per serving	Amount per serving
Calories 90	**Cholesterol** NA	**Total Carbohydrate** 24g
Total Fat 0g	**Sodium** 5mg	Dietary Fiber NA
Saturated Fat NA	**Protein** NA	Sugars 23g

Santa Cruz Organic, Red Tart Cherry Juice

8 fl oz (240 ml)

Amount per serving	Amount per serving	Amount per serving
Calories 120	**Cholesterol** 0mg	**Total Carbohydrate** 30g
Total Fat 0g	**Sodium** 20mg	Dietary Fiber <1g
Saturated Fat 0g	**Protein** 0g	Sugars 25g

Santa Cruz Organic, Strawberry Lemonade

8 fl oz (240 ml)

Amount per serving	Amount per serving	Amount per serving
Calories 90	**Cholesterol** NA	**Total Carbohydrate** 23g
Total Fat 0g	**Sodium** 5mg	Dietary Fiber NA
Saturated Fat NA	**Protein** 0g	Sugars 22g

Santa Cruz Organic, White Grape Juice

8 fl oz (240 ml)

Amount per serving	Amount per serving	Amount per serving
Calories 160	**Cholesterol** NA	**Total Carbohydrate** 39g
Total Fat 0g	**Sodium** 20mg	Dietary Fiber NA
Saturated Fat NA	**Protein** <1g	Sugars 39g

Uncle Matt's, Organic Apple Juice

8 fl oz

Amount per serving	Amount per serving	Amount per serving
Calories 120	**Cholesterol** NA	**Total Carbohydrate** 30g
Total Fat 0g	**Sodium** 60mg	Dietary Fiber NA
Saturated Fat NA	**Protein** 1g	Sugars 28g

Uncle Matt's, Organic Grapefruit Juice

8 fl oz

Amount per serving	Amount per serving	Amount per serving
Calories 90	**Cholesterol** NA	**Total Carbohydrate** 22g
Total Fat 0g	**Sodium** 0mg	Dietary Fiber NA
Saturated Fat NA	**Protein** 1g	Sugars 17g

Uncle Matt's, Organic Lemonade

8 fl oz

Amount per serving	Amount per serving	Amount per serving
Calories 120	**Cholesterol** NA	**Total Carbohydrate** 30g
Total Fat 0g	**Sodium** 15mg	Dietary Fiber NA
Saturated Fat NA	**Protein** 0g	Sugars 27g

Uncle Matt's, Organic Orange Juice Pulp Free

8 fl oz

Amount per serving	Amount per serving	Amount per serving
Calories 110	**Cholesterol** NA	**Total Carbohydrate** 26g
Total Fat 0g	**Sodium** 0mg	Dietary Fiber NA
Saturated Fat NA	**Protein** 2g	Sugars 22g

Uncle Matt's, Organic Orange Juice with Pulp

8 fl oz

Amount per serving	Amount per serving	Amount per serving
Calories 110	**Cholesterol** NA	**Total Carbohydrate** 26g
Total Fat 0g	**Sodium** 0mg	Dietary Fiber NA
Saturated Fat NA	**Protein** 2g	Sugars 22g

Uncle Matt's, Organic Orange Juice, Calcium & Vitamin D

8 fl oz

Amount per serving	Amount per serving	Amount per serving
Calories 110	**Cholesterol** NA	**Total Carbohydrate** 26g
Total Fat 0g	**Sodium** 10mg	Dietary Fiber NA
Saturated Fat NA	**Protein** 2g	Sugars 22g

Uncle Matt's, Organic Orange Mango Juice

8 fl oz (240 ml)

Amount per serving	Amount per serving	Amount per serving
Calories 100	**Cholesterol** NA	**Total Carbohydrate** 24g
Total Fat 0g	**Sodium** 0mg	Dietary Fiber 2g
Saturated Fat 0g	**Protein** 1g	Sugars 23g

Uncle Matt's, Organic Orange Tangerine Juice

8 fl oz (240 ml)

Amount per serving	Amount per serving	Amount per serving
Calories 100	**Cholesterol** NA	**Total Carbohydrate** 23g
Total Fat 0g	**Sodium** 0mg	Dietary Fiber 0g
Saturated Fat 0g	**Protein** 2g	Sugars 23g

Soda

Honest Fizz, Root Beer, Organic Zero Calorie Soda

12 fl oz

Amount per serving	Amount per serving	Amount per serving
Calories 0	**Cholesterol** NA	**Total Carbohydrate** 5g
Total Fat 0g	**Sodium** 7mg	Dietary Fiber NA
Saturated Fat NA	**Protein** 0g	Sugars 0g

Teas

AriZona, Organic Green Tea with Ginseng and Honey

1 cup

Amount per serving	Amount per serving	Amount per serving
Calories 50	**Cholesterol** 0rng	**Total Carbohydrate** 14g
Total Fat 0g	**Sodium** 10mg	Dietary Fiber 0g
Saturated Fat 0g	**Protein** 0g	Sugars 13g

AriZona, Organic Pomegranate Green Tea

1 cup

Amount per serving	Amount per serving	Amount per serving
Calories 50	**Cholesterol** 0mg	**Total Carbohydrate** 13g
Total Fat 0g	**Sodium** 10mg	Dietary Fiber 0g
Saturated Fat 0g	**Protein** 0g	Sugars 13g

AriZona, Organic Yumberry Green Tea

1 cup

Amount per serving	Amount per serving	Amount per serving
Calories 50	**Cholesterol** 0mg	**Total Carbohydrate** 13g
Total Fat 0g	**Sodium** 10mg	Dietary Fiber 0g
Saturated Fat 0g	**Protein** 0g	Sugars 13g

Bigelow Teas, Organic Breakfast Blend Decaffeinated Tea, Brewed

8 fl oz

Amount per serving	Amount per serving	Amount per serving
Calories 0	**Cholesterol** 0mg	**Total Carbohydrate** NA
Total Fat 0g	**Sodium** NA	Dietary Fiber NA
Saturated Fat NA	**Protein** 0g	Sugars 0g

Bigelow Teas, Organic Ceylon-Fair Trade Tea, Brewed, Prepared with Tap Water

8 fl oz

Amount per serving	Amount per serving	Amount per serving
Calories 0	**Cholesterol** 0mg	**Total Carbohydrate** NA
Total Fat 0g	**Sodium** NA	Dietary Fiber NA
Saturated Fat NA	**Protein** 0g	Sugars 0g

Bigelow Teas, Organic Chamomile Citrus Herb Tea, Brewed, Prepared with Tap Water

8 fl oz

Amount per serving	Amount per serving	Amount per serving
Calories 0	**Cholesterol** 0mg	**Total Carbohydrate** NA
Total Fat 0g	**Sodium** NA	Dietary Fiber NA
Saturated Fat NA	**Protein** 0g	Sugars 0g

Bigelow Teas, Organic Green Decaffeinated Tea, Brewed, Prepared with Tap Water

8 fl oz

Amount per serving	Amount per serving	Amount per serving
Calories 0	**Cholesterol** 0mg	**Total Carbohydrate** NA
Total Fat 0g	**Sodium** NA	Dietary Fiber NA
Saturated Fat NA	**Protein** 0g	Sugars 0g

Bigelow Teas, Organic Green Tea Pomegranate & Acai, Brewed

8 fl oz

Amount per serving	Amount per serving	Amount per serving
Calories 0	**Cholesterol** 0mg	**Total Carbohydrate** NA
Total Fat 0g	**Sodium** NA	Dietary Fiber NA
Saturated Fat NA	**Protein** 0g	Sugars 0g

Bigelow Teas, Organic Green Tea, Brewed, Prepared with Tap Water

8 fl oz

Amount per serving	Amount per serving	Amount per serving
Calories 0	**Cholesterol** 0mg	**Total Carbohydrate** NA
Total Fat 0g	**Sodium** NA	Dietary Fiber NA
Saturated Fat NA	**Protein** 0g	Sugars 0g

Bigelow Teas, Organic Imperial Earl Grey Tea, Brewed, Prepared with Tap Water

8 fl oz

Amount per serving	Amount per serving	Amount per serving
Calories 0	**Cholesterol** 0mg	**Total Carbohydrate** NA
Total Fat 0g	**Sodium** NA	Dietary Fiber NA
Saturated Fat NA	**Protein** 0g	Sugars 0g

Bigelow Teas, Organic Moroccan Mint Herb Tea, Brewed, Prepared with Tap Water

8 fl oz

Amount per serving	Amount per serving	Amount per serving
Calories 0	**Cholesterol** 0mg	**Total Carbohydrate** NA
Total Fat 0g	**Sodium** NA	Dietary Fiber NA
Saturated Fat NA	**Protein** 0g	Sugars 0g

Bigelow Teas, Organic Pure Green Decaffeinated Tea, Brewed

8 fl oz

Amount per serving	Amount per serving	Amount per serving
Calories 0	**Cholesterol** 0mg	**Total Carbohydrate** NA
Total Fat 0g	**Sodium** NA	Dietary Fiber NA
Saturated Fat NA	**Protein** 0g	Sugars 0g

Bigelow Teas, Organic Pure Green Tea, Brewed, Prepared with Tap Water

8 fl oz

Amount per serving	Amount per serving	Amount per serving
Calories 0	**Cholesterol** 0mg	**Total Carbohydrate** NA
Total Fat 0g	**Sodium** NA	Dietary Fiber NA
Saturated Fat NA	**Protein** 0g	Sugars 0g

Bigelow Teas, Organic Rooibos with Asian Pear Tea, Brewed, Prepared with Tap Water

8 fl oz

Amount per serving	Amount per serving	Amount per serving
Calories 0	**Cholesterol** 0mg	**Total Carbohydrate** NA
Total Fat 0g	**Sodium** NA	Dietary Fiber NA
Saturated Fat NA	**Protein** 0g	Sugars 0g

Bigelow Teas, Organic White Tea with Raspberry & Chrysanthemum, Brewed

8 fl oz

Amount per serving	Amount per serving	Amount per serving
Calories 0	**Cholesterol** 0mg	**Total Carbohydrate** NA
Total Fat 0g	**Sodium** NA	Dietary Fiber NA
Saturated Fat NA	**Protein** 0g	Sugars 0g

Celestial Seasonings®, Organic Earl Grey Estate Tea

1 tea bag (2g)

Amount per serving	Amount per serving	Amount per serving
Calories 0	**Cholesterol** NA	**Total Carbohydrate** 0g
Total Fat 0g	**Sodium** 0mg	Dietary Fiber NA
Saturated Fat NA	**Protein** 0g	Sugars 0g

Celestial Seasonings®, Organic English Breakfast Tea

1 tea bag (2g)

Amount per serving	Amount per serving	Amount per serving
Calories 0	**Cholesterol** NA	**Total Carbohydrate** 0g
Total Fat 0g	**Sodium** 0mg	Dietary Fiber NA
Saturated Fat NA	**Protein** 0g	Sugars 0g

Celestial Seasonings®, Organic Jasmine Green Tea

1 tea bag (1g)

Amount per serving	Amount per serving	Amount per serving
Calories 0	**Cholesterol** NA	**Total Carbohydrate** 0g
Total Fat 0g	**Sodium** 0mg	Dietary Fiber NA
Saturated Fat NA	**Protein** 0g	Sugars 0g

Celestial Seasonings®, Organic Perfect Trio Estate Tea, Green, Black, & White Tea

1 tea bag (2g)

Amount per serving	Amount per serving	Amount per serving
Calories 0	**Cholesterol** NA	**Total Carbohydrate** 0g
Total Fat 0g	**Sodium** 0mg	Dietary Fiber NA
Saturated Fat NA	**Protein** 0g	Sugars 0g

Celestial Seasonings®, Organic Pure Green Estate Tea

1 tea bag (2g)

Amount per serving	Amount per serving	Amount per serving
Calories 0	**Cholesterol** NA	**Total Carbohydrate** 0g
Total Fat 0g	**Sodium** 0mg	Dietary Fiber NA
Saturated Fat NA	**Protein** 0g	Sugars 0g

Eden Foods, Organic Matcha, Green Tea Powder

1g

Amount per serving	Amount per serving	Amount per serving
Calories 3	**Cholesterol** 0mg	**Total Carbohydrate** <1g
Total Fat 0g	**Sodium** 0mg	Dietary Fiber 0g
Saturated Fat 0g	**Protein** 0g	Sugars <1g

Honest Tea, (Not Too) Sweet Tea

16.9 fl oz

Amount per serving	Amount per serving	Amount per serving
Calories 100	**Cholesterol** NA	**Total Carbohydrate** 25g
Total Fat 0g	**Sodium** 10mg	Dietary Fiber NA
Saturated Fat NA	**Protein** 0g	Sugars 25g

Honest Tea, Assam Black Tea

8 fl oz

Amount per serving	Amount per serving	Amount per serving
Calories 17	**Cholesterol** NA	**Total Carbohydrate** 5g
Total Fat 0g	**Sodium** 5mg	Dietary Fiber NA
Saturated Fat NA	**Protein** 0g	Sugars 5g

Honest Tea, Berry Good Lemonade

12 fl oz

Amount per serving	Amount per serving	Amount per serving
Calories 70	**Cholesterol** NA	**Total Carbohydrate** 17g
Total Fat 0g	**Sodium** 15mg	Dietary Fiber NA
Saturated Fat NA	**Protein** 0g	Sugars 16g

Honest Tea, Black Forest Berry

8 fl oz

Amount per serving	Amount per serving	Amount per serving
Calories 30	**Cholesterol** NA	**Total Carbohydrate** 8g
Total Fat 0g	**Sodium** 5mg	Dietary Fiber NA
Saturated Fat NA	**Protein** 0g	Sugars 8g

Honest Tea, Classic Green Tea

8 fl oz

Amount per serving	Amount per serving	Amount per serving
Calories 30	**Cholesterol** NA	**Total Carbohydrate** 9g
Total Fat 0g	**Sodium** 5mg	Dietary Fiber NA
Saturated Fat NA	**Protein** 0g	Sugars 9g

Honest Tea, Community Green Tea with Maltese Orange

8 fl oz

Amount per serving	Amount per serving	Amount per serving
Calories 17	**Cholesterol** NA	**Total Carbohydrate** 5g
Total Fat 0g	**Sodium** 5mg	Dietary Fiber NA
Saturated Fat NA	**Protein** 0g	Sugars 5g

Honest Tea, Green Dragon Tea with Passion Fruit

8 fl oz

Amount per serving	Amount per serving	Amount per serving
Calories 30	**Cholesterol** NA	**Total Carbohydrate** 8g
Total Fat 0g	**Sodium** 5mg	Dietary Fiber NA
Saturated Fat NA	**Protein** 0g	Sugars 8g

Honest Tea, Half & Half, Organic Tea with Lemonade

16.9 fl oz

Amount per serving	Amount per serving	Amount per serving
Calories 100	**Cholesterol** NA	**Total Carbohydrate** 25g
Total Fat 0g	**Sodium** 10mg	Dietary Fiber NA
Saturated Fat NA	**Protein** 0g	Sugars 24g

Honest Tea, Heavenly Lemon Tulsi

8 fl oz

Amount per serving	Amount per serving	Amount per serving
Calories 30	**Cholesterol** NA	**Total Carbohydrate** 8g
Total Fat 0g	**Sodium** 5mg	Dietary Fiber NA
Saturated Fat NA	**Protein** 0g	Sugars 8g

Honest Tea, Honey Green Tea

16.9 fl oz

Amount per serving	Amount per serving	Amount per serving
Calories 70	**Cholesterol** NA	**Total Carbohydrate** 18g
Total Fat 0g	**Sodium** 10mg	Dietary Fiber NA
Saturated Fat NA	**Protein** 0g	Sugars 18g

Honest Tea, Jasmine Green Energy Tea

8 fl oz

Amount per serving	Amount per serving	Amount per serving
Calories 17	**Cholesterol** NA mg	**Total Carbohydrate** 5g
Total Fat 0g	**Sodium** 5mg	Dietary Fiber NA
Saturated Fat NA	**Protein** 0g	Sugars 5g

Honest Tea, Just Black Tea

8 fl oz

Amount per serving	Amount per serving	Amount per serving
Calories 0	**Cholesterol** NA	**Total Carbohydrate** 0g
Total Fat 0g	**Sodium** 5mg	Dietary Fiber NA
Saturated Fat NA	**Protein** 0g	Sugars 0g

Honest Tea, Just Green Tea

8 fl oz

Amount per serving	Amount per serving	Amount per serving
Calories 0	**Cholesterol** NA	**Total Carbohydrate** 0g
Total Fat 0g	**Sodium** 5mg	Dietary Fiber NA
Saturated Fat NA	**Protein** 0g	Sugars 0g

Honest Tea, Lemon Tea

16.9 fl oz

Amount per serving	Amount per serving	Amount per serving
Calories 80	**Cholesterol** NA	**Total Carbohydrate** 21g
Total Fat 0g	**Sodium** 5mg	Dietary Fiber NA
Saturated Fat NA	**Protein** 0g	Sugars 21g

Honest Tea, Lori's Lemon Tea

8 fl oz

Amount per serving	Amount per serving	Amount per serving
Calories 30	**Cholesterol** NA	**Total Carbohydrate** 8g
Total Fat 0g	**Sodium** 5mg	Dietary Fiber NA
Saturated Fat NA	**Protein** 0g	Sugars 8g

Honest Tea, Mango Acai White Tea

8 fl oz

Amount per serving	Amount per serving	Amount per serving
Calories 35	**Cholesterol** NA	**Total Carbohydrate** 9g
Total Fat 0g	**Sodium** 5mg	Dietary Fiber NA
Saturated Fat NA	**Protein** 0g	Sugars 9g

Honest Tea, Moroccan Mint Green Tea

8 fl oz

Amount per serving	Amount per serving	Amount per serving
Calories 17	**Cholesterol** NA	**Total Carbohydrate** 5g
Total Fat 0g	**Sodium** 5mg	Dietary Fiber NA
Saturated Fat NA	**Protein** 0g	Sugars 5g

Honest Tea, Peach Oo-La-Long

8 fl oz

Amount per serving	Amount per serving	Amount per serving
Calories 30	**Cholesterol** NA	**Total Carbohydrate** 8g
Total Fat 0g	**Sodium** 5mg	Dietary Fiber NA
Saturated Fat NA	**Protein** 0g	Sugars 8g

Honest Tea, Peach White Tea

16.9 fl oz

Amount per serving	Amount per serving	Amount per serving
Calories 80	**Cholesterol** NA	**Total Carbohydrate** 20g
Total Fat 0g	**Sodium** 10mg	Dietary Fiber NA
Saturated Fat NA	**Protein** 0g	Sugars 20g

Honest Tea, Pomegranate Red Tea with Goji Berry

8 fl oz

Amount per serving	Amount per serving	Amount per serving
Calories 35	**Cholesterol** NA	**Total Carbohydrate** 9g
Total Fat 0g	**Sodium** 5mg	Dietary Fiber NA
Saturated Fat NA	**Protein** 0g	Sugars 9g

Honest Tea, Raspberry Fields

16 fl oz

Amount per serving	Amount per serving	Amount per serving
Calories 70	**Cholesterol** NA	**Total Carbohydrate** 18g
Total Fat 0g	**Sodium** 10mg	Dietary Fiber NA
Saturated Fat NA	**Protein** 0g	Sugars 18g

Honest Tea, Raspberry Tea

16.9 fl oz

Amount per serving	Amount per serving	Amount per serving
Calories 100	**Cholesterol** NA	**Total Carbohydrate** 25g
Total Fat 0g	**Sodium** 10mg	Dietary Fiber NA
Saturated Fat NA	**Protein** 0g	Sugars 25g

Honest Tea, Unsweet Lemon Tea

16.9 fl oz

Amount per serving	Amount per serving	Amount per serving
Calories 0	**Cholesterol** NA	**Total Carbohydrate** 1g
Total Fat 0g	**Sodium** 25mg	Dietary Fiber NA
Saturated Fat NA	**Protein** 0g	Sugars 0g

Honest Zero, Zero Calorie Passion Fruit Green Tea

16 fl oz

Amount per serving	Amount per serving	Amount per serving
Calories 0	**Cholesterol** NA	**Total Carbohydrate** 0g
Total Fat 0g	**Sodium** 10mg	Dietary Fiber NA
Saturated Fat NA	**Protein** 0g	Sugars 0g

Organic Valley, Heavy Whipping Cream, Pasteurized

1 tbsp (15 ml)

Amount per serving	Amount per serving	Amount per serving
Calories 50	**Cholesterol** 20mg	**Total Carbohydrate** 0g
Total Fat 6g	**Sodium** 5mg	Dietary Fiber 0g
Saturated Fat 3.5g	**Protein** 0g	Sugars 0g

Organic Valley, Heavy Whipping Cream, Ultra Pasteurized

1 tbsp (15 ml)

Amount per serving

Amount per serving

Amount per serving

Calories 50
Total Fat 6g
  Saturated Fat 3.5g

Cholesterol 20mg
Sodium 5mg
Protein 0g

Total Carbohydrate 0g
  Dietary Fiber NA
  Sugars NA

Organic Valley, Organic Fuel, High Protein Milk Shake, Chocolate

1 bottle (325 ml)

Amount per serving

Amount per serving

Amount per serving

Calories 260
Total Fat 6g
  Saturated Fat 3g

Cholesterol 35mg
Sodium 190mg
Protein 26g

Total Carbohydrate 27g
  Dietary Fiber 1g
  Sugars 26g

Pyure, O.E.O., Organic Green Tea Yerba Mate & Guayusa Extracts 2 fl oz (60 ml)

1 bottle (2 fl oz/60 ml)

Amount per serving

Amount per serving

Amount per serving

Calories 0
Total Fat NA
  Saturated Fat NA

Cholesterol NA
Sodium NA
Protein NA

Total Carbohydrate NA
  Dietary Fiber NA
  Sugars NA

Third Street, Third Street Half & Half Lemonade

8 fl oz

Amount per serving

Amount per serving

Amount per serving

Calories 80
Total Fat 0g
  Saturated Fat NA

Cholesterol 0mg
Sodium 10mg
Protein 0g

Total Carbohydrate 19g
  Dietary Fiber 0g
  Sugars 19g

Third Street, Third Street Mint & Honey Ready-to-Drink Green Iced Tea

8 fl oz

Amount per serving

Amount per serving

Amount per serving

Calories 50
Total Fat 0g
  Saturated Fat NA

Cholesterol 0mg
Sodium 10mg
Protein 0g

Total Carbohydrate 13g
  Dietary Fiber 0g
  Sugars 13g

Third Street, Third Street Peach Ready-to-Drink Black Iced Tea

8 fl oz

Amount per serving

Amount per serving

Amount per serving

Calories 60
Total Fat 0g
  Saturated Fat NA

Cholesterol 0mg
Sodium 10mg
Protein 0g

Total Carbohydrate 13g
  Dietary Fiber 0g
  Sugars 12g

Third Street, Third Street Pucker-Up Lemonade

8 fl oz

Amount per serving	Amount per serving	Amount per serving
Calories 90	**Cholesterol** 0mg	**Total Carbohydrate** 22g
Total Fat 0g	**Sodium** 10mg	Dietary Fiber 0g
Saturated Fat NA	**Protein** 0g	Sugars 22g

Third Street, Third Street Raspberry Ready-to-Drink Black Iced Tea

8 fl oz

Amount per serving	Amount per serving	Amount per serving
Calories 50	**Cholesterol** 0mg	**Total Carbohydrate** 12g
Total Fat 0g	**Sodium** 10mg	Dietary Fiber 0g
Saturated Fat NA	**Protein** 0g	Sugars 12g

Third Street, Third Street Slightly Sweet Ready-to-Drink Black Iced Tea

8 fl oz

Amount per serving	Amount per serving	Amount per serving
Calories 50	**Cholesterol** 0mg	**Total Carbohydrate** 12g
Total Fat 0g	**Sodium** 10mg	Dietary Fiber 0g
Saturated Fat NA	**Protein** 0g	Sugars 12g

Third Street, Third Street Slightly Sweet Ready-to-Drink Green Iced Tea

8 fl oz

Amount per serving	Amount per serving	Amount per serving
Calories 50	**Cholesterol** 0mg	**Total Carbohydrate** 12g
Total Fat 0g	**Sodium** 10mg	Dietary Fiber 0g
Saturated Fat NA	**Protein** 0g	Sugars 12g

Third Street, Third Street Unsweetened Ready-to-Drink Black Iced Tea

8 fl oz

Amount per serving	Amount per serving	Amount per serving
Calories 0	**Cholesterol** 0mg	**Total Carbohydrate** 0g
Total Fat 0g	**Sodium** 10mg	Dietary Fiber 0g
Saturated Fat NA	**Protein** 0g	Sugars 0g

Third Street, Third Street Unsweetened Ready-to-Drink Green Iced Tea

8 fl oz

Amount per serving	Amount per serving	Amount per serving
Calories 0	**Cholesterol** 0mg	**Total Carbohydrate** 0g
Total Fat 0g	**Sodium** 10mg	Dietary Fiber 0g
Saturated Fat NA	**Protein** 0g	Sugars 0g

Prepared Foods

Why Eat Prepared Foods?

Prepared foods are convenient and enjoyable to eat, but they don't fit neatly into one food group. For example, a cheese pizza counts in several groups—the crust in the grains group, the tomato sauce in the vegetable group, and the cheese in the dairy group. For the nutrient benefits of mixed foods, you need to look at each food component. Frozen and shelf-stable partially prepared foods are convenient and can be healthy, depending on their ingredients.

Why Choose Organic Prepared Foods?

Organic prepared foods are made with organic ingredients—meat, fish, dairy, eggs, grains, and produce raised or grown without the use of synthetic fertilizers, pesticides, or herbicides. Organic prepared foods contain no artificial ingredients such as synthetic food coloring, additives, or preservatives.

Daily Goal

There is no daily goal for prepared foods. Compare each component of the prepared food with the daily goal for that food.

A prepared entrée should provide:

300 to 500 calories

10 grams or more protein

30% or less fat calories (10 to 28 grams total fat)

10% or less saturated fat (1 to 2 grams)

480 milligrams or less sodium

USDA Organic Nutrients in Prepared Foods

See the USDA organic nutrients for each individual food ingredient found in each prepared dish.

Condiments

Annie's, Organic Dijon Mustard

1 tsp

Amount per serving	Amount per serving	Amount per serving
Calories 5	**Cholesterol** NA	**Total Carbohydrate** 1g
Total Fat 0g	**Sodium** 120mg	Dietary Fiber NA
Saturated Fat NA	**Protein** 0g	Sugars NA

Annie's, Organic Honey Mustard

1 tsp

Amount per serving	Amount per serving	Amount per serving
Calories 10	**Cholesterol** NA	**Total Carbohydrate** 2g
Total Fat 0g	**Sodium** 45mg	Dietary Fiber NA
Saturated Fat NA	**Protein** 0g	Sugars 2g

Annie's, Organic Horseradish Mustard

1 tsp

Amount per serving	Amount per serving	Amount per serving
Calories 5	**Cholesterol** NA	**Total Carbohydrate** 1g
Total Fat 0g	**Sodium** 60mg	Dietary Fiber NA
Saturated Fat 0g	**Protein** 0g	Sugars NA

Annie's, Organic Hot Chipotle BBQ Sauce

2 tbsp (34g)

Amount per serving	Amount per serving	Amount per serving
Calories 35	**Cholesterol** NA	**Total Carbohydrate** 7g
Total Fat 1g	**Sodium** 220mg	Dietary Fiber NA
Saturated Fat NA	**Protein** 0g	Sugars 5g

Annie's, Organic Ketchup

1 tbsp

Amount per serving	Amount per serving	Amount per serving
Calories 15	**Cholesterol** NA	**Total Carbohydrate** 5g
Total Fat 0g	**Sodium** 170mg	Dietary Fiber NA
Saturated Fat 0g	**Protein** 0g	Sugars 4g

Annie's, Organic Original Recipe BBQ Sauce

2 tbsp (34g)

Amount per serving	Amount per serving	Amount per serving
Calories 35	**Cholesterol** NA	**Total Carbohydrate** 6g
Total Fat 1g	**Sodium** 200mg	Dietary Fiber NA
Saturated Fat NA	**Protein** 0g	Sugars 4g

Annie's, Organic Smoky Maple BBQ Sauce

2 tbsp (34g)

Amount per serving	Amount per serving	Amount per serving
Calories 35	**Cholesterol** NA	**Total Carbohydrate** 7g
Total Fat 1g	**Sodium** 210mg	Dietary Fiber NA
Saturated Fat NA	**Protein** 0g	Sugars 5g

Annie's, Organic Sweet & Spicy BBQ Sauce

2 tbsp (34g)

Amount per serving	Amount per serving	Amount per serving
Calories 40	**Cholesterol** NA	**Total Carbohydrate** 10g
Total Fat 0g	**Sodium** 300mg	Dietary Fiber 1g
Saturated Fat NA	**Protein** 0g	Sugars 8g

Annie's, Organic Vegan Worcestershire Sauce

1 tsp (5g)

Amount per serving	Amount per serving	Amount per serving
Calories 5	**Cholesterol** NA	**Total Carbohydrate** 1g
Total Fat 0g	**Sodium** 60mg	Dietary Fiber NA
Saturated Fat NA	**Protein** 0g	Sugars NA

Annie's, Organic Yellow Mustard

1 tsp

Amount per serving	Amount per serving	Amount per serving
Calories 5	**Cholesterol** NA	**Total Carbohydrate** 1g
Total Fat 0g	**Sodium** 50mg	Dietary Fiber NA
Saturated Fat NA	**Protein** 0g	Sugars NA

Eden Foods, Brown Mustard, Organic Jar

1 tsp

Amount per serving	Amount per serving	Amount per serving
Calories 0	**Cholesterol** 0mg	**Total Carbohydrate** <1g
Total Fat 0g	**Sodium** 80mg	Dietary Fiber NA
Saturated Fat 0g	**Protein** 0g	Sugars 0g

Eden Foods, Brown Mustard, Organic, Squeeze Bottle

1 tsp

Amount per serving	Amount per serving	Amount per serving
Calories 0	**Cholesterol** 0mg	**Total Carbohydrate** 1g
Total Fat 0g	**Sodium** 80mg	Dietary Fiber 0g
Saturated Fat 0g	**Protein** 0g	Sugars 0g

Eden Foods, Brown Rice Vinegar, Organic, Imported

1 tbsp

Amount per serving	Amount per serving	Amount per serving
Calories 2	**Cholesterol** NA	**Total Carbohydrate** 0g
Total Fat 0g	**Sodium** 0mg	Dietary Fiber NA
Saturated Fat NA	**Protein** 0g	Sugars 0g

Eden Foods, Sauerkraut, Organic

1/4 cup

Amount per serving	Amount per serving	Amount per serving
Calories 5	**Cholesterol** 0mg	**Total Carbohydrate** 2g
Total Fat 0g	**Sodium** 150mg	Dietary Fiber 1g
Saturated Fat NA	**Protein** 0g	Sugars 0g

Eden Foods, Shoyu Soy Sauce, Organic (Imported)

1 tbsp

Amount per serving	Amount per serving	Amount per serving
Calories 15	**Cholesterol** 0mg	**Total Carbohydrate** 2g
Total Fat 0g	**Sodium** 1040mg	Dietary Fiber 0g
Saturated Fat 0g	**Protein** 2g	Sugars 0g

Eden Foods, Tamari Soy Sauce, Brewed in U.S., Organic

1 tbsp

Amount per serving	Amount per serving	Amount per serving
Calories 15	**Cholesterol** 0mg	**Total Carbohydrate** 2g
Total Fat 0g	**Sodium** 860mg	Dietary Fiber 0g
Saturated Fat 0g	**Protein** 2g	Sugars 0g

Eden Foods, Tamari Soy Sauce, Organic (Imported)

1 tbsp

Amount per serving	Amount per serving	Amount per serving
Calories 10	**Cholesterol** 0mg	**Total Carbohydrate** 2g
Total Fat 0g	**Sodium** 990mg	Dietary Fiber 0g
Saturated Fat 0g	**Protein** 2g	Sugars 0g

Eden Foods, Yellow Mustard, Organic, Jar

1 tsp

Amount per serving	Amount per serving	Amount per serving
Calories 0	**Cholesterol** 0mg	**Total Carbohydrate** 0g
Total Fat 0g	**Sodium** 80mg	Dietary Fiber NA
Saturated Fat NA	**Protein** 0g	Sugars 0g

Eden Foods, Yellow Mustard, Organic, Squeeze Bottle

1 tsp

Amount per serving	Amount per serving	Amount per serving
Calories 0	Cholesterol 0mg	Total Carbohydrate 0g
Total Fat 0g	Sodium 80mg	Dietary Fiber 0g
Saturated Fat 0g	Protein 0g	Sugars 0g

Muir Glen Organic, Tomato Ketchup, 24 oz

1 tbsp (17g)

Amount per serving	Amount per serving	Amount per serving
Calories 20	Cholesterol 0mg	Total Carbohydrate 4g
Total Fat 0g	Sodium 230mg	Dietary Fiber 0g
Saturated Fat 0g	Protein 0g	Sugars 3g

OrganicVille®, Enchilada Sauce

1/4 cup (62g)

Amount per serving	Amount per serving	Amount per serving
Calories 20	Cholesterol 0mg	Total Carbohydrate 4g
Total Fat 0g	Sodium 270mg	Dietary Fiber 1g
Saturated Fat 0g	Protein 1g	Sugars 2g

OrganicVille®, Hot Sauce

1 tsp (5 ml)

Amount per serving	Amount per serving	Amount per serving
Calories 0	Cholesterol 0mg	Total Carbohydrate 0g
Total Fat 0g	Sodium 80mg	Dietary Fiber 0g
Saturated Fat 0g	Protein 0g	Sugars 0g

OrganicVille®, Mole Sauce

1 tbsp (15g)

Amount per serving	Amount per serving	Amount per serving
Calories 10	Cholesterol 0mg	Total Carbohydrate 1g
Total Fat 0.5g	Sodium 70mg	Dietary Fiber 0g
Saturated Fat 0g	Protein 0g	Sugars 1g

OrganicVille®, Organic Ketchup

1 tbsp (17g)

Amount per serving	Amount per serving	Amount per serving
Calories 20	Cholesterol 0mg	Total Carbohydrate 4g
Total Fat 0g	Sodium 125mg	Dietary Fiber 0g
Saturated Fat 0g	Protein 0g	Sugars 3g

OrganicVille®, Original Chili Sauce

2 tbsp (30g)

Amount per serving	Amount per serving	Amount per serving
Calories 30	**Cholesterol** 0mg	**Total Carbohydrate** 7g
Total Fat 0g	**Sodium** 270mg	Dietary Fiber <1g
Saturated Fat 0g	**Protein** 0g	Sugars 4g

OrganicVille®, Original Organic BBQ Sauce

2 tbsp (30g)

Amount per serving	Amount per serving	Amount per serving
Calories 50	**Cholesterol** 0mg	**Total Carbohydrate** 13g
Total Fat 0g	**Sodium** 200mg	Dietary Fiber <1g
Saturated Fat 0g	**Protein** 0g	Sugars 11g

OrganicVille®, Sky Valley Sriracha Sauce

1 tsp

Amount per serving	Amount per serving	Amount per serving
Calories 5	**Cholesterol** 0mg	**Total Carbohydrate** 1g
Total Fat 0g	**Sodium** 150mg	Dietary Fiber 0g
Saturated Fat 0g	**Protein** 0g	Sugars 1g

OrganicVille®, Taco Sauce

1 tbsp (15g)

Amount per serving	Amount per serving	Amount per serving
Calories 5	**Cholesterol** 0mg	**Total Carbohydrate** 1g
Total Fat 0g	**Sodium** 65mg	Dietary Fiber 0g
Saturated Fat 0g	**Protein** 0g	Sugars 1g

OrganicVille®, Tangy Organic BBQ Sauce

2 tbsp (30g)

Amount per serving	Amount per serving	Amount per serving
Calories 35	**Cholesterol** 0mg	**Total Carbohydrate** 8g
Total Fat 0g	**Sodium** 200mg	Dietary Fiber <1g
Saturated Fat 0g	**Protein** 0g	Sugars 6g

Premier Japan, Organic Wheat-Free Hoisin Sauce

1 tsp

Amount per serving	Amount per serving	Amount per serving
Calories 15	**Cholesterol** 0mg	**Total Carbohydrate** 3g
Total Fat 0g	**Sodium** 160mg	Dietary Fiber 0g
Saturated Fat 0g	**Protein** 0g	Sugars 2g

Premier Japan, Organic Wheat-Free Teriyaki Sauce

1 tsp

Amount per serving	Amount per serving	Amount per serving
Calories 15	**Cholesterol** 0mg	**Total Carbohydrate** 3g
Total Fat 0g	**Sodium** 250mg	Dietary Fiber 0g
Saturated Fat 0g	**Protein** 0g	Sugars 2g

San-J, Organic Gluten-Free Tamari Travel Packs

2 packs

Amount per serving	Amount per serving	Amount per serving
Calories 10	**Cholesterol** 0mg	**Total Carbohydrate** <1g
Total Fat 0g	**Sodium** 940mg	Dietary Fiber 0g
Saturated Fat 0g	**Protein** 2g	Sugars 0g

San-J, Organic Tamari Gluten-Free Reduced Sodium Soy Sauce

1 tbsp

Amount per serving	Amount per serving	Amount per serving
Calories 15	**Cholesterol** 0mg	**Total Carbohydrate** 1g
Total Fat 0g	**Sodium** 700mg	Dietary Fiber 0g
Saturated Fat 0g	**Protein** 2g	Sugars 0g

San-J, Organic Tamari Gluten-Free Soy Sauce

1 tbsp

Amount per serving	Amount per serving	Amount per serving
Calories 10	**Cholesterol** 0mg	**Total Carbohydrate** <1g
Total Fat 0g	**Sodium** 940mg	Dietary Fiber 0g
Saturated Fat 0g	**Protein** 2g	Sugars 0g

Spectrum®, Mayonnaise with Cage Free Eggs, Organic

1 tbsp (14g)

Amount per serving	Amount per serving	Amount per serving
Calories 100	**Cholesterol** 10mg	**Total Carbohydrate** 0g
Total Fat 11g	**Sodium** 85mg	Dietary Fiber NA
Saturated Fat 1.5g	**Protein** 0g	Sugars NA

Spectrum®, Mayonnaise with Cage Free Eggs, Organic (Squeeze)

1 tbsp (14g)

Amount per serving	Amount per serving	Amount per serving
Calories 100	**Cholesterol** 10mg	**Total Carbohydrate** 0g
Total Fat 11g	**Sodium** 85mg	Dietary Fiber NA
Saturated Fat 1.5g	**Protein** 0g	Sugars NA

Spectrum®, Mayonnaise with Olive Oil, Organic

1 tbsp (14g)

Amount per serving	Amount per serving	Amount per serving
Calories 100	**Cholesterol** 10mg	**Total Carbohydrate** 1g
Total Fat 11g	**Sodium** 75mg	Dietary Fiber NA
Saturated Fat 1.5g	**Protein** 0g	Sugars NA

Spectrum®, Omega-3 Mayonnaise with Flax Oil, Organic

1 tbsp (14g)

Amount per serving	Amount per serving	Amount per serving
Calories 100	**Cholesterol** 10mg	**Total Carbohydrate** >1g
Total Fat 11g	**Sodium** 90mg	Dietary Fiber NA
Saturated Fat 1.5g	**Protein** 0g	Sugars NA

The Wizard's, Organic Wheat-Free Vegan Worcestershire

1 tsp

Amount per serving	Amount per serving	Amount per serving
Calories 5	**Cholesterol** 0mg	**Total Carbohydrate** 1g
Total Fat 0g	**Sodium** 130mg	Dietary Fiber 0g
Saturated Fat 0g	**Protein** 0g	Sugars 1g

Wan Ja Shan, Organic Gluten Free Ponzu Sauce (Citrus Seasoned Soy Sauce), 10 oz

1 tbsp (15 ml)

Amount per serving	Amount per serving	Amount per serving
Calories 12.5	**Cholesterol** 0mg	**Total Carbohydrate** 2.3g
Total Fat 0g	**Sodium** 524mg	Dietary Fiber 0g
Saturated Fat 0g	**Protein** 0.9g	Sugars 1.5g

Wan Ja Shan, Organic Gluten Free Shiitake Stir Fry Sauce, 10 oz

1 tbsp (15 ml)

Amount per serving	Amount per serving	Amount per serving
Calories 15	**Cholesterol** 0mg	**Total Carbohydrate** 3g
Total Fat 0g	**Sodium** 337mg	Dietary Fiber 0g
Saturated Fat 0g	**Protein** 1g	Sugars 3g

Wan Ja Shan, Organic Gluten Free Tamari Soy Sauce, 10 oz

1 tbsp (15 ml)

Amount per serving	Amount per serving	Amount per serving
Calories 11	**Cholesterol** 0mg	**Total Carbohydrate** 1g
Total Fat 0g	**Sodium** 910mg	Dietary Fiber 0g
Saturated Fat 0g	**Protein** 1g	Sugars 1g

Wan Ja Shan, Organic Gluten Free Tamari Soy Sauce, Less Sodium, 10 oz

1 tbsp (15 ml)

Amount per serving	Amount per serving	Amount per serving
Calories 9	**Cholesterol** 0mg	**Total Carbohydrate** 1g
Total Fat 0g	**Sodium** 680mg	Dietary Fiber 0g
Saturated Fat 0g	**Protein** 1g	Sugars 1g

Wan Ja Shan, Organic Gluten Free Worchestershire Sauce, 10 oz

1 tbsp (15 ml)

Amount per serving	Amount per serving	Amount per serving
Calories 4	**Cholesterol** 0mg	**Total Carbohydrate** 1g
Total Fat 0g	**Sodium** 150mg	Dietary Fiber 0g
Saturated Fat 0g	**Protein** 0g	Sugars 1g

Wan Ja Shan, Organic Soy Sauce, 10 oz

1 tbsp (15 ml)

Amount per serving	Amount per serving	Amount per serving
Calories 11	**Cholesterol** 0mg	**Total Carbohydrate** 1g
Total Fat 0g	**Sodium** 910mg	Dietary Fiber 0g
Saturated Fat 0g	**Protein** 1g	Sugars 1g

Wan Ja Shan, Organic Soy Sauce, Less Sodium, 10 oz

1 tbsp (15 ml)

Amount per serving	Amount per serving	Amount per serving
Calories 9	**Cholesterol** 0mg	**Total Carbohydrate** 1g
Total Fat 0g	**Sodium** 680mg	Dietary Fiber 0g
Saturated Fat 0g	**Protein** 1g	Sugars 1g

Wan Ja Shan, Organic Tamari Soy Sauce, 10 oz

1 tbsp (15 ml)

Amount per serving	Amount per serving	Amount per serving
Calories 11	**Cholesterol** 0mg	**Total Carbohydrate** 1g
Total Fat 0g	**Sodium** 910mg	Dietary Fiber 0g
Saturated Fat 0g	**Protein** 1g	Sugars 1g

Wan Ja Shan, Organic Teriyaki Sauce, 10 oz

1 tbsp (15 ml)

Amount per serving	Amount per serving	Amount per serving
Calories 11	**Cholesterol** 0mg	**Total Carbohydrate** 2g
Total Fat 0g	**Sodium** 735mg	Dietary Fiber 0g
Saturated Fat 0g	**Protein** 1g	Sugars 1g

Entrées

Alexia All Natural, Organic Hashed Browns

2/3 cup/84g

Amount per serving	Amount per serving	Amount per serving
Calories 60	**Cholesterol** 0mg	**Total Carbohydrate** 13g
Total Fat 0g	**Sodium** 310mg	Dietary Fiber 2g
Saturated Fat 0g	**Protein** 2g	Sugars <1g

Alexia All Natural, Organic Oven Crinkles with Sea Salt

84g/about 13 pieces

Amount per serving	Amount per serving	Amount per serving
Calories 120	**Cholesterol** 0mg	**Total Carbohydrate** 19g
Total Fat 4g	**Sodium** 170mg	Dietary Fiber 3g
Saturated Fat 0g	**Protein** 2g	Sugars 0g

Alexia All Natural, Organic Oven Crinkles with Sea Salt and Pepper

84g/about 13 pieces

Amount per serving	Amount per serving	Amount per serving
Calories 120	**Cholesterol** 0mg	**Total Carbohydrate** 20g
Total Fat 4g	**Sodium** 310mg	Dietary Fiber 3g
Saturated Fat 0g	**Protein** 2g	Sugars 0g

Alexia All Natural, Organic Yukon Select Fries

84g/about 24 pieces

Amount per serving	Amount per serving	Amount per serving
Calories 35	**Cholesterol** 0mg	**Total Carbohydrate** 18g
Total Fat 4g	**Sodium** 200mg	Dietary Fiber 3g
Saturated Fat 0g	**Protein** 2g	Sugars 0g

Ancient Harvest, Gluten-Free Culinary Ancient Grains Organic Spicy Curry

54g dry/about 1 cup prepared

Amount per serving	Amount per serving	Amount per serving
Calories 210	**Cholesterol** 0mg	**Total Carbohydrate** 39g
Total Fat 3g	**Sodium** 350mg	Dietary Fiber 5g
Saturated Fat 0.5g	**Protein** 7g	Sugars 2g

Ancient Harvest, Gluten-Free Culinary Ancient Grains Organic Butter & Parmesan

54g dry/about 1 cup prepared

Amount per serving	Amount per serving	Amount per serving
Calories 210	**Cholesterol** 0mg	**Total Carbohydrate** 38g
Total Fat 3.5g	**Sodium** 470mg	Dietary Fiber 4g
Saturated Fat 1g	**Protein** 8g	Sugars 2g

Ancient Harvest, Gluten-Free Culinary Ancient Grains Organic Sea Salt & Herb

54g dry/about 1 cup prepared

Amount per serving	Amount per serving	Amount per serving
Calories 210	**Cholesterol** 0mg	**Total Carbohydrate** 38g
Total Fat 3.5g	**Sodium** 340mg	Dietary Fiber 5g
Saturated Fat 0.5g	**Protein** 7g	Sugars 2g

Ancient Harvest, Gluten-Free Culinary Ancient Grains Organic Spanish Style

54g dry/about 1 cup prepared

Amount per serving	Amount per serving	Amount per serving
Calories 200	**Cholesterol** 0mg	**Total Carbohydrate** 38g
Total Fat 3.5g	**Sodium** 390mg	Dietary Fiber 5g
Saturated Fat 0g	**Protein** 7g	Sugars 3g

Ancient Harvest, Supergrain Mac & Cheese™ Mild Cheddar with Elbows

74g dry/about 1 cup prepared

Amount per serving	Amount per serving	Amount per serving
Calories 270	**Cholesterol** 5mg	**Total Carbohydrate** 58g
Total Fat 2g	**Sodium** 430mg	Dietary Fiber 2g
Saturated Fat 1g	**Protein** 4g	Sugars 2g

Ancient Harvest, Supergrain Mac & Cheese™ Mild Cheddar with Llamas

74g dry/about 1 cup prepared

Amount per serving	Amount per serving	Amount per serving
Calories 270	**Cholesterol** 5mg	**Total Carbohydrate** 58g
Total Fat 2g	**Sodium** 430mg	Dietary Fiber 2g
Saturated Fat 1g	**Protein** 4g	Sugars 2g

Ancient Harvest, Supergrain Mac & Cheese™ Sharp Cheddar with Shells

74g dry/about 1 cup prepared

Amount per serving	Amount per serving	Amount per serving
Calories 270	**Cholesterol** 5mg	**Total Carbohydrate** 58g
Total Fat 2g	**Sodium** 430mg	Dietary Fiber 2g
Saturated Fat 0.5g	**Protein** 4g	Sugars 2g

Ancient Harvest, Supergrain Mac & Cheese™ White Cheddar with Shells

74g dry/about 1 cup prepared

Amount per serving	Amount per serving	Amount per serving
Calories 270	**Cholesterol** 5mg	**Total Carbohydrate** 59g
Total Fat 2g	**Sodium** 400mg	Dietary Fiber 2g
Saturated Fat 0.5g	**Protein** 4g	Sugars 2g

Annie Chun's, Organic Chicken & Vegetable Potstickers

7 pieces

Amount per serving	Amount per serving	Amount per serving
Calories 220	**Cholesterol** 25mg	**Total Carbohydrate** 32g
Total Fat 3.5g	**Sodium** 620mg	Dietary Fiber 2g
Saturated Fat 0.5g	**Protein** 14g	Sugars 3g

Annie Chun's, Organic Chow Mein, Asian Meal Starter

1/3 box

Amount per serving	Amount per serving	Amount per serving
Calories 220	**Cholesterol** 0mg	**Total Carbohydrate** 42g
Total Fat 1.5g	**Sodium** 570mg	Dietary Fiber 1g
Saturated Fat 0g	**Protein** 8g	Sugars 6g

Annie Chun's, Organic Peanut Sesame, Asian Meal Starter

1/3 box

Amount per serving	Amount per serving	Amount per serving
Calories 250	**Cholesterol** 0mg	**Total Carbohydrate** 41g
Total Fat 5g	**Sodium** 360mg	Dietary Fiber 2g
Saturated Fat 0g	**Protein** 9g	Sugars 5g

Annie Chun's, Organic Pork & Vegetable Potstickers

7 pieces

Amount per serving	Amount per serving	Amount per serving
Calories 260	**Cholesterol** 30mg	**Total Carbohydrate** 32g
Total Fat 10g	**Sodium** 600mg	Dietary Fiber 2g
Saturated Fat 3g	**Protein** 12g	Sugars 3g

Annie Chun's, Organic Shiitake & Vegetable Potstickers

7 pieces

Amount per serving	Amount per serving	Amount per serving
Calories 240	**Cholesterol** 0mg	**Total Carbohydrate** 44g
Total Fat 3.5g	**Sodium** 640mg	Dietary Fiber 3g
Saturated Fat 0.5g	**Protein** 8g	Sugars 4g

Annie Chun's, Organic Soy Ginger, Asian Meal Starter

1/3 box

Amount per serving	Amount per serving	Amount per serving
Calories 220	**Cholesterol** 0mg	**Total Carbohydrate** 41g
Total Fat 1.5g	**Sodium** 600mg	Dietary Fiber 1g
Saturated Fat 0g	**Protein** 8g	Sugars 5g

Annie Chun's, Organic Teriyaki, Asian Meal Starter

1/3 box

Amount per serving	Amount per serving	Amount per serving
Calories 220	**Cholesterol** 0mg	**Total Carbohydrate** 43g
Total Fat 1.5g	**Sodium** 590mg	Dietary Fiber 1g
Saturated Fat 0g	**Protein** 8g	Sugars 7g

Annie's, Organic Family Size Four Cheese Pizza

1/5 pizza (133g)

Amount per serving	Amount per serving	Amount per serving
Calories 320	**Cholesterol** 25mg	**Total Carbohydrate** 42g
Total Fat 11g	**Sodium** 720mg	Dietary Fiber 3g
Saturated Fat 5g	**Protein** 14g	Sugars 4g

Annie's, Organic Family Size Pepperoni Pizza

1/5 pizza (134g)

Amount per serving	Amount per serving	Amount per serving
Calories 340	**Cholesterol** 25mg	**Total Carbohydrate** 42g
Total Fat 12g	**Sodium** 770mg	Dietary Fiber 3g
Saturated Fat 5g	**Protein** 14g	Sugars 4g

Annie's, Organic Family Size Spinach & Mushroom Pizza

1/5 pizza (142g)

Amount per serving	Amount per serving	Amount per serving
Calories 310	**Cholesterol** 25mg	**Total Carbohydrate** 42g
Total Fat 10g	**Sodium** 620mg	Dietary Fiber 3g
Saturated Fat 5g	**Protein** 11g	Sugars 3g

Annie's, Organic Family Size Supreme Pizza

1/5 pizza (144g)

Amount per serving	Amount per serving	Amount per serving
Calories 340	**Cholesterol** 25mg	**Total Carbohydrate** 43g
Total Fat 12g	**Sodium** 760mg	Dietary Fiber 3g
Saturated Fat 5g	**Protein** 13g	Sugars 5g

Annie's, Organic Grass Fed Classic Mild Cheddar Macaroni & Cheese

2.5 oz (71g) About 1 cup prepared

Amount per serving	Amount per serving	Amount per serving
Calories 270	**Cholesterol** 15mg	**Total Carbohydrate** 46g
Total Fat 5g	**Sodium** 520mg	Dietary Fiber 3g
Saturated Fat 2.5g	**Protein** 10g	Sugars 5g

Annie's, Organic Grass Fed Shells & Real Aged Cheddar

2.5 oz (71g) About 1 cup prepared

Amount per serving	Amount per serving	Amount per serving
Calories 260	**Cholesterol** 10mg	**Total Carbohydrate** 47g
Total Fat 3.5g	**Sodium** 590mg	Dietary Fiber 3g
Saturated Fat 1.5g	**Protein** 10g	Sugars 5g

Annie's, Organic Grass Fed Shells & White Cheddar

2.5 oz (71g) About 1 cup prepared

Amount per serving	Amount per serving	Amount per serving
Calories 260	**Cholesterol** 10mg	**Total Carbohydrate** 47g
Total Fat 3.5g	**Sodium** 590mg	Dietary Fiber 3g
Saturated Fat 1.5g	**Protein** 10g	Sugars 5g

Back to Nature, Organic Macaroni & Cheese Dinner

3/4 cup

Amount per serving	Amount per serving	Amount per serving
Calories 240	**Cholesterol** 5mg	**Total Carbohydrate** 49g
Total Fat 2.5g	**Sodium** 630mg	Dietary Fiber 2g
Saturated Fat 1g	**Protein** 10g	Sugars 8g

Back to Nature, Organic Shells & Cheddar Dinner

3/4 cup

Amount per serving	Amount per serving	Amount per serving
Calories 290	**Cholesterol** 5mg	**Total Carbohydrate** 58g
Total Fat 2.5g	**Sodium** 750mg	Dietary Fiber 2g
Saturated Fat 1g	**Protein** 12g	Sugars 10g

Back to Nature, Organic Shells & White Cheddar Dinner

3/4 cup

Amount per serving	Amount per serving	Amount per serving
Calories 240	**Cholesterol** 5mg	**Total Carbohydrate** 49g
Total Fat 2.5g	**Sodium** 630mg	Dietary Fiber 2g
Saturated Fat 1g	**Protein** 10g	Sugars 8g

Blake's, Chicken Pot Pie made with Organic vegetables and a flaky organic crust

One package (227g)

Amount per serving	Amount per serving	Amount per serving
Calories 340	**Cholesterol** 30mg	**Total Carbohydrate** 34g
Total Fat 17g	**Sodium** 470mg	Dietary Fiber 5g
Saturated Fat 8g	**Protein** 15g	Sugars 1g

Blake's, Farmhouse Mac & Cheese made with Organic pasta with breadcrumb topping

8 oz (227g)

Amount per serving	Amount per serving	Amount per serving
Calories 370	**Cholesterol** 50mg	**Total Carbohydrate** 45g
Total Fat 18g	**Sodium** 480mg	Dietary Fiber 4g
Saturated Fat 5g	**Protein** 7g	Sugars 0g

Blake's, Gluten-Free Chicken Pot Pie made with Organic vegetables

One package (227g)

Amount per serving	Amount per serving	Amount per serving
Calories 310	**Cholesterol** 75mg	**Total Carbohydrate** 32g
Total Fat 13g	**Sodium** 540mg	Dietary Fiber 2g
Saturated Fat 4g	**Protein** 15g	Sugars 2g

Blake's, Harvest Vegetable Pie made with Organic vegetables

One package (227g)

Amount per serving	Amount per serving	Amount per serving
Calories 420	**Cholesterol** 0mg	**Total Carbohydrate** 46g
Total Fat 25g	**Sodium** 540mg	Dietary Fiber 7g
Saturated Fat 10g	**Protein** 8g	Sugars 2g

Blake's, Mac & Cheese with Chicken made with Organic chicken

8 oz (227g)

Amount per serving	Amount per serving	Amount per serving
Calories 360	**Cholesterol** 80mg	**Total Carbohydrate** 34g
Total Fat 17g	**Sodium** 320mg	Dietary Fiber 3g
Saturated Fat 5g	**Protein** 18g	Sugars 5g

Blake's, Mac & Cheese with Veggies made with organic vegetables

8 oz (227g)

Amount per serving	Amount per serving	Amount per serving
Calories 300	**Cholesterol** 35mg	**Total Carbohydrate** 40g
Total Fat 12g	**Sodium** 510mg	Dietary Fiber 5g
Saturated Fat 3.5g	**Protein** 7g	Sugars 1g

Blake's, Macaroni & Beef made with Organic pasta in an organic tomato sauce

1 cup (227g)

Amount per serving	Amount per serving	Amount per serving
Calories 220	**Cholesterol** 30mg	**Total Carbohydrate** 22g
Total Fat 8g	**Sodium** 620mg	Dietary Fiber 2g
Saturated Fat 2g	**Protein** 15g	Sugars 5g

Blake's, Shepherd's Pie made with Organic corn and organic mashed potatoes

One package (227g)

Amount per serving	Amount per serving	Amount per serving
Calories 240	**Cholesterol** 30mg	**Total Carbohydrate** 26g
Total Fat 9g	**Sodium** 520mg	Dietary Fiber 2g
Saturated Fat 3g	**Protein** 14g	Sugars 2g

Blake's, Upside Down Chicken & Waffle Pie made with Organic sweet mashed potatoes

One package (227g)

Amount per serving	Amount per serving	Amount per serving
Calories 280	**Cholesterol** 30mg	**Total Carbohydrate** 35g
Total Fat 10g	**Sodium** 300mg	Dietary Fiber 4g
Saturated Fat 2.5g	**Protein** 14g	Sugars 9g

Blake's, White Meat Chicken Pie made with Organic chicken

One package (227g)

Amount per serving	Amount per serving	Amount per serving
Calories 290	**Cholesterol** 45mg	**Total Carbohydrate** 25g
Total Fat 13g	**Sodium** 650mg	Dietary Fiber 3g
Saturated Fat 6g	**Protein** 18g	Sugars NA

Bold Organic, Deluxe

1/2 pizza

Amount per serving	Amount per serving	Amount per serving
Calories 460	**Cholesterol** 10mg	**Total Carbohydrate** 56g
Total Fat 24g	**Sodium** 790mg	Dietary Fiber 5g
Saturated Fat 4.5g	**Protein** 8g	Sugars 12g

Bold Organic, Meat Lovers Pizza

1/2 pizza

Amount per serving	Amount per serving	Amount per serving
Calories 450	**Cholesterol** 10mg	**Total Carbohydrate** 54g
Total Fat 24g	**Sodium** 790mg	Dietary Fiber 5g
Saturated Fat 4.5g	**Protein** 7g	Sugars 11g

Bold Organic, Vegan Cheese Pizza

1/2 pizza

Amount per serving	Amount per serving	Amount per serving
Calories 380	**Cholesterol** 0mg	**Total Carbohydrate** 54g
Total Fat 18g	**Sodium** 580mg	Dietary Fiber 5g
Saturated Fat 2.5g	**Protein** 4g	Sugars 11g

Bold Organic, Veggie Lovers Pizza

1/2 pizza

Amount per serving	Amount per serving	Amount per serving
Calories 390	**Cholesterol** 10mg	**Total Carbohydrate** 55g
Total Fat 18g	**Sodium** 580mg	Dietary Fiber 5g
Saturated Fat 2.5g	**Protein** 5g	Sugars 12g

Dr. McDougall's Right Foods, Hot & Sour with Organic Noodles Big Cup

27g

Amount per serving	Amount per serving	Amount per serving
Calories 100	**Cholesterol** 0mg	**Total Carbohydrate** 19g
Total Fat 0.5g	**Sodium** 320mg	Dietary Fiber 2g
Saturated Fat 0g	**Protein** 4g	Sugars 1g

Dr. McDougall's Right Foods, Miso Soup with Organic Noodles Big Cup

27g

Amount per serving	Amount per serving	Amount per serving
Calories 100	**Cholesterol** 0mg	**Total Carbohydrate** 18g
Total Fat 0.5g	**Sodium** 390mg	Dietary Fiber 1g
Saturated Fat 0g	**Protein** 5g	Sugars 1g

Dr. McDougall's Right Foods, Pistachio Citrus Quinoa Salad

66g

Amount per serving	Amount per serving	Amount per serving
Calories 240	**Cholesterol** 0mg	**Total Carbohydrate** 42g
Total Fat 4g	**Sodium** 360mg	Dietary Fiber 4g
Saturated Fat 0g	**Protein** 9g	Sugars 3g

Dr. McDougall's Right Foods, Ramen Soup Vegan Chicken Made with Organic Ramen

26g

Amount per serving	Amount per serving	Amount per serving
Calories 100	**Cholesterol** 0mg	**Total Carbohydrate** 20g
Total Fat 0.5g	**Sodium** 340mg	Dietary Fiber 1g
Saturated Fat 0g	**Protein** 4g	Sugars 0.5g

Dr. McDougall's Right Foods, Tomato Pine Nut Quinoa

68g

Amount per serving	Amount per serving	Amount per serving
Calories 260	**Cholesterol** 0mg	**Total Carbohydrate** 44g
Total Fat 5g	**Sodium** 480mg	Dietary Fiber 4g
Saturated Fat 0g	**Protein** 10g	Sugars 4g

Earthbound Farm Organic, Frozen Roasted Organic Red Potatoes

2/3 cup (110g)

Amount per serving	Amount per serving	Amount per serving
Calories 100	**Cholesterol** 0mg	**Total Carbohydrate** 23g
Total Fat 0g	**Sodium** 10mg	Dietary Fiber 2g
Saturated Fat 0g	**Protein** 3g	Sugars 1g

Earthbound Farm Organic, Frozen Roasted Organic Sweet Potato Slices

2/3 cup (110g)

Amount per serving	Amount per serving	Amount per serving
Calories 140	**Cholesterol** 0mg	**Total Carbohydrate** 32g
Total Fat 1g	**Sodium** 170mg	Dietary Fiber 4g
Saturated Fat 0g	**Protein** 2g	Sugars 23g

Earthbound Farm Organic, Frozen Roasted Organic Yukon Gold Wedges

2/3 cup (110g)

Amount per serving	Amount per serving	Amount per serving
Calories 110	**Cholesterol** 0mg	**Total Carbohydrate** 23g
Total Fat 1.5g	**Sodium** 1mg	Dietary Fiber 3g
Saturated Fat 0g	**Protein** 3g	Sugars 1g

Eden Foods, Brown Rice & Chick Peas, Organic

1/2 cup

Amount per serving	Amount per serving	Amount per serving
Calories 110	**Cholesterol** NA	**Total Carbohydrate** 23g
Total Fat 1g	**Sodium** 135mg	Dietary Fiber 2g
Saturated Fat 0g	**Protein** 3g	Sugars 0g

Eden Foods, Cajun Rice & Small Red Beans, Organic

1/2 cup

Amount per serving	Amount per serving	Amount per serving
Calories 110	**Cholesterol** NA	**Total Carbohydrate** 23g
Total Fat 1g	**Sodium** 115mg	Dietary Fiber 3g
Saturated Fat 0g	**Protein** 3g	Sugars <1g

Eden Foods, Caribbean Rice & Black Beans, Organic

1/2 cup

Amount per serving	Amount per serving	Amount per serving
Calories 120	**Cholesterol** NA	**Total Carbohydrate** 23g
Total Fat 1g	**Sodium** 100mg	Dietary Fiber 4g
Saturated Fat 0g	**Protein** 4g	Sugars <1g

Eden Foods, Curried Rice & Lentils, Organic

1/2 cup

Amount per serving	Amount per serving	Amount per serving
Calories 130	**Cholesterol** NA	**Total Carbohydrate** 21g
Total Fat 1g	**Sodium** 200mg	Dietary Fiber 1g
Saturated Fat 0g	**Protein** 4g	Sugars <1g

Eden Foods, Genmai (Brown Rice) Miso, Organic

1 tbsp

Amount per serving	Amount per serving	Amount per serving
Calories 25	**Cholesterol** 0mg	**Total Carbohydrate** 3g
Total Fat 0.5g	**Sodium** 780mg	Dietary Fiber 2g
Saturated Fat 0g	**Protein** 2g	Sugars 1g

Eden Foods, Mexican Rice & Black Beans, Organic

1/2 cup

Amount per serving	Amount per serving	Amount per serving
Calories 110	**Cholesterol** NA	**Total Carbohydrate** 22g
Total Fat 1g	**Sodium** 270mg	Dietary Fiber 3g
Saturated Fat 0g	**Protein** 5g	Sugars 1g

Eden Foods, Moroccan Rice & Garbanzo Beans, Organic

1/2 cup

Amount per serving	Amount per serving	Amount per serving
Calories 110	**Cholesterol** NA	**Total Carbohydrate** 22g
Total Fat 1g	**Sodium** 230mg	Dietary Fiber 3g
Saturated Fat 0g	**Protein** 4g	Sugars <1g

Eden Foods, Spanish Rice & Pinto Beans, Organic

1/2 cup

Amount per serving	Amount per serving	Amount per serving
Calories 120	**Cholesterol** NA	**Total Carbohydrate** 22g
Total Fat 1g	**Sodium** 260mg	Dietary Fiber 3g
Saturated Fat 0g	**Protein** 4g	Sugars <1g

Edward & Sons, Miso-Cup, Organic Traditional with Tofu

1 cup

Amount per serving	Amount per serving	Amount per serving
Calories 35	**Cholesterol** 0mg	**Total Carbohydrate** 4g
Total Fat 1g	**Sodium** 480mg	Dietary Fiber <1g
Saturated Fat 0g	**Protein** 2g	Sugars <1g

Edward & Sons, Organic Home Style Mashed Potatoes

1/2 cup / prepared

Amount per serving	Amount per serving	Amount per serving
Calories 150	**Cholesterol** 0mg	**Total Carbohydrate** 20g
Total Fat 0g	**Sodium** 190mg	Dietary Fiber 2g
Saturated Fat 0g	**Protein** 2g	Sugars 1g

Edward & Sons, Organic Roasted Garlic Mashed Potatoes

1/2 cup / prepared

Amount per serving	Amount per serving	Amount per serving
Calories 150	**Cholesterol** 0mg	**Total Carbohydrate** 20g
Total Fat 0g	**Sodium** 190mg	Dietary Fiber 2g
Saturated Fat 0g	**Protein** 2g	Sugars 1g

Edward & Sons, Road's End Organics, Organic GF Alfredo Mac & Cheese

1 cup / prepared

Amount per serving	Amount per serving	Amount per serving
Calories 330	**Cholesterol** 0mg	**Total Carbohydrate** 63g
Total Fat 2.5g	**Sodium** 310mg	Dietary Fiber 5g
Saturated Fat 0g	**Protein** 8g	Sugars <1g

Edward & Sons, Road's End Organics, Organic GF Cheddar Penne & Cheese

3/4 cup

Amount per serving	Amount per serving	Amount per serving
Calories 330	**Cholesterol** 0mg	**Total Carbohydrate** 63g
Total Fat 2.5g	**Sodium** 340mg	Dietary Fiber 5g
Saturated Fat 0g	**Protein** 8g	Sugars 1g

Horizon®, Macaroni & Mild Cheddar Cheese

2.5 oz (71g) About 1 cup prepared

Amount per serving	Amount per serving	Amount per serving
Calories 270	**Cholesterol** 10mg	**Total Carbohydrate** 47g
Total Fat 4.5g	**Sodium** 600mg	Dietary Fiber 1g
Saturated Fat 2.5g	**Protein** 10g	Sugars 4g

Horizon®, Pasta Shells & White Cheddar Cheese

2.5 oz (71g) About 1 cup prepared

Amount per serving	Amount per serving	Amount per serving
Calories 270	**Cholesterol** 10mg	**Total Carbohydrate** 47g
Total Fat 4.5g	**Sodium** 600mg	Dietary Fiber 1g
Saturated Fat 2.5g	**Protein** 10g	Sugars 3g

KOYO, Asian Vegetable Ramen, 2 oz

1 package (60g)

Amount per serving	Amount per serving	Amount per serving
Calories 210	**Cholesterol** 0mg	**Total Carbohydrate** 43g
Total Fat 1g	**Sodium** 910mg	Dietary Fiber 2g
Saturated Fat 0.5g	**Protein** 8g	Sugars 5g

KOYO, Garlic Pepper Ramen, 2 oz

1 package (60g)

Amount per serving	Amount per serving	Amount per serving
Calories 210	**Cholesterol** 0mg	**Total Carbohydrate** 42g
Total Fat 1g	**Sodium** 880mg	Dietary Fiber 2g
Saturated Fat 0.5g	**Protein** 8g	Sugars 5g

KOYO, Lemongrass Ginger Ramen, 2 oz

1 package (60g)

Amount per serving	Amount per serving	Amount per serving
Calories 210	**Cholesterol** 0mg	**Total Carbohydrate** 43g
Total Fat 1g	**Sodium** 620mg	Dietary Fiber 2g
Saturated Fat 0.5g	**Protein** 8g	Sugars 4g

KOYO, Mushroom Ramen, 2 oz

1 package (57g)

Amount per serving	Amount per serving	Amount per serving
Calories 200	**Cholesterol** 0mg	**Total Carbohydrate** 41g
Total Fat 1g	**Sodium** 810mg	Dietary Fiber 2g
Saturated Fat 0.5g	**Protein** 7g	Sugars 4g

KOYO, Seaweed Ramen, 2 oz

1 package (57g)

Amount per serving	Amount per serving	Amount per serving
Calories 200	**Cholesterol** 0mg	**Total Carbohydrate** 41g
Total Fat 1g	**Sodium** 760mg	Dietary Fiber 2g
Saturated Fat 0.5g	**Protein** 7g	Sugars 4g

KOYO, Soba Ramen, 2 oz

1 package (60g)

Amount per serving	Amount per serving	Amount per serving
Calories 210	**Cholesterol** 0mg	**Total Carbohydrate** 44g
Total Fat 1g	**Sodium** 840mg	Dietary Fiber 2g
Saturated Fat 0.5g	**Protein** 7g	Sugars 6g

KOYO, Tofu Miso Ramens, 2 oz

1 package (57g)

Amount per serving	Amount per serving	Amount per serving
Calories 200	**Cholesterol** 0mg	**Total Carbohydrate** 40g
Total Fat 1g	**Sodium** 840mg	Dietary Fiber 2g
Saturated Fat 0.5g	**Protein** 7g	Sugars 4g

Lundberg Family Farms, Organic Alfredo Risotto

54g/about 1/4 cup rice and 2 tsp seasoning mix (1 cup prepared)

Amount per serving	Amount per serving	Amount per serving
Calories 190	**Cholesterol** 0mg	**Total Carbohydrate** 39g
Total Fat 1.5g	**Sodium** 490mg	Dietary Fiber 1g
Saturated Fat 0.5g	**Protein** 6g	Sugars 1g

Lundberg Family Farms, Organic Brown Rice Pasta & Sauce Mix—Garlic & Olive Oil

1 cup as prepared (64g dry)

Amount per serving	Amount per serving	Amount per serving
Calories 220	**Cholesterol** 0mg	**Total Carbohydrate** 46g
Total Fat 3.5g	**Sodium** 440mg	Dietary Fiber 4g
Saturated Fat 0.5g	**Protein** 5g	Sugars 2g

Lundberg Family Farms, Organic Brown Rice Pasta & Sauce Mix—Leek & Mushroom

1 cup as prepared (64g dry)

Amount per serving	Amount per serving	Amount per serving
Calories 220	**Cholesterol** 0mg	**Total Carbohydrate** 47g
Total Fat 3.5g	**Sodium** 530mg	Dietary Fiber 4g
Saturated Fat 0.5g	**Protein** 5g	Sugars 2g

Lundberg Family Farms, Organic Brown Rice Pasta & Sauce Mix—Roasted Red Pepper

1 cup as prepared (65g dry)

Amount per serving	Amount per serving	Amount per serving
Calories 220	**Cholesterol** 0mg	**Total Carbohydrate** 47g
Total Fat 3.5g	**Sodium** 440mg	Dietary Fiber 4g
Saturated Fat 0.5g	**Protein** 5g	Sugars 3g

Lundberg Family Farms, Organic Brown Rice Pasta & Sauce Mix—Spinach & Rosemary

1 cup as prepared (64g dry)

Amount per serving	Amount per serving	Amount per serving
Calories 220	**Cholesterol** 0mg	**Total Carbohydrate** 46g
Total Fat 3.5g	**Sodium** 470mg	Dietary Fiber 4g
Saturated Fat 0.5g	**Protein** 5g	Sugars 3g

Lundberg Family Farms, Organic Crabby Rice—Chesapeake Bay Style Seasoning

2 oz (57g/about 1/4 cup rice blend and 1 tbsp seasoning mix) (1 cup prepared)

Amount per serving	Amount per serving	Amount per serving
Calories 200	**Cholesterol** 0mg	**Total Carbohydrate** 45g
Total Fat 0.5g	**Sodium** 470mg	Dietary Fiber 1g
Saturated Fat 0g	**Protein** 4g	Sugars 1g

Lundberg Family Farms, Organic Florentine Risotto, Cooked

56g (about 1/4 cup rice and 2 1/2 tsp seasoning mix) (1 cup prepared)

Amount per serving	Amount per serving	Amount per serving
Calories 200	**Cholesterol** 0mg	**Total Carbohydrate** 42g
Total Fat 1g	**Sodium** 610mg	Dietary Fiber 1g
Saturated Fat 0g	**Protein** 6g	Sugars 2g

Lundberg Family Farms, Organic Porcini Mushroom Risotto, Cooked

58g (about 1/4 cup rice and 2 tsp seasoning mix) (1 cup prepared)

Amount per serving	Amount per serving	Amount per serving
Calories 200	**Cholesterol** 0mg	**Total Carbohydrate** 43g
Total Fat 1g	**Sodium** 660mg	Dietary Fiber 1g
Saturated Fat 0g	**Protein** 5g	Sugars 2g

Lundberg Family Farms, Organic Rice & Durum Wheat Pasta Pilaf—Original

2 oz (56g/about 1/3 cup rice blend and 1 1/2 tsp seasoning mix) (1 cup prepared)

Amount per serving	Amount per serving	Amount per serving
Calories 210	**Cholesterol** 0mg	**Total Carbohydrate** 45g
Total Fat 2g	**Sodium** 470mg	Dietary Fiber 3g
Saturated Fat 0g	**Protein** 4g	Sugars 1g

Lundberg Family Farms, Organic Whole Grain Brown Rice Pilaf, Original

2 oz (57g/about 1/4 cup rice blend and 1 tbsp seasoning and orzo mix) (1 cup prepared)

Amount per serving	Amount per serving	Amount por serving
Calories 210	**Cholesterol** 0mg	**Total Carbohydrate** 44g
Total Fat 1.5g	**Sodium** 470mg	Dietary Fiber 2g
Saturated Fat 0g	**Protein** 5g	Sugars 1g

Lundberg Family Farms, Organic Whole Grain Brown Rice Pilaf, Toasted Almond

2 oz (57g/about 1/4 cup rice, 1 tsp seasoning mix and 1 tsp almonds) (1 cup prepared)

Amount per serving	Amount per serving	Amount per serving
Calories 220	**Cholesterol** 0mg	**Total Carbohydrate** 42g
Total Fat 3.5g	**Sodium** 470mg	Dietary Fiber 3g
Saturated Fat 0.5g	**Protein** 5g	Sugars 1g

Lundberg Family Farms, Organic Whole Grain Jambalaya

2 oz (56g/about 1/3 cup rice blend and 2 tsp seasoning mix) (1 cup prepared)

Amount per serving	Amount per serving	Amount per serving
Calories 220	**Cholesterol** 0mg	**Total Carbohydrate** 46g
Total Fat 2g	**Sodium** 470mg	Dietary Fiber 3g
Saturated Fat 0g	**Protein** 4g	Sugars 2g

Lundberg Family Farms, Organic Whole Grain Rice & Black Beans

2 oz (56g/about 1/4 cup rice and 1 1/3 tbsp seasoning mix) (1 cup prepared)

Amount per serving	Amount per serving	Amount per serving
Calories 210	**Cholesterol** 0mg	**Total Carbohydrate** 44g
Total Fat 2g	**Sodium** 480mg	Dietary Fiber 5g
Saturated Fat 0g	**Protein** 6g	Sugars 2g

Lundberg Family Farms, Organic Whole Grain Rice & Lentils—Mild Curry

2 oz (56g/about 1/4 cup rice blend and 1 1/2 tsp seasoning mix) (1 cup prepared)

Amount per serving	Amount per serving	Amount per serving
Calories 210	**Cholesterol** 0mg	**Total Carbohydrate** 43g
Total Fat 2g	**Sodium** 460mg	Dietary Fiber 3g
Saturated Fat 0g	**Protein** 6g	Sugars 0g

Lundberg Family Farms, Organic Whole Grain Rice & Lentils—Original

2 oz (56g/about 1/4 cup rice blend and 1 1/2 tsp seasoning mix) (1 cup prepared)

Amount per serving	Amount per serving	Amount per serving
Calories 210	**Cholesterol** 0mg	**Total Carbohydrate** 43g
Total Fat 1.5g	**Sodium** 470mg	Dietary Fiber 3g
Saturated Fat 0g	**Protein** 6g	Sugars 1g

Lundberg Family Farms, Organic Whole Grain Rice & Quinoa—Basil & Bell Pepper

2 oz (57g/about 1/4 cup rice and 1 tbsp quinoa and seasoning mix) (1 cup prepared)

Amount per serving	Amount per serving	Amount per serving
Calories 210	**Cholesterol** 0mg	**Total Carbohydrate** 43g
Total Fat 2g	**Sodium** 480mg	Dietary Fiber 3g
Saturated Fat 0g	**Protein** 5g	Sugars 1g

Lundberg Family Farms, Organic Whole Grain Rice & Quinoa—Peruvian Style

2 oz (57g/about 1/4 cup rice and 1 tbsp quinoa and seasoning mix) (1 cup prepared)

Amount per serving	Amount per serving	Amount per serving
Calories 210	**Cholesterol** 0mg	**Total Carbohydrate** 43g
Total Fat 2g	**Sodium** 470mg	Dietary Fiber 3g
Saturated Fat 0g	**Protein** 5g	Sugars 1g

Lundberg Family Farms, Organic Whole Grain Rice & Quinoa—Rosemary Blend

2 oz (57g/about 1/4 cup rice and 1 tbsp quinoa and seasoning mix) (1 cup prepared)

Amount per serving	Amount per serving	Amount per serving
Calories 210	**Cholesterol** 0mg	**Total Carbohydrate** 43g
Total Fat 2g	**Sodium** 470mg	Dietary Fiber 3g
Saturated Fat 0g	**Protein** 5g	Sugars 1g

Lundberg Family Farms, Organic Whole Grain Rice & Red Beans

2 oz (56g/about 1/4 cup rice and 1 1/3 tbsp seasoning mix) (1 cup prepared)

Amount per serving	Amount per serving	Amount per serving
Calories 210	**Cholesterol** 0mg	**Total Carbohydrate** 44g
Total Fat 2g	**Sodium** 470mg	Dietary Fiber 4g
Saturated Fat 0g	**Protein** 6g	Sugars 2g

Lundberg Family Farms, Whole Grain Rice & Quinoa—Spanish Style

2 oz (57g/about 1/4 cup rice and 1 tbsp quinoa and seasoning mix) (1 cup prepared)

Amount per serving	Amount per serving	Amount per serving
Calories 210	**Cholesterol** 0mg	**Total Carbohydrate** 43g
Total Fat 2g	**Sodium** 460mg	Dietary Fiber 3g
Saturated Fat 0g	**Protein** 5g	Sugars 2g

Lundberg Family Farms, Whole Grain Spanish Rice

2 oz (56g/about 1/3 cup rice blend and 2 tsp seasoning mix) (1 cup prepared)

Amount per serving	Amount per serving	Amount per serving
Calories 220	**Cholesterol** 0mg	**Total Carbohydrate** 46g
Total Fat 2g	**Sodium** 460mg	Dietary Fiber 3g
Saturated Fat 0g	**Protein** 5g	Sugars 2g

Lundberg Family Farms, Whole Grain Yellow Rice

2 oz (56g/about 1/3 cup rice blend and 1 1/2 tsp seasoning mix) (1 cup prepared)

Amount per serving	Amount per serving	Amount per serving
Calories 210	**Cholesterol** 0mg	**Total Carbohydrate** 45g
Total Fat 2g	**Sodium** 470mg	Dietary Fiber 3g
Saturated Fat 0g	**Protein** 4g	Sugars 1g

PJ's Organics, Breakfast Burritos, Denver-Style Breakfast

1 burrito

Amount per serving	Amount per serving	Amount per serving
Calories 340	**Cholesterol** 30mg	**Total Carbohydrate** 41g
Total Fat 13g	**Sodium** 530mg	Dietary Fiber 2g
Saturated Fat 4.5g	**Protein** 14g	Sugars 1g

PJ's Organics, Breakfast Burritos, Skinny Breakfast

1 burrito

Amount per serving	Amount per serving	Amount per serving
Calories 300	**Cholesterol** 5mg	**Total Carbohydrate** 41g
Total Fat 8g	**Sodium** 570mg	Dietary Fiber 2g
Saturated Fat 1g	**Protein** 15g	Sugars 2g

PJ's Organics, Breakfast Burritos, Surf's Up Breakfast

1 burrito

Amount per serving	Amount per serving	Amount per serving
Calories 330	**Cholesterol** 130mg	**Total Carbohydrate** 42g
Total Fat 12g	**Sodium** 560mg	Dietary Fiber 3g
Saturated Fat 2.5g	**Protein** 14g	Sugars 1g

PJ's Organics, Breakfast Burritos, Turkey & Eggs Breakfast

1 burrito

Amount per serving	Amount per serving	Amount per serving
Calories 340	**Cholesterol** 35mg	**Total Carbohydrate** 45g
Total Fat 12g	**Sodium** 600mg	Dietary Fiber 2g
Saturated Fat 2.5g	**Protein** 13g	Sugars 1g

PJ's Organics, Classic Burritos, Chicken & Cheese with Green Chiles

1 burrito

Amount per serving	Amount per serving	Amount per serving
Calories 320	**Cholesterol** 20mg	**Total Carbohydrate** 47g
Total Fat 9g	**Sodium** 540mg	Dietary Fiber 4g
Saturated Fat 2g	**Protein** 13g	Sugars 1g

PJ's Organics, Classic Burritos, Skinny Chicken

1 burrito

Amount per serving	Amount per serving	Amount per serving
Calories 290	**Cholesterol** 15mg	**Total Carbohydrate** 53g
Total Fat 2.5g	**Sodium** 510mg	Dietary Fiber 4g
Saturated Fat 0.5g	**Protein** 14g	Sugars 1g

PJ's Organics, Classic Burritos, Southwestern-Style Chicken

1 burrito

Amount per serving	Amount per serving	Amount per serving
Calories 340	**Cholesterol** 30mg	**Total Carbohydrate** 47g
Total Fat 9g	**Sodium** 700mg	Dietary Fiber 3g
Saturated Fat 3g	**Protein** 17g	Sugars 1g

PJ's Organics, Classic Burritos, Steak & Cheese

1 burrito

Amount per serving	Amount per serving	Amount per serving
Calories 340	**Cholesterol** 20mg	**Total Carbohydrate** 51g
Total Fat 9g	**Sodium** 600mg	Dietary Fiber 4g
Saturated Fat 2g	**Protein** 14g	Sugars 1g

PJ's Organics, Classic Burritos, Traditional Chicken

1 burrito

Amount per serving	Amount per serving	Amount per serving
Calories 340	**Cholesterol** 25mg	**Total Carbohydrate** 50g
Total Fat 8g	**Sodium** 570mg	Dietary Fiber 4g
Saturated Fat 2g	**Protein** 17g	Sugars 1g

Seeds of Change, Ready-To-Heat, Brown Basmati Rice

1 cup (137g)

Amount per serving	Amount per serving	Amount per serving
Calories 220	**Cholesterol** 0mg	**Total Carbohydrate** 43g
Total Fat 3.5g	**Sodium** 10mg	Dietary Fiber 2g
Saturated Fat 0.5g	**Protein** 5g	Sugars 0g

Seeds of Change, Ready-To-Heat, Caribbean Style Rice

1 cup (152g)

Amount per serving	Amount per serving	Amount per serving
Calories 250	**Cholesterol** 0mg	**Total Carbohydrate** 50g
Total Fat 3g	**Sodium** 360mg	Dietary Fiber 5g
Saturated Fat 0g	**Protein** 6g	Sugars 1g

Seeds of Change, Ready-To-Heat, Indian Rice Blend

1 cup (143g)

Amount per serving	Amount per serving	Amount per serving
Calories 230	**Cholesterol** 0mg	**Total Carbohydrate** 41g
Total Fat 3.5g	**Sodium** 480mg	Dietary Fiber 4g
Saturated Fat 0g	**Protein** 8g	Sugars 1g

Seeds of Change, Ready-To-Heat, Quinoa & Brown Rice

1 cup (142g)

Amount per serving	Amount per serving	Amount per serving
Calories 240	**Cholesterol** 0mg	**Total Carbohydrate** 47g
Total Fat 3.5g	**Sodium** 400mg	Dietary Fiber 3g
Saturated Fat 0.5g	**Protein** 6g	Sugars 1g

Seeds of Change, Ready-To-Heat, Seven Whole Grains

1 cup (145g)

Amount per serving	Amount per serving	Amount per serving
Calories 240	Cholesterol 0mg	Total Carbohydrate 47g
Total Fat 3g	Sodium 340mg	Dietary Fiber 4g
Saturated Fat 0g	Protein 6g	Sugars 1g

Seeds of Change, Ready-To-Heat, Spanish Style Rice

1 cup (150g)

Amount per serving	Amount per serving	Amount per serving
Calories 260	Cholesterol 0mg	Total Carbohydrate 52g
Total Fat 4g	Sodium 480mg	Dietary Fiber 3g
Saturated Fat 0.5g	Protein 5g	Sugars 1g

Seeds of Change, Rice and Grain Blends, Brown Rice Blend

1/4 cup dry grains and 1 tbsp seasoning mix (50g) (About 1 cup cooked)

Amount per serving	Amount per serving	Amount per serving
Calories 180	Cholesterol 0mg	Total Carbohydrate 36g
Total Fat 1.5g	Sodium 450mg	Dietary Fiber 2g
Saturated Fat 0g	Protein 5g	Sugars 3g

Seeds of Change, Rice and Grain Blends, Cuban Style Rice

1/3 cup dry rice/bean blend and 1 tbsp seasoning mix (58g) (About 1 cup cooked)

Amount per serving	Amount per serving	Amount per serving
Calories 210	Cholesterol 0mg	Total Carbohydrate 42g
Total Fat 2g	Sodium 350mg	Dietary Fiber 3g
Saturated Fat 0g	Protein 6g	Sugars 2g

Seeds of Change, Rice and Grain Blends, Mediterranean Style Rice

1/4 cup dry rice/pea blend and 1 tsp seasoning mix (47g) (About 1 cup cooked)

Amount per serving	Amount per serving	Amount per serving
Calories 170	Cholesterol 0mg	Total Carbohydrate 34g
Total Fat 1.5g	Sodium 420mg	Dietary Fiber 2g
Saturated Fat 0g	Protein 4g	Sugars 1g

Seeds of Change, Rice and Grain Blends, Moroccan Style Rice

1/4 cup dry grains and 1/2 tsp seasoning mix (51g) (About 1 cup cooked)

Amount per serving	Amount per serving	Amount per serving
Calories 180	Cholesterol 0mg	Total Carbohydrate 38g
Total Fat 1.5g	Sodium 240mg	Dietary Fiber 2g
Saturated Fat 0g	Protein 4g	Sugars 1g

Seeds of Change, Rice and Grain Blends, Quinoa & Brown Rice

1 cup (142g)

Amount per serving	Amount per serving	Amount per serving
Calories 240	**Cholesterol** 0mg	**Total Carbohydrate** 47g
Total Fat 3.5g	**Sodium** 460mg	Dietary Fiber 3g
Saturated Fat 0.5g	**Protein** 6g	Sugars 1g

Seeds of Change, Rice and Grain Blends, Seven Whole Grains

1 cup (145g)

Amount per serving	Amount per serving	Amount per serving
Calories 240	**Cholesterol** 0mg	**Total Carbohydrate** 47g
Total Fat 3g	**Sodium** 340mg	Dietary Fiber 4g
Saturated Fat 0g	**Protein** 6g	Sugars 1g

Gravies

Imagine®, Natural Creations, Organic Roasted Turkey Flavored Gravy

1/4 cup (60 ml)

Amount per serving	Amount per serving	Amount per serving
Calories 20	**Cholesterol** 0mg	**Total Carbohydrate** 4g
Total Fat 0.5g	**Sodium** 210mg	Dietary Fiber 0g
Saturated Fat 0g	**Protein** 0g	Sugars 0g

Imagine®, Natural Creations, Organic Savory Beef Flavored Gravy

1/4 cup (60 ml)

Amount per serving	Amount per serving	Amount per serving
Calories 20	**Cholesterol** 0mg	**Total Carbohydrate** 4g
Total Fat 0g	**Sodium** 240mg	Dietary Fiber 0g
Saturated Fat 0g	**Protein** 0g	Sugars 0g

Imagine®, Natural Creations, Organic Vegetarian Wild Mushroom Gravy

1/4 cup (60 ml)

Amount per serving	Amount per serving	Amount per serving
Calories 15	**Cholesterol** 0mg	**Total Carbohydrate** 4g
Total Fat 0g	**Sodium** 170mg	Dietary Fiber 0g
Saturated Fat 0g	**Protein** 0g	Sugars 0g

Road's End Organics, Organic Savory Herb Gravy Mix, Dry

1 tbsp

Amount per serving	Amount per serving	Amount per serving
Calories 25	**Cholesterol** 0mg	**Total Carbohydrate** 5g
Total Fat 0g	**Sodium** 210mg	Dietary Fiber 0g
Saturated Fat 0g	**Protein** <1g	Sugars 0g

Road's End Organics, Organic Shiitake Gravy Mix, Dry

1 tbsp

Amount per serving	Amount per serving	Amount per serving
Calories 25	Cholesterol 0mg	Total Carbohydrate 5g
Total Fat 0g	Sodium 200mg	Dietary Fiber <1g
Saturated Fat 0g	Protein <1g	Sugars 0g

Simply Organic Foods, Brown Gravy Mix

2 tsp

Amount per serving	Amount per serving	Amount per serving
Calories 20	Cholesterol 0mg	Total Carbohydrate 5g
Total Fat 0g	Sodium 290mg	Dietary Fiber 0g
Saturated Fat 0g	Protein 0g	Sugars 0g

Simply Organic Foods, Vegetarian Brown Gravy

2 tsp

Amount per serving	Amount per serving	Amount per serving
Calories 20	Cholesterol 0mg	Total Carbohydrate 5g
Total Fat 0g	Sodium 330mg	Dietary Fiber 0g
Saturated Fat 0g	Protein 0g	Sugars 0g

Meal Products

Garden of Eatin', Blue Corn Taco Dinner Kit

2 taco shells, 7.5g (3 tsp) seasoning mix, 14g (3 tsp) taco sauce

Amount per serving	Amount per serving	Amount per serving
Calories 150	Cholesterol 0mg	Total Carbohydrate 20g
Total Fat 6g	Sodium 600mg	Dietary Fiber 1g
Saturated Fat 0g	Protein 2g	Sugars 2g

Garden of Eatin', Blue Corn Taco Shells

2 taco shells (about 27g)

Amount per serving	Amount per serving	Amount per serving
Calories 140	Cholesterol 0mg	Total Carbohydrate 17g
Total Fat 7g	Sodium 5mg	Dietary Fiber 1g
Saturated Fat 0.5g	Protein 2g	Sugars 0g

Garden of Eatin', Organic Whole Wheat Tortillas

1 tortilla (47g)

Amount per serving	Amount per serving	Amount per serving
Calories 110	Cholesterol 0mg	Total Carbohydrate 22g
Total Fat 1g	Sodium 130mg	Dietary Fiber 3g
Saturated Fat 0g	Protein 4g	Sugars 0g

Garden of Eatin', Yellow Corn Taco Dinner Kit

2 taco shells, 7.5g (3 tsp) seasoning mix, 14g (3 tsp) taco sauce

Amount per serving	Amount per serving	Amount per serving
Calories 150	**Cholesterol** 0mg	**Total Carbohydrate** 20g
Total Fat 6g	**Sodium** 600mg	Dietary Fiber 1g
Saturated Fat 0g	**Protein** 2g	Sugars 2g

Garden of Eatin', Yellow Corn Taco Shells

2 taco shells (about 27g)

Amount per serving	Amount per serving	Amount per serving
Calories 140	**Cholesterol** 0mg	**Total Carbohydrate** 17g
Total Fat 7g	**Sodium** 5mg	Dietary Fiber 1g
Saturated Fat 0.5g	**Protein** 2g	Sugars 0g

La Tortilla Factory, Organic Non-GMO Tortillas Traditional Flour, Burrito Size

1 tortilla (67g)

Amount per serving	Amount per serving	Amount per serving
Calories 160	**Cholesterol** 0mg	**Total Carbohydrate** 28g
Total Fat 3.5g	**Sodium** 340mg	Dietary Fiber 1g
Saturated Fat 1.5g	**Protein** 4g	Sugars 1g

La Tortilla Factory, Organic Non-GMO Tortillas Traditional Flour, Soft Tacot

1 tortilla (43g)

Amount per serving	Amount per serving	Amount per serving
Calories 120	**Cholesterol** 0mg	**Total Carbohydrate** 21g
Total Fat 3g	**Sodium** 260mg	Dietary Fiber 1g
Saturated Fat 1g	**Protein** 3g	Sugars 1g

La Tortilla Factory, Organic Non-GMO Tortillas Whole Wheat, Burrito Size

1 tortilla (67g)

Amount per serving	Amount per serving	Amount per serving
Calories 190	**Cholesterol** 0mg	**Total Carbohydrate** 32g
Total Fat 5g	**Sodium** 390mg	Dietary Fiber 3g
Saturated Fat 2g	**Protein** 5g	Sugars 1g

La Tortilla Factory, Organic Non-GMO Tortillas, Yellow Corn

1 tortilla (34g)

Amount per serving	Amount per serving	Amount per serving
Calories 70	**Cholesterol** 0mg	**Total Carbohydrate** 14g
Total Fat 0.5g	**Sodium** 0mg	Dietary Fiber 1g
Saturated Fat 0g	**Protein** 1g	Sugars 0g

La Tortilla Factory, Sonoma Organic Tortillas, Yellow Corn

2 tortillas (68g)

Amount per serving	Amount per serving	Amount per serving
Calories 120	**Cholesterol** 0mg	**Total Carbohydrate** 25g
Total Fat 1.5g	**Sodium** 0mg	Dietary Fiber 2g
Saturated Fat 0g	**Protein** 3g	Sugars 0g

La Tortilla Factory, Sonoma Organic Wraps, Traditional

1 wrap (67g)

Amount per serving	Amount per serving	Amount per serving
Calories 180	**Cholesterol** 0mg	**Total Carbohydrate** 28g
Total Fat 6g	**Sodium** 360mg	Dietary Fiber 2g
Saturated Fat 1g	**Protein** 5g	Sugars 2g

Rudi's Organic Bakery, 7 Grain with Flax Wraps

1 slice = 2.2 oz (62g)

Amount per serving	Amount per serving	Amount per serving
Calories 160	**Cholesterol** 0mg	**Total Carbohydrate** 27g
Total Fat 3g	**Sodium** 330mg	Dietary Fiber 3g
Saturated Fat 1g	**Protein** 5g	Sugars 2g

Rudi's Organic Bakery, Multigrain Wraps

1 slice = 2.2 oz (62g)

Amount per serving	Amount per serving	Amount per serving
Calories 150	**Cholesterol** 0mg	**Total Carbohydrate** 26g
Total Fat 2.5g	**Sodium** 320mg	Dietary Fiber 3g
Saturated Fat 1g	**Protein** 5g	Sugars 2g

Rudi's Organic Bakery, Spelt Tortillas

1 slice = 2 oz (57g)

Amount per serving	Amount per serving	Amount per serving
Calories 150	**Cholesterol** 0mg	**Total Carbohydrate** 26g
Total Fat 3.5g	**Sodium** 260mg	Dietary Fiber 1g
Saturated Fat 1.5g	**Protein** 4g	Sugars 2g

Rudi's Organic Bakery, Whole Spelt Tortillas

1 slice = 2 oz (57g)

Amount per serving	Amount per serving	Amount per serving
Calories 150	**Cholesterol** 0mg	**Total Carbohydrate** 26g
Total Fat 3.5g	**Sodium** 250mg	Dietary Fiber 2g
Saturated Fat 1.5g	**Protein** 4g	Sugars 2g

Sauces

Annie's, Organic Annie's, Original BBQ Sauce

2 tbsp

Amount per serving	Amount per serving	Amount per serving
Calories 45	**Cholesterol** NA	**Total Carbohydrate** 9g
Total Fat 1g	**Sodium** 240mg	Dietary Fiber NA
Saturated Fat NA	**Protein** 0g	Sugars 5g

Annie's, Organic Hot Chipotle BBQ Sauce

2 tbsp

Amount per serving	Amount per serving	Amount per serving
Calories 45	**Cholesterol** NA	**Total Carbohydrate** 9g
Total Fat 1g	**Sodium** 250mg	Dietary Fiber 1g
Saturated Fat NA	**Protein** 0g	Sugars 5g

Annie's, Organic Smokey Maple BBQ Sauce

2 tbsp

Amount per serving	Amount per serving	Amount per serving
Calories 45	**Cholesterol** NA	**Total Carbohydrate** 9g
Total Fat 1g	**Sodium** 240mg	Dietary Fiber NA
Saturated Fat NA	**Protein** 0g	Sugars 5g

Annie's, Organic Sweet & Spicy BBQ Sauce

2 tbsp

Amount per serving	Amount per serving	Amount per serving
Calories 40	**Cholesterol** NA	**Total Carbohydrate** 10g
Total Fat 0g	**Sodium** 310mg	Dietary Fiber 1g
Saturated Fat NA	**Protein** 0g	Sugars 9g

Classico, Red Sauce, Organic Spinach and Garlic

1/2 cup

Amount per serving	Amount per serving	Amount per serving
Calories 70	**Cholesterol** 0mg	**Total Carbohydrate** 11g
Total Fat 1.5g	**Sodium** 330mg	Dietary Fiber 2g
Saturated Fat 0g	**Protein** 2g	Sugars 7g

Classico, Red Sauce, Organic Tomato, Herbs and Spices

1/2 cup

Amount per serving	Amount per serving	Amount per serving
Calories 70	**Cholesterol** 0mg	**Total Carbohydrate** 12g
Total Fat 1g	**Sodium** 400mg	Dietary Fiber 2g
Saturated Fat 0g	**Protein** 2g	Sugars 7g

Eden Foods, Crushed Tomatoes with Basil, Organic

1/4 cup

Amount per serving	Amount per serving	Amount per serving
Calories 20	**Cholesterol** 0mg	**Total Carbohydrate** 3g
Total Fat 0g	**Sodium** 0mg	Dietary Fiber 1g
Saturated Fat 0g	**Protein** 1g	Sugars 2g

Eden Foods, Crushed Tomatoes with Onions and Garlic, Organic

1/4 cup

Amount per serving	Amount per serving	Amount per serving
Calories 20	**Cholesterol** 0mg	**Total Carbohydrate** 3g
Total Fat 0g	**Sodium** 0mg	Dietary Fiber 1g
Saturated Fat 0g	**Protein** 1g	Sugars 2g

Eden Foods, Crushed Tomatoes with Roasted Onion, Organic

1/4 cup

Amount per serving	Amount per serving	Amount per serving
Calories 20	**Cholesterol** 0mg	**Total Carbohydrate** 3g
Total Fat 0g	**Sodium** 0mg	Dietary Fiber 1g
Saturated Fat 0g	**Protein** 1g	Sugars 2g

Eden Foods, Crushed Tomatoes with Sweet Basil, Organic

1/4 cup

Amount per serving	Amount per serving	Amount per serving
Calories 20	**Cholesterol** 0mg	**Total Carbohydrate** 3g
Total Fat 0g	**Sodium** 0mg	Dietary Fiber 1g
Saturated Fat 0g	**Protein** 1g	Sugars 2g

Eden Foods, Crushed Tomatoes, Organic

1/4 cup

Amount per serving	Amount per serving	Amount per serving
Calories 20	**Cholesterol** 0mg	**Total Carbohydrate** 3g
Total Fat 0g	**Sodium** 0mg	Dietary Fiber 1g
Saturated Fat 0g	**Protein** 1g	Sugars 2g

Eden Foods, Diced Tomatoes with Basil, Organic

1/2 cup

Amount per serving	Amount per serving	Amount per serving
Calories 30	**Cholesterol** 0mg	**Total Carbohydrate** 6g
Total Fat 0g	**Sodium** 5mg	Dietary Fiber 2g
Saturated Fat 0g	**Protein** 1g	Sugars 4g

Eden Foods, Diced Tomatoes with Green Chiles, Organic

1/2 cup

Amount per serving	Amount per serving	Amount per serving
Calories 30	**Cholesterol** 0mg	**Total Carbohydrate** 5g
Total Fat 0g	**Sodium** 35mg	Dietary Fiber 2g
Saturated Fat 0g	**Protein** 2g	Sugars 3g

Eden Foods, Diced Tomatoes with Roasted Onion, Organic

1/2 cup

Amount per serving	Amount per serving	Amount per serving
Calories 30	**Cholesterol** 0mg	**Total Carbohydrate** 6g
Total Fat 0g	**Sodium** 5mg	Dietary Fiber 2g
Saturated Fat 0g	**Protein** 1g	Sugars 4g

Eden Foods, Diced Tomatoes, Organic

1/2 cup

Amount per serving	Amount per serving	Amount per serving
Calories 30	**Cholesterol** 0mg	**Total Carbohydrate** 6g
Total Fat 0g	**Sodium** 5mg	Dietary Fiber 2g
Saturated Fat 0g	**Protein** 1g	Sugars 4g

Eden Foods, Pizza-Pasta Sauce, Organic

1/4 cup

Amount per serving	Amount per serving	Amount per serving
Calories 35	**Cholesterol** 0mg	**Total Carbohydrate** 4g
Total Fat 1g	**Sodium** 150mg	Dietary Fiber 2g
Saturated Fat 0g	**Protein** 1g	Sugars 2g

Eden Foods, Spaghetti Sauce, No Salt Added, Organic

1/2 cup

Amount per serving	Amount per serving	Amount per serving
Calories 70	**Cholesterol** 0mg	**Total Carbohydrate** 9g
Total Fat 2.5g	**Sodium** 10mg	Dietary Fiber 5g
Saturated Fat 0g	**Protein** 2g	Sugars 4g

Eden Foods, Spaghetti Sauce, Organic

1/2 cup

Amount per serving	Amount per serving	Amount per serving
Calories 70	**Cholesterol** 0mg	**Total Carbohydrate** 9g
Total Fat 2.5g	**Sodium** 300mg	Dietary Fiber 5g
Saturated Fat 0g	**Protein** 2g	Sugars 4g

Imagine®, Natural Creations, Organic Latin Veracruz Culinary Simmer Sauce

1/4 cup (60g)

Amount per serving	Amount per serving	Amount per serving
Calories 30	Cholesterol 0mg	Total Carbohydrate 5g
Total Fat 1g	Sodium 150mg	Dietary Fiber 1g
Saturated Fat 0g	Protein <1g	Sugars 2g

Imagine®, Natural Creations, Organic Louisiana Creole Culinary Simmer Sauce

1/4 cup (60g)

Amount per serving	Amount per serving	Amount per serving
Calories 25	Cholesterol 0mg	Total Carbohydrate 5g
Total Fat 0.5g	Sodium 130mg	Dietary Fiber 1g
Saturated Fat 0g	Protein <1g	Sugars 2g

Imagine®, Natural Creations, Organic Portobello Red Wine Culinary Simmer Sauce

1/4 cup (60g)

Amount per serving	Amount per serving	Amount per serving
Calories 20	Cholesterol <5mg	Total Carbohydrate 3g
Total Fat 1g	Sodium 160mg	Dietary Fiber NA
Saturated Fat 0.5g	Protein 0g	Sugars 0g

Imagine®, Natural Creations, Organic Thai Coconut Curry Culinary Simmer Sauce

1/4 cup (60g)

Amount per serving	Amount per serving	Amount per serving
Calories 45	Cholesterol 0mg	Total Carbohydrate 3g
Total Fat 3g	Sodium 240mg	Dietary Fiber 1g
Saturated Fat 2.5g	Protein <1g	Sugars <1g

Jovial Foods, Jovial 100% Organic Crushed Tomatoes

1/2 cup (124g)

Amount per serving	Amount per serving	Amount per serving
Calories 30	Cholesterol NA	Total Carbohydrate 6g
Total Fat 0g	Sodium 30mg	Dietary Fiber 1g
Saturated Fat NA	Protein 1g	Sugars 4g

Jovial Foods, Jovial 100% Organic Diced Tomatoes

1/2 cup (124g)

Amount per serving	Amount per serving	Amount per serving
Calories 30	Cholesterol NA	Total Carbohydrate 6g
Total Fat 0g	Sodium 30mg	Dietary Fiber 1g
Saturated Fat NA	Protein 1g	Sugars 4g

Jovial Foods, Jovial 100% Organic Whole Peeled Tomatoes

1/2 cup (124g)

Amount per serving	Amount per serving	Amount per serving
Calories 30	**Cholesterol** NA	**Total Carbohydrate** 6g
Total Fat 0g	**Sodium** 30mg	Dietary Fiber 1g
Saturated Fat NA	**Protein** 1g	Sugars 4g

KOYO, Organic Reduced Sodium Shoyu Soy Sauce, 10 fl oz

1 tbsp (15 ml)

Amount per serving	Amount per serving	Amount per serving
Calories 10	**Cholesterol** 0mg	**Total Carbohydrate** 1g
Total Fat 0g	**Sodium** 690mg	Dietary Fiber 0g
Saturated Fat 0g	**Protein** <1g	Sugars 0g

KOYO, Organic Shoyu Soy Sauce, 10 fl oz

1 tbsp (15 ml)

Amount per serving	Amount per serving	Amount per serving
Calories 10	**Cholesterol** 0mg	**Total Carbohydrate** 1g
Total Fat 0g	**Sodium** 920mg	Dietary Fiber 0g
Saturated Fat 0g	**Protein** 1g	Sugars 0g

KOYO, Organic Tamari Soy Sauce, 10 fl oz

1 tbsp (15 ml)

Amount per serving	Amount per serving	Amount per serving
Calories 10	**Cholesterol** 0mg	**Total Carbohydrate** 1g
Total Fat 0g	**Sodium** 920mg	Dietary Fiber 0g
Saturated Fat 0g	**Protein** 1g	Sugars 0g

Muir Glen Organic, Cabernet Marinara Organic Pasta Sauce, 25.5 oz

1/2 cup (125g)

Amount per serving	Amount per serving	Amount per serving
Calories 50	**Cholesterol** 0mg	**Total Carbohydrate** 10g
Total Fat 0.5g	**Sodium** 280mg	Dietary Fiber 2g
Saturated Fat 0g	**Protein** 2g	Sugars 6g

Muir Glen Organic, Chunky Tomato & Herb Pasta Sauce, 25.5 oz

1/2 cup (125g)

Amount per serving	Amount per serving	Amount per serving
Calories 50	**Cholesterol** 0mg	**Total Carbohydrate** 10g
Total Fat 0.5g	**Sodium** 280mg	Dietary Fiber 2g
Saturated Fat 0g	**Protein** 2g	Sugars 6g

Muir Glen Organic, Chunky Tomato Sauce, 28 oz

1/4 cup (65g)

Amount per serving	Amount per serving	Amount per serving
Calories 25	**Cholesterol** 0mg	**Total Carbohydrate** 5g
Total Fat 0g	**Sodium** 190mg	Dietary Fiber 1g
Saturated Fat 0g	**Protein** 1g	Sugars 3g

Muir Glen Organic, Crushed Tomatoes with Basil, 28 oz

1/4 cup (65g)

Amount per serving	Amount per serving	Amount per serving
Calories 25	**Cholesterol** 0mg	**Total Carbohydrate** 5g
Total Fat 0g	**Sodium** 190mg	Dietary Fiber 1g
Saturated Fat 0g	**Protein** 1g	Sugars 3g

Muir Glen Organic, Crushed Tomatoes, Fire Roasted, 14.5 oz

1/4 cup (65g)

Amount per serving	Amount per serving	Amount per serving
Calories 20	**Cholesterol** 0mg	**Total Carbohydrate** 5g
Total Fat 0g	**Sodium** 160mg	Dietary Fiber 1g
Saturated Fat 0g	**Protein** 1g	Sugars 3g

Muir Glen Organic, Crushed Tomatoes, Fire Roasted, 14.5 oz

1/4 cup (65g)

Amount per serving	Amount per serving	Amount per serving
Calories 20	**Cholesterol** 0mg	**Total Carbohydrate** 5g
Total Fat 0g	**Sodium** 160mg	Dietary Fiber 1g
Saturated Fat 0g	**Protein** 1g	Sugars 3g

Muir Glen Organic, Crushed Tomatoes, Fire Roasted, 28 oz

1/4 cup (65g)

Amount per serving	Amount per serving	Amount per serving
Calories 20	**Cholesterol** 0mg	**Total Carbohydrate** 4g
Total Fat 0g	**Sodium** 160mg	Dietary Fiber 1g
Saturated Fat 0g	**Protein** <1g	Sugars 2g

Muir Glen Organic, Crushed Tomatoes, Fire Roasted, 28 oz

1/4 cup (65g)

Amount per serving	Amount per serving	Amount per serving
Calories 20	**Cholesterol** 0mg	**Total Carbohydrate** 4g
Total Fat 0g	**Sodium** 160mg	Dietary Fiber 1g
Saturated Fat 0g	**Protein** <1g	Sugars 2g

Muir Glen Organic, Diced Tomatoes with Basil and Garlic, 14.5 oz

1/2 cup (130g)

Amount per serving	Amount per serving	Amount per serving
Calories 30	**Cholesterol** 0mg	**Total Carbohydrate** 6g
Total Fat 0g	**Sodium** 290mg	Dietary Fiber 1g
Saturated Fat 0g	**Protein** 1g	Sugars 4g

Muir Glen Organic, Diced Tomatoes with Garlic and Onion, 14.5 oz

1/2 cup (130g)

Amount per serving	Amount per serving	Amount per serving
Calories 30	**Cholesterol** 0mg	**Total Carbohydrate** 6g
Total Fat 0g	**Sodium** 290mg	Dietary Fiber 1g
Saturated Fat 0g	**Protein** 1g	Sugars 4g

Muir Glen Organic, Diced Tomatoes with Italian Herbs, 14.5 oz

1/2 cup (130g)

Amount per serving	Amount per serving	Amount per serving
Calories 30	**Cholesterol** 0mg	**Total Carbohydrate** 6g
Total Fat 0g	**Sodium** 350mg	Dietary Fiber 1g
Saturated Fat 0g	**Protein** 1g	Sugars 4g

Muir Glen Organic, Diced Tomatoes, 14.5 oz

1/2 cup (130g)

Amount per serving	Amount per serving	Amount per serving
Calories 30	**Cholesterol** 0mg	**Total Carbohydrate** 6g
Total Fat 0g	**Sodium** 290mg	Dietary Fiber 1g
Saturated Fat 0g	**Protein** 1g	Sugars 4g

Muir Glen Organic, Diced Tomatoes, 28 oz

1/2 cup (130g)

Amount per serving	Amount per serving	Amount per serving
Calories 30	**Cholesterol** 0mg	**Total Carbohydrate** 6g
Total Fat 0g	**Sodium** 290mg	Dietary Fiber 1g
Saturated Fat 0g	**Protein** 1g	Sugars 4g

Muir Glen Organic, Diced Tomatoes, Fire Roasted

1/2 cup (130g)

Amount per serving	Amount per serving	Amount per serving
Calories 30	**Cholesterol** 0mg	**Total Carbohydrate** 6g
Total Fat 0g	**Sodium** 290mg	Dietary Fiber 1g
Saturated Fat 0g	**Protein** 1g	Sugars 4g

Muir Glen Organic, Diced Tomatoes, Fire Roasted with Green Chilies, 14.5 oz

1/2 cup (120g)

Amount per serving	Amount per serving	Amount per serving
Calories 30	Cholesterol 0mg	Total Carbohydrate 6g
Total Fat 0g	Sodium 420mg	Dietary Fiber 1g
Saturated Fat 0g	Protein 1g	Sugars 0g

Muir Glen Organic, Diced Tomatoes, Fire Roasted, 14.5 oz

1/2 cup (130g)

Amount per serving	Amount per serving	Amount per serving
Calories 30	Cholesterol 0mg	Total Carbohydrate 6g
Total Fat 0g	Sodium 290mg	Dietary Fiber 1g
Saturated Fat 0g	Protein 1g	Sugars 4g

Muir Glen Organic, Diced Tomatoes, Fire Roasted, 14.5 oz

1/2 cup (130g)

Amount per serving	Amount per serving	Amount per serving
Calories 30	Cholesterol 0mg	Total Carbohydrate 6g
Total Fat 0g	Sodium 290mg	Dietary Fiber 1g
Saturated Fat 0g	Protein 1g	Sugars 4g

Muir Glen Organic, Diced Tomatoes, Fire Roasted, 28 oz

1/2 cup (130g)

Amount per serving	Amount per serving	Amount per serving
Calories 30	Cholesterol 0mg	Total Carbohydrate 6g
Total Fat 0g	Sodium 290mg	Dietary Fiber 1g
Saturated Fat 0g	Protein 1g	Sugars 4g

Muir Glen Organic, Diced Tomatoes, Fire Roasted, No Salt Added, 14.5 oz

1/2 cup (130g)

Amount per serving	Amount per serving	Amount per serving
Calories 30	Cholesterol 0mg	Total Carbohydrate 5g
Total Fat 0g	Sodium 25mg	Dietary Fiber 1g
Saturated Fat 0g	Protein 1g	Sugars 3g

Muir Glen Organic, Diced Tomatoes, No Salt Added

1/2 cup (130g)

Amount per serving	Amount per serving	Amount per serving
Calories 30	Cholesterol 0mg	Total Carbohydrate 6g
Total Fat 0g	Sodium 15mg	Dietary Fiber 1g
Saturated Fat 0g	Protein 1g	Sugars 4g

Muir Glen Organic, Fire Roasted Tomato Organic Pasta Sauce, 25.5 oz

1/2 cup (125g)

Amount per serving	Amount per serving	Amount per serving
Calories 70	**Cholesterol** 0mg	**Total Carbohydrate** 12g
Total Fat 2g	**Sodium** 390mg	Dietary Fiber 2g
Saturated Fat 0g	**Protein** 2g	Sugars 5g

Muir Glen Organic, Garden Vegetable Organic Pasta Sauce, 25.5 oz

1/2 cup (125g)

Amount per serving	Amount per serving	Amount per serving
Calories 50	**Cholesterol** 0mg	**Total Carbohydrate** 10g
Total Fat 0.5g	**Sodium** 290mg	Dietary Fiber 2g
Saturated Fat 0g	**Protein** 2g	Sugars 6g

Muir Glen Organic, Garlic Roasted Organic Pasta Sauce, 25.5 oz

1/2 cup (125g)

Amount per serving	Amount per serving	Amount per serving
Calories 60	**Cholesterol** 0mg	**Total Carbohydrate** 11g
Total Fat 0g	**Sodium** 260mg	Dietary Fiber 2g
Saturated Fat 0g	**Protein** 2g	Sugars 6g

Muir Glen Organic, Ground Peeled Tomatoes, 28 oz

1/4 cup (65g)

Amount per serving	Amount per serving	Amount per serving
Calories 20	**Cholesterol** 0mg	**Total Carbohydrate** 4g
Total Fat 0g	**Sodium** 190mg	Dietary Fiber 1g
Saturated Fat 0g	**Protein** <1g	Sugars 2g

Muir Glen Organic, Italian Herb Organic Pasta Sauce, 25.5 oz

1/2 cup (125g)

Amount per serving	Amount per serving	Amount per serving
Calories 50	**Cholesterol** 0mg	**Total Carbohydrate** 10g
Total Fat 0.5g	**Sodium** 280mg	Dietary Fiber 2g
Saturated Fat 0g	**Protein** 2g	Sugars 6g

Muir Glen Organic, Pizza Sauce, 15 oz

1/4 cup (62g)

Amount per serving	Amount per serving	Amount per serving
Calories 40	**Cholesterol** 0mg	**Total Carbohydrate** 6g
Total Fat 1g	**Sodium** 230mg	Dietary Fiber 2g
Saturated Fat 0g	**Protein** 1g	Sugars 3g

Muir Glen Organic, Portabello Mushroom Pasta Sauce, 25.5 oz

1/2 cup (125g)

Amount per serving	Amount per serving	Amount per serving
Calories 50	Cholesterol 0mg	Total Carbohydrate 9g
Total Fat 0g	Sodium 280mg	Dietary Fiber 2g
Saturated Fat 0g	Protein 2g	Sugars 5g

Muir Glen Organic, Stewed Tomatoes, 14.5 oz

1/2 cup (128g)

Amount per serving	Amount per serving	Amount per serving
Calories 30	Cholesterol 0mg	Total Carbohydrate 6g
Total Fat 0g	Sodium 290mg	Dietary Fiber 1g
Saturated Fat 0g	Protein 1g	Sugars 3g

Muir Glen Organic, Tomato Basil Organic Pasta Sauce, 25.5 oz

1/2 cup (125g)

Amount per serving	Amount per serving	Amount per serving
Calories 60	Cholesterol 0mg	Total Carbohydrate 10g
Total Fat 0.5g	Sodium 260mg	Dietary Fiber 2g
Saturated Fat 0g	Protein 2g	Sugars 6g

Muir Glen Organic, Tomato Paste, 6 oz

2 tbsp (33g)

Amount per serving	Amount per serving	Amount per serving
Calories 30	Cholesterol 0mg	Total Carbohydrate 6g
Total Fat 0g	Sodium 20mg	Dietary Fiber 1g
Saturated Fat 0g	Protein 2g	Sugars 3g

Muir Glen Organic, Tomato Puree, 28 oz

1/4 cup (63g)

Amount per serving	Amount per serving	Amount per serving
Calories 20	Cholesterol 0mg	Total Carbohydrate 5g
Total Fat 0g	Sodium 20mg	Dietary Fiber 1g
Saturated Fat 0g	Protein 1g	Sugars 3g

Muir Glen Organic, Tomato Sauce, 15 oz

1/4 cup (62g)

Amount per serving	Amount per serving	Amount per serving
Calories 20	Cholesterol 0mg	Total Carbohydrate 5g
Total Fat 0g	Sodium 260mg	Dietary Fiber 1g
Saturated Fat 0g	Protein <1g	Sugars 3g

Muir Glen Organic, Tomato Sauce, 8 oz

1/4 cup (62g)

Amount per serving	Amount per serving	Amount per serving
Calories 20	**Cholesterol** 0mg	**Total Carbohydrate** 5g
Total Fat 0g	**Sodium** 260mg	Dietary Fiber 1g
Saturated Fat 0g	**Protein** <1g	Sugars 3g

Muir Glen Organic, Tomato Sauce, No Salt Added, 15 oz

1/4 cup (62g)

Amount per serving	Amount per serving	Amount per serving
Calories 20	**Cholesterol** 0mg	**Total Carbohydrate** 5g
Total Fat 0g	**Sodium** 30mg	Dietary Fiber 1g
Saturated Fat 0g	**Protein** <1g	Sugars 3g

Muir Glen Organic, Whole Peeled Plum Tomatoes, 28 oz

1/2 cup (120g)

Amount per serving	Amount per serving	Amount per serving
Calories 25	**Cholesterol** 0mg	**Total Carbohydrate** 5g
Total Fat 0g	**Sodium** 260mg	Dietary Fiber 1g
Saturated Fat 0g	**Protein** 1g	Sugars 3g

Muir Glen Organic, Whole Peeled Tomatoes with Basil, 28 oz

1/2 cup (122g)

Amount per serving	Amount per serving	Amount per serving
Calories 25	**Cholesterol** 0mg	**Total Carbohydrate** 5g
Total Fat 0g	**Sodium** 260mg	Dietary Fiber 1g
Saturated Fat 0g	**Protein** 1g	Sugars 3g

Muir Glen Organic, Whole Peeled Tomatoes, 14.5 oz

1/2 cup (120g)

Amount per serving	Amount per serving	Amount per serving
Calories 25	**Cholesterol** 0mg	**Total Carbohydrate** 5g
Total Fat 0g	**Sodium** 260mg	Dietary Fiber 1g
Saturated Fat 0g	**Protein** 1g	Sugars 3g

Muir Glen Organic, Whole Peeled Tomatoes, 28 oz

1/2 cup (120g)

Amount per serving	Amount per serving	Amount per serving
Calories 25	**Cholesterol** 0mg	**Total Carbohydrate** 5g
Total Fat 0g	**Sodium** 260mg	Dietary Fiber 1g
Saturated Fat 0g	**Protein** 1g	Sugars 3g

Muir Glen Organic, Whole Tomatoes, Fire Roasted, 28 oz

1/2 cup (122g)

Amount per serving	Amount per serving	Amount per serving
Calories 25	**Cholesterol** 0mg	**Total Carbohydrate** 5g
Total Fat 0g	**Sodium** 290mg	Dietary Fiber 1g
Saturated Fat 0g	**Protein** 1g	Sugars 3g

Newman's Own, Organic Marinara Pasta Sauce

1/2 cup

Amount per serving	Amount per serving	Amount per serving
Calories 70	**Cholesterol** 0mg	**Total Carbohydrate** 12g
Total Fat 2g	**Sodium** 550mg	Dietary Fiber 3g
Saturated Fat 0g	**Protein** 2g	Sugars 8g

OrganicVille®, Brown Rice Miso

3/4 tbsp (12g)

Amount per serving	Amount per serving	Amount per serving
Calories 25	**Cholesterol** 0mg	**Total Carbohydrate** 3g
Total Fat 1g	**Sodium** 540mg	Dietary Fiber 0g
Saturated Fat 0g	**Protein** 1g	Sugars 3g

OrganicVille®, Island Organic Teriyaki

1 tbsp (15g)

Amount per serving	Amount per serving	Amount per serving
Calories 25	**Cholesterol** 0mg	**Total Carbohydrate** 4g
Total Fat 1g	**Sodium** 240mg	Dietary Fiber 0g
Saturated Fat 0g	**Protein** <1g	Sugars 3g

OrganicVille®, Italian Herb Organic Pasta Sauce

1/2 cup (113g)

Amount per serving	Amount per serving	Amount per serving
Calories 60	**Cholesterol** 0mg	**Total Carbohydrate** 2g
Total Fat 1.5g	**Sodium** 490mg	Dietary Fiber 2g
Saturated Fat 0g	**Protein** 2g	Sugars 3g

OrganicVille®, Marinara Organic Pasta Sauce

1/2 cup (113g)

Amount per serving	Amount per serving	Amount per serving
Calories 50	**Cholesterol** 0mg	**Total Carbohydrate** 9g
Total Fat 1g	**Sodium** 460mg	Dietary Fiber 2g
Saturated Fat 0g	**Protein** 1g	Sugars 3g

OrganicVille®, Mushroom Organic Pasta Sauce

1/2 cup (113g)

Amount per serving	Amount per serving	Amount per serving
Calories 45	**Cholesterol** 0mg	**Total Carbohydrate** 8g
Total Fat 1g	**Sodium** 450mg	Dietary Fiber 2g
Saturated Fat 0g	**Protein** 1g	Sugars 3g

OrganicVille®, Organic Pizza Sauce

1/2 cup (56g)

Amount per serving	Amount per serving	Amount per serving
Calories 25	**Cholesterol** 0mg	**Total Carbohydrate** 3g
Total Fat 1g	**Sodium** 245mg	Dietary Fiber 1g
Saturated Fat <1g	**Protein** 1g	Sugars 2g

OrganicVille®, Red Miso

3/4 tbsp (12g)

Amount per serving	Amount per serving	Amount per serving
Calories 25	**Cholesterol** 0mg	**Total Carbohydrate** 4g
Total Fat 1g	**Sodium** 560mg	Dietary Fiber 0g
Saturated Fat 0g	**Protein** 2g	Sugars 4g

OrganicVille®, Saikyo Sweet Miso

3/4 tbsp (12g)

Amount per serving	Amount per serving	Amount per serving
Calories 25	**Cholesterol** 0mg	**Total Carbohydrate** 5g
Total Fat 0.5g	**Sodium** 310mg	Dietary Fiber <1g
Saturated Fat 0g	**Protein** <1g	Sugars 4g

OrganicVille®, Sesame Organic Teriyaki

1 tbsp (15g)

Amount per serving	Amount per serving	Amount per serving
Calories 25	**Cholesterol** 0mg	**Total Carbohydrate** 4g
Total Fat 1g	**Sodium** 280mg	Dietary Fiber 0g
Saturated Fat 0g	**Protein** <1g	Sugars 3g

OrganicVille®, Tomato Basil Organic Pasta Sauce

1/2 cup (113g)

Amount per serving	Amount per serving	Amount per serving
Calories 50	**Cholesterol** 0mg	**Total Carbohydrate** 9g
Total Fat 1g	**Sodium** 460mg	Dietary Fiber 2g
Saturated Fat 0g	**Protein** 1g	Sugars 3g

OrganicVille®, White Miso

3/4 tbsp (12g)

Amount per serving	Amount per serving	Amount per serving
Calories 25	**Cholesterol** 0mg	**Total Carbohydrate** 3g
Total Fat 1g	**Sodium** 530mg	Dietary Fiber <1g
Saturated Fat 0g	**Protein** 1g	Sugars 3g

Seeds of Change, Indian Simmer Sauce, Jalfrezi

1/3 cup (85g)

Amount per serving	Amount per serving	Amount per serving
Calories 90	**Cholesterol** 350mg	**Total Carbohydrate** 9g
Total Fat 6g	**Sodium** 310mg	Dietary Fiber 1g
Saturated Fat 2g	**Protein** 1g	Sugars 1g

Seeds of Change, Indian Simmer Sauce, Korma

1/3 cup (85g)

Amount per serving	Amount per serving	Amount per serving
Calories 130	**Cholesterol** 10mg	**Total Carbohydrate** 11g
Total Fat 9g	**Sodium** 370mg	Dietary Fiber 1g
Saturated Fat 6g	**Protein** 1g	Sugars 1g

Seeds of Change, Indian Simmer Sauce, Madras

1/3 cup (85g)

Amount per serving	Amount per serving	Amount per serving
Calories 60	**Cholesterol** 0mg	**Total Carbohydrate** 8g
Total Fat 3g	**Sodium** 310mg	Dietary Fiber 1g
Saturated Fat 0g	**Protein** 1g	Sugars 1g

Seeds of Change, Indian Simmer Sauce, Tikka Masala

1/3 cup (85g)

Amount per serving	Amount per serving	Amount per serving
Calories 90	**Cholesterol** 5mg	**Total Carbohydrate** 8g
Total Fat 6g	**Sodium** 350mg	Dietary Fiber 1g
Saturated Fat 1.5g	**Protein** 1g	Sugars 1g

Simply Organic Foods, Alfredo Sauce

1 tbsp

Amount per serving	Amount per serving	Amount per serving
Calories 35	**Cholesterol** 0mg	**Total Carbohydrate** 7g
Total Fat 0g	**Sodium** 310mg	Dietary Fiber 0g
Saturated Fat 0g	**Protein** 2g	Sugars 2g

Simply Organic Foods, Enchilada Sauce

1 tsp

Amount per serving	Amount per serving	Amount per serving
Calories 15	**Cholesterol** 0mg	**Total Carbohydrate** 3g
Total Fat 0g	**Sodium** 340mg	Dietary Fiber 1g
Saturated Fat 0g	**Protein** 0g	Sugars 0g

Simply Organic Foods, Garden Vegetable Spaghetti Sauce

1 tbsp

Amount per serving	Amount per serving	Amount per serving
Calories 30	**Cholesterol** 0mg	**Total Carbohydrate** 7g
Total Fat 0g	**Sodium** 300mg	Dietary Fiber 1g
Saturated Fat 0g	**Protein** 0g	Sugars 2g

Simply Organic Foods, Hollandaise Sauce Mix

3/4 tsp

Amount per serving	Amount per serving	Amount per serving
Calories 10	**Cholesterol** 10mg	**Total Carbohydrate** 2g
Total Fat 0g	**Sodium** 95mg	Dietary Fiber 0g
Saturated Fat 0g	**Protein** 0g	Sugars <1g

Simply Organic Foods, Mushroom Sauce Mix

2 tsp

Amount per serving	Amount per serving	Amount per serving
Calories 20	**Cholesterol** 0mg	**Total Carbohydrate** 4g
Total Fat 0g	**Sodium** 300mg	Dietary Fiber 0g
Saturated Fat 0g	**Protein** 0g	Sugars 0g

Seasonings

Eden Foods, Black & Tan Gomasio (Sesame Salt), Organic

1 tsp

Amount per serving	Amount per serving	Amount per serving
Calories 20	**Cholesterol** 0mg	**Total Carbohydrate** <1g
Total Fat 1.5g	**Sodium** 80mg	Dietary Fiber 0g
Saturated Fat 0g	**Protein** <1g	Sugars 0g

Eden Foods, Black Gomasio (Sesame Salt), Organic

1 tsp

Amount per serving	Amount per serving	Amount per serving
Calories 20	**Cholesterol** 0mg	**Total Carbohydrate** <1g
Total Fat 1.5g	**Sodium** 80mg	Dietary Fiber 0g
Saturated Fat 0g	**Protein** <1g	Sugars 0g

Eden Foods, Dulse Flakes, Sea Vegetable, Organic, Wild, Hand Harvested, Raw

1 tsp

Amount per serving	Amount per serving	Amount per serving
Calories 3	**Cholesterol** 0mg	**Total Carbohydrate** 0g
Total Fat 0g	**Sodium** 15mg	Dietary Fiber 0g
Saturated Fat 0g	**Protein** 0g	Sugars 0g

Eden Foods, Dulse Whole Leaf, Sea Vegetable, Organic, Wild, Hand Harvested

1/4 cup

Amount per serving	Amount per serving	Amount per serving
Calories 10	**Cholesterol** 0mg	**Total Carbohydrate** 2g
Total Fat 0g	**Sodium** 60mg	Dietary Fiber 1g
Saturated Fat 0g	**Protein** <1g	Sugars 0g

Eden Foods, Garlic Gomasio (Sesame Salt), Organic

1 tsp

Amount per serving	Amount per serving	Amount per serving
Calories 15	**Cholesterol** 0mg	**Total Carbohydrate** <1g
Total Fat 1.5g	**Sodium** 80mg	Dietary Fiber 0g
Saturated Fat 0g	**Protein** <1g	Sugars 0g

Eden Foods, Gomasio (Sesame Salt), Organic

1 tsp

Amount per serving	Amount per serving	Amount per serving
Calories 15	**Cholesterol** 0mg	**Total Carbohydrate** <1g
Total Fat 1.5g	**Sodium** 80mg	Dietary Fiber 0g
Saturated Fat 0g	**Protein** <1g	Sugars 0g

Eden Foods, Seaweed Gomasio (Sesame Salt), Organic

1 tsp

Amount per serving	Amount per serving	Amount per serving
Calories 15	**Cholesterol** 0mg	**Total Carbohydrate** <1g
Total Fat 1.5g	**Sodium** 80mg	Dietary Fiber 0g
Saturated Fat 0g	**Protein** <1g	Sugars 0g

Manna Organics, Himalayan Pink Salt

1/2 tsp (1g)

Amount per serving	Amount per serving	Amount per serving
Calories 0	**Cholesterol** 0mg	**Total Carbohydrate** 0g
Total Fat 0g	**Sodium** 390mg	Dietary Fiber 0g
Saturated Fat 0g	**Protein** 0g	Sugars 0g

Manna Organics, Untreated Sea Salt

1/2 tsp (1g)

Amount per serving	Amount per serving	Amount per serving
Calories 0	**Cholesterol** 0mg	**Total Carbohydrate** 0g
Total Fat 0g	**Sodium** 390mg	Dietary Fiber 0g
Saturated Fat 0g	**Protein** 0g	Sugars 0g

Manna Organics, Xanthan Gum, GMO Free

1 tbsp (6g)

Amount per serving	Amount per serving	Amount per serving
Calories 20	**Cholesterol** 0mg	**Total Carbohydrate** 5g
Total Fat 0g	**Sodium** 105mg	Dietary Fiber 5g
Saturated Fat 0g	**Protein** 0g	Sugars 0g

Simply Organic Foods, Black Bean Seasoning Mix

2 tsp

Amount per serving	Amount per serving	Amount per serving
Calories 15	**Cholesterol** 0mg	**Total Carbohydrate** 3g
Total Fat 0g	**Sodium** 260mg	Dietary Fiber 0g
Saturated Fat 0g	**Protein** 0g	Sugars 0g

Simply Organic Foods, Citrus 'n Herb Seasoning

1/4 tsp

Amount per serving	Amount per serving	Amount per serving
Calories 5	**Cholesterol** 0mg	**Total Carbohydrate** 0g
Total Fat 0g	**Sodium** 0mg	Dietary Fiber 0g
Saturated Fat 0g	**Protein** 0g	Sugars 0g

Simply Organic Foods, Dirty Rice Seasoning Mix

2 tsp

Amount per serving	Amount per serving	Amount per serving
Calories 20	**Cholesterol** 0mg	**Total Carbohydrate** 4g
Total Fat 0g	**Sodium** 410mg	Dietary Fiber 1g
Saturated Fat 0g	**Protein** 1g	Sugars 0g

Simply Organic Foods, Fajita Seasoning

2 tsp

Amount per serving	Amount per serving	Amount per serving
Calories 20	**Cholesterol** 0mg	**Total Carbohydrate** 5g
Total Fat 0g	**Sodium** 270mg	Dietary Fiber 1g
Saturated Fat 0g	**Protein** 0g	Sugars 0g

Simply Organic Foods, Fish Taco Seasoning Mix

1 tbsp

Amount per serving	Amount per serving	Amount per serving
Calories 25	Cholesterol 0mg	Total Carbohydrate 5g
Total Fat 0g	Sodium 370mg	Dietary Fiber 1g
Saturated Fat 0g	Protein 1g	Sugars 0g

Simply Organic Foods, French Onion Dip

1/2 tsp

Amount per serving	Amount per serving	Amount per serving
Calories 5	Cholesterol 0mg	Total Carbohydrate 1g
Total Fat 0g	Sodium 125mg	Dietary Fiber 0g
Saturated Fat 0g	Protein 0g	Sugars 0g

Simply Organic Foods, Gumbo Base Seasoning Mix

1 tbsp

Amount per serving	Amount per serving	Amount per serving
Calories 25	Cholesterol 0mg	Total Carbohydrate 6g
Total Fat 0g	Sodium 410mg	Dietary Fiber 1g
Saturated Fat 0g	Protein 1g	Sugars 0g

Simply Organic Foods, Jambalaya Seasoning Mix

2 tsp

Amount per serving	Amount per serving	Amount per serving
Calories 15	Cholesterol 0mg	Total Carbohydrate 3g
Total Fat 0g	Sodium 460mg	Dietary Fiber 1g
Saturated Fat 0g	Protein 1g	Sugars 0g

Simply Organic Foods, Mild Chili Seasoning Mix

2 tsp

Amount per serving	Amount per serving	Amount per serving
Calories 15	Cholesterol 0mg	Total Carbohydrate 3g
Total Fat 0g	Sodium 280mg	Dietary Fiber 1g
Saturated Fat 0g	Protein 0g	Sugars 1g

Simply Organic Foods, Orange Ginger Seasoning

1/4 tsp

Amount per serving	Amount per serving	Amount per serving
Calories 5	Cholesterol 0mg	Total Carbohydrate <1g
Total Fat 0g	Sodium 60mg	Dietary Fiber 0g
Saturated Fat 0g	Protein 0g	Sugars 0g

Simply Organic Foods, Red Bean Seasoning Mix

2 tsp

Amount per serving	Amount per serving	Amount per serving
Calories 15	**Cholesterol** 0mg	**Total Carbohydrate** 3g
Total Fat 0g	**Sodium** 250mg	Dietary Fiber 1g
Saturated Fat 0g	**Protein** 0g	Sugars 0g

Simply Organic Foods, Roasted Chicken Gravy Seasoning Mix

2 tsp

Amount per serving	Amount per serving	Amount per serving
Calories 20	**Cholesterol** 0mg	**Total Carbohydrate** 4g
Total Fat 0g	**Sodium** 290mg	Dietary Fiber 0g
Saturated Fat 0g	**Protein** 0g	Sugars 0g

Simply Organic Foods, Roasted Turkey Gravy Seasoning Mix

2 tsp

Amount per serving	Amount per serving	Amount per serving
Calories 20	**Cholesterol** 0mg	**Total Carbohydrate** 4g
Total Fat 0g	**Sodium** 290mg	Dietary Fiber 0g
Saturated Fat 0g	**Protein** 0g	Sugars 0g

Simply Organic Foods, Salsa Mix

1/2 tsp

Amount per serving	Amount per serving	Amount per serving
Calories 5	**Cholesterol** 0mg	**Total Carbohydrate** 1g
Total Fat 0g	**Sodium** 60mg	Dietary Fiber 0g
Saturated Fat 0g	**Protein** 0g	Sugars 0g

Simply Organic Foods, Seafood Seasoning

1/4 tsp

Amount per serving	Amount per serving	Amount per serving
Calories 0	**Cholesterol** 0mg	**Total Carbohydrate** 0g
Total Fat 0g	**Sodium** 40mg	Dietary Fiber 0g
Saturated Fat 0g	**Protein** 0g	Sugars 0g

Simply Organic Foods, Southwest Taco seasoning mix

1 tbsp

Amount per serving	Amount per serving	Amount per serving
Calories 25	**Cholesterol** 0mg	**Total Carbohydrate** 5g
Total Fat 0.5g	**Sodium** 360mg	Dietary Fiber 1g
Saturated Fat 0g	**Protein** 1g	Sugars 0g

Simply Organic Foods, Spicy Chili Seasoning Mix

2 tsp

Amount per serving	Amount per serving	Amount per serving
Calories 15	**Cholesterol** 0mg	**Total Carbohydrate** 3g
Total Fat 0g	**Sodium** 210mg	Dietary Fiber 1g
Saturated Fat 0g	**Protein** 1g	Sugars 0g

Simply Organic Foods, Spicy Steak Seasoning

1/4 tsp

Amount per serving	Amount per serving	Amount per serving
Calories 0	**Cholesterol** 0mg	**Total Carbohydrate** 0g
Total Fat 0g	**Sodium** 35mg	Dietary Fiber 0g
Saturated Fat 0g	**Protein** 0g	Sugars 0g

Simply Organic Foods, Steak Seasoning

1/4 tsp

Amount per serving	Amount per serving	Amount per serving
Calories 0	**Cholesterol** 0mg	**Total Carbohydrate** 0g
Total Fat 0g	**Sodium** 85mg	Dietary Fiber 0g
Saturated Fat 0g	**Protein** 0g	Sugars 0g

Simply Organic Foods, Vegetable Seasoning

1/4 tsp

Amount per serving	Amount per serving	Amount per serving
Calories 0	**Cholesterol** 0mg	**Total Carbohydrate** 0g
Total Fat 0g	**Sodium** 40mg	Dietary Fiber 0g
Saturated Fat 0g	**Protein** 0g	Sugars 0g

Simply Organic Foods, Vegetarian Chili Seasoning Mix

2 tsp

Amount per serving	Amount per serving	Amount per serving
Calories 15	**Cholesterol** 0mg	**Total Carbohydrate** 3g
Total Fat 0g	**Sodium** 210mg	Dietary Fiber 1g
Saturated Fat 0g	**Protein** 1g	Sugars 0g

Soups

Amy's, Organic Black Bean Vegetable Soup

1 cup

Amount per serving	Amount per serving	Amount per serving
Calories 140	**Cholesterol** 0mg	**Total Carbohydrate** 26g
Total Fat 1.5g	**Sodium** 620mg	Dietary Fiber 5g
Saturated Fat 0g	**Protein** 6g	Sugars 7g

Amy's, Organic Chunky Tomato Bisque

1 cup

Amount per serving	Amount per serving	Amount per serving
Calories 130	**Cholesterol** 10mg	**Total Carbohydrate** 21g
Total Fat 3.5g	**Sodium** 680mg	Dietary Fiber 3g
Saturated Fat 2g	**Protein** 3g	Sugars 14g

Amy's, Organic Chunky Vegetable Soup

1 cup

Amount per serving	Amount per serving	Amount per serving
Calories 60	**Cholesterol** 0mg	**Total Carbohydrate** 13g
Total Fat 0g	**Sodium** 680mg	Dietary Fiber 3g
Saturated Fat 0g	**Protein** 3g	Sugars 5g

Amy's, Organic Cream of Tomato Soup

1 cup

Amount per serving	Amount per serving	Amount per serving
Calories 110	**Cholesterol** 10mg	**Total Carbohydrate** 19g
Total Fat 2.5g	**Sodium** 690mg	Dietary Fiber 3g
Saturated Fat 1.5g	**Protein** 3g	Sugars 13g

Amy's, Organic Curried Lentil Soup

1 cup

Amount per serving	Amount per serving	Amount per serving
Calories 230	**Cholesterol** 0mg	**Total Carbohydrate** 30g
Total Fat 8g	**Sodium** 680mg	Dietary Fiber 11g
Saturated Fat 1g	**Protein** 9g	Sugars 4g

Amy's, Organic Fire Roasted Southwestern Vegetable Soup

1 cup

Amount per serving	Amount per serving	Amount per serving
Calories 140	**Cholesterol** 0mg	**Total Carbohydrate** 21g
Total Fat 4g	**Sodium** 680mg	Dietary Fiber 4g
Saturated Fat 0.5g	**Protein** 4g	Sugars 4g

Amy's, Organic Hearty French Country Vegetable Soup

1 cup

Amount per serving	Amount per serving	Amount per serving
Calories 180	**Cholesterol** 0mg	**Total Carbohydrate** 23g
Total Fat 8g	**Sodium** 640mg	Dietary Fiber 5g
Saturated Fat 1g	**Protein** 5g	Sugars 4g

Amy's, Organic Hearty Rustic Italian Vegetable Soup

1 cup

Amount per serving	Amount per serving	Amount per serving
Calories 140	Cholesterol 0mg	Total Carbohydrate 18g
Total Fat 6g	Sodium 680mg	Dietary Fiber 4g
Saturated Fat 1g	Protein 4g	Sugars 4g

Amy's, Organic Hearty Spanish Rice & Red Bean Soup

1/2 can

Amount per serving	Amount per serving	Amount per serving
Calories 140	Cholesterol 0mg	Total Carbohydrate 24g
Total Fat 2.5g	Sodium 690mg	Dietary Fiber 5g
Saturated Fat 0g	Protein 5g	Sugars 3g

Amy's, Organic Lentil Soup

1 cup

Amount per serving	Amount per serving	Amount per serving
Calories 180	Cholesterol 0mg	Total Carbohydrate 25g
Total Fat 5g	Sodium 590mg	Dietary Fiber 6g
Saturated Fat 1g	Protein 8g	Sugars 3g

Amy's, Organic Lentil Vegetable Soup

1 cup

Amount per serving	Amount per serving	Amount per serving
Calories 160	Cholesterol 0mg	Total Carbohydrate 24g
Total Fat 4g	Sodium 680mg	Dietary Fiber 8g
Saturated Fat 0.5g	Protein 7g	Sugars 5g

Amy's, Organic Light in Sodium, Chunky Tomato Bisque

1 cup

Amount per serving	Amount per serving	Amount per serving
Calories 130	Cholesterol 10mg	Total Carbohydrate 21g
Total Fat 3.5g	Sodium 340mg	Dietary Fiber 3g
Saturated Fat 2g	Protein 3g	Sugars 14g

Amy's, Organic Light in Sodium, Cream of Tomato Soup

1 cup

Amount per serving	Amount per serving	Amount per serving
Calories 110	Cholesterol 10mg	Total Carbohydrate 19g
Total Fat 2.5g	Sodium 340mg	Dietary Fiber 3g
Saturated Fat 1.5g	Protein 3g	Sugars 13g

Amy's, Organic Light in Sodium, Lentil Vegetable Soup

1 cup

Amount per serving	Amount per serving	Amount per serving
Calories 160	**Cholesterol** 0mg	**Total Carbohydrate** 24g
Total Fat 4g	**Sodium** 340mg	Dietary Fiber 8g
Saturated Fat 0.5g	**Protein** 7g	Sugars 5g

Amy's, Organic Light in Sodium, Split Pea Soup

1 cup

Amount per serving	Amount per serving	Amount per serving
Calories 100	**Cholesterol** 0mg	**Total Carbohydrate** 19g
Total Fat 0g	**Sodium** 330mg	Dietary Fiber 6g
Saturated Fat 0g	**Protein** 7g	Sugars 4g

Amy's, Organic Split Pea Soup

1 cup

Amount per serving	Amount per serving	Amount per serving
Calories 100	**Cholesterol** 0mg	**Total Carbohydrate** 19g
Total Fat 0g	**Sodium** 670mg	Dietary Fiber 6g
Saturated Fat 0g	**Protein** 7g	Sugars 4g

Amy's, Organic Summer Corn & Vegetable Soup

1 cup

Amount per serving	Amount per serving	Amount per serving
Calories 150	**Cholesterol** 15mg	**Total Carbohydrate** 23g
Total Fat 3g	**Sodium** 560mg	Dietary Fiber 2g
Saturated Fat 2.5g	**Protein** 4g	Sugars 6g

Amy's, Organic Tuscan Bean & Rice Soup

1 cup

Amount per serving	Amount per serving	Amount per serving
Calories 160	**Cholesterol** 0mg	**Total Carbohydrate** 25g
Total Fat 4.5g	**Sodium** 680mg	Dietary Fiber 5g
Saturated Fat 0.5g	**Protein** 5g	Sugars 4g

Andean Dream, Gluten & Corn Free, Vegan Vegetarian Quinoa Noodle Soup

1 cup

Amount per serving	Amount per serving	Amount per serving
Calories 100	**Cholesterol** 0mg	**Total Carbohydrate** 22g
Total Fat 0.5g	**Sodium** 580mg	Dietary Fiber 1g
Saturated Fat 0g	**Protein** 3g	Sugars <1g

Andean Dream, Gluten & Corn Free, Vegan Vegetarian Tomato Quinoa Noodle Soup

1 cup

Amount per serving	Amount per serving	Amount per serving
Calories 130	**Cholesterol** 0mg	**Total Carbohydrate** 27g
Total Fat 0.5g	**Sodium** 580mg	Dietary Fiber 2g
Saturated Fat 0g	**Protein** 3g	Sugars 1g

Dr. McDougall's Right Foods, Organic Gluten-Free Black Bean Soup

245g

Amount per serving	Amount per serving	Amount per serving
Calories 150	**Cholesterol** 0mg	**Total Carbohydrate** 29g
Total Fat 1g	**Sodium** 480mg	Dietary Fiber 6g
Saturated Fat 0g	**Protein** 8g	Sugars 1g

Dr. McDougall's Right Foods, Organic Gluten-Free Butternut Azteca Soup

245g

Amount per serving	Amount per serving	Amount per serving
Calories 70	**Cholesterol** 0mg	**Total Carbohydrate** 17g
Total Fat 0g	**Sodium** 480mg	Dietary Fiber 1g
Saturated Fat 0g	**Protein** 2g	Sugars 1g

Dr. McDougall's Right Foods, Organic Gluten-Free French Lentil Soup

245g

Amount per serving	Amount per serving	Amount per serving
Calories 130	**Cholesterol** 0mg	**Total Carbohydrate** 23g
Total Fat 0.5g	**Sodium** 480mg	Dietary Fiber 9g
Saturated Fat 0g	**Protein** 8g	Sugars 2g

Dr. McDougall's Right Foods, Organic Gluten-Free Lentil Vegetable Soup

245g

Amount per serving	Amount per serving	Amount per serving
Calories 130	**Cholesterol** 0mg	**Total Carbohydrate** 24g
Total Fat 0.5g	**Sodium** 480mg	Dietary Fiber 10g
Saturated Fat 0g	**Protein** 8g	Sugars 3g

Dr. McDougall's Right Foods, Organic Gluten-Free Lower Sodium Black Bean Soup

245g

Amount per serving	Amount per serving	Amount per serving
Calories 150	**Cholesterol** 0mg	**Total Carbohydrate** 28g
Total Fat 1g	**Sodium** 290mg	Dietary Fiber 6g
Saturated Fat 0g	**Protein** 8g	Sugars 3g

Dr. McDougall's Right Foods, Organic Gluten-Free Lower Sodium French Lentil Soup

245g

Amount per serving	Amount per serving	Amount per serving
Calories 130	**Cholesterol** 0mg	**Total Carbohydrate** 23g
Total Fat 0g	**Sodium** 290mg	Dietary Fiber 9g
Saturated Fat 0g	**Protein** 8g	Sugars 2g

Dr. McDougall's Right Foods, Organic Gluten-Free Minestrone Soup

245g

Amount per serving	Amount per serving	Amount per serving
Calories 90	**Cholesterol** 0mg	**Total Carbohydrate** 19g
Total Fat 0.5g	**Sodium** 480mg	Dietary Fiber 5g
Saturated Fat 0g	**Protein** 5g	Sugars 3g

Dr. McDougall's Right Foods, Organic Gluten-Free Split Pea Soup

245g

Amount per serving	Amount per serving	Amount per serving
Calories 120	**Cholesterol** 0mg	**Total Carbohydrate** 22g
Total Fat 0g	**Sodium** 480mg	Dietary Fiber 7g
Saturated Fat 0g	**Protein** 7g	Sugars 1g

Dr. McDougall's Right Foods, Organic Gluten-Free Vegetable Soup

245g

Amount per serving	Amount per serving	Amount per serving
Calories 90	**Cholesterol** 0mg	**Total Carbohydrate** 17g
Total Fat 1.5g	**Sodium** 480mg	Dietary Fiber 3g
Saturated Fat 0g	**Protein** 4g	Sugars 4g

Dr. McDougall's Right Foods, Organic Lower Sodium Chunky Tomato Soup

245g

Amount per serving	Amount per serving	Amount per serving
Calories 80	**Cholesterol** 0mg	**Total Carbohydrate** 18g
Total Fat 0g	**Sodium** 290mg	Dietary Fiber 2g
Saturated Fat 0g	**Protein** 2g	Sugars 1g

Dr. McDougall's Right Foods, Organic Lower Sodium Vegetable Soup

245g

Amount per serving	Amount per serving	Amount per serving
Calories 90	**Cholesterol** 0mg	**Total Carbohydrate** 17g
Total Fat 1.5g	**Sodium** 290mg	Dietary Fiber 3g
Saturated Fat 0g	**Protein** 4g	Sugars 4g

Dr. McDougall's Right Foods, Organic Tortilla Soup

245g

Amount per serving	Amount per serving	Amount per serving
Calories 100	**Cholesterol** 0mg	**Total Carbohydrate** 20g
Total Fat 0.5g	**Sodium** 530mg	Dietary Fiber 4g
Saturated Fat 0g	**Protein** 5g	Sugars 2g

Health Valley, Organic 40% Less Sodium Lentil & Carrot Soup

1 cup (240g)

Amount per serving	Amount per serving	Amount per serving
Calories 110	**Cholesterol** 0mg	**Total Carbohydrate** 24g
Total Fat 0g	**Sodium** 450mg	Dietary Fiber 8g
Saturated Fat 0g	**Protein** 8g	Sugars 4g

Health Valley, Organic 40% Less Sodium, 14 Garden Vegetable Soup

1 cup (240g)

Amount per serving	Amount per serving	Amount per serving
Calories 80	**Cholesterol** 0mg	**Total Carbohydrate** 18g
Total Fat 0g	**Sodium** 480mg	Dietary Fiber 4g
Saturated Fat 0g	**Protein** 3g	Sugars 6g

Health Valley, Organic 40% Less Sodium, 5 Bean Vegetable Soup

1 cup (240g)

Amount per serving	Amount per serving	Amount per serving
Calories 100	**Cholesterol** 0mg	**Total Carbohydrate** 23g
Total Fat 0g	**Sodium** 480mg	Dietary Fiber 6g
Saturated Fat 0g	**Protein** 5g	Sugars 4g

Health Valley, Organic 40% Less Sodium, Black Bean Vegetable Soup

1 cup (240g)

Amount per serving	Amount per serving	Amount per serving
Calories 110	**Cholesterol** 0mg	**Total Carbohydrate** 25g
Total Fat 0g	**Sodium** 480mg	Dietary Fiber 5g
Saturated Fat 0g	**Protein** 5g	Sugars 5g

Health Valley, Organic 40% Less Sodium, Corn & Vegetable Soup

1 cup (240g)

Amount per serving	Amount per serving	Amount per serving
Calories 100	**Cholesterol** 0mg	**Total Carbohydrate** 22g
Total Fat 0g	**Sodium** 460mg	Dietary Fiber 4g
Saturated Fat 0g	**Protein** 3g	Sugars 5g

Health Valley, Organic 40% Less Sodium, Minestrone Soup

1 cup (240g)

Amount per serving	Amount per serving	Amount per serving
Calories 110	**Cholesterol** 0mg	**Total Carbohydrate** 26g
Total Fat 0g	**Sodium** 470mg	Dietary Fiber 7g
Saturated Fat 0g	**Protein** 6g	Sugars 6g

Health Valley, Organic 40% Less Sodium, Split Pea & Carrots Soup

1 cup (240g)

Amount per serving	Amount per serving	Amount per serving
Calories 120	**Cholesterol** 0mg	**Total Carbohydrate** 26g
Total Fat 0g	**Sodium** 480mg	Dietary Fiber 7g
Saturated Fat 0g	**Protein** 7g	Sugars 4g

Health Valley, Organic 40% Less Sodium, Tomato Vegetable Soup

1 cup (240g)

Amount per serving	Amount per serving	Amount per serving
Calories 70	**Cholesterol** 0mg	**Total Carbohydrate** 17g
Total Fat 0g	**Sodium** 470mg	Dietary Fiber 5g
Saturated Fat 0g	**Protein** 3g	Sugars 7g

Health Valley, Organic 40% Less Sodium, Vegetable Barley Soup

1 cup (240g)

Amount per serving	Amount per serving	Amount per serving
Calories 90	**Cholesterol** 0mg	**Total Carbohydrate** 20g
Total Fat 0.5g	**Sodium** 480mg	Dietary Fiber 4g
Saturated Fat 0g	**Protein** 3g	Sugars 3g

Health Valley, Organic Chicken Noodle Soup

1 cup (240g)

Amount per serving	Amount per serving	Amount per serving
Calories 80	**Cholesterol** 15mg	**Total Carbohydrate** 11g
Total Fat 2.5g	**Sodium** 480mg	Dietary Fiber 3g
Saturated Fat 0g	**Protein** 4g	Sugars 1g

Health Valley, Organic Cream of Celery Soup

1 cup (240g)

Amount per serving	Amount per serving	Amount per serving
Calories 100	**Cholesterol** 10mg	**Total Carbohydrate** 17g
Total Fat 2g	**Sodium** 410mg	Dietary Fiber 3g
Saturated Fat 1g	**Protein** 4g	Sugars 5g

Health Valley, Organic Cream of Chicken Soup

1 cup (240g)

Amount per serving	Amount per serving	Amount per serving
Calories 110	**Cholesterol** 5mg	**Total Carbohydrate** 15g
Total Fat 3g	**Sodium** 480mg	Dietary Fiber 3g
Saturated Fat 1g	**Protein** 7g	Sugars 5g

Health Valley, Organic Cream of Mushroom Soup

1 cup (240g)

Amount per serving	Amount per serving	Amount per serving
Calories 90	**Cholesterol** 10mg	**Total Carbohydrate** 14g
Total Fat 2g	**Sodium** 480mg	Dietary Fiber 3g
Saturated Fat 1g	**Protein** 4g	Sugars 3g

Health Valley, Organic No Salt Added Black Bean Soup

1 cup (240g)

Amount per serving	Amount per serving	Amount per serving
Calories 140	**Cholesterol** 0mg	**Total Carbohydrate** 29g
Total Fat 1.5g	**Sodium** 30mg	Dietary Fiber 6g
Saturated Fat 0g	**Protein** 7g	Sugars 4g

Health Valley, Organic No Salt Added Butternut Squash Soup

1 cup (240g)

Amount per serving	Amount per serving	Amount per serving
Calories 100	**Cholesterol** <5mg	**Total Carbohydrate** 20g
Total Fat 2g	**Sodium** 75mg	Dietary Fiber 3g
Saturated Fat 0.5g	**Protein** 3g	Sugars 3g

Health Valley, Organic No Salt Added Chicken Noodle Soup

1 cup (240g)

Amount per serving	Amount per serving	Amount per serving
Calories 80	**Cholesterol** 15mg	**Total Carbohydrate** 12g
Total Fat 2.5g	**Sodium** 135mg	Dietary Fiber 3g
Saturated Fat 0g	**Protein** 5g	Sugars 1g

Health Valley, Organic No Salt Added Chicken Rice Soup

1 cup (240g)

Amount per serving	Amount per serving	Amount per serving
Calories 110	**Cholesterol** 10mg	**Total Carbohydrate** 19g
Total Fat 1.5g	**Sodium** 120mg	Dietary Fiber 3g
Saturated Fat 0g	**Protein** 5g	Sugars 1g

Health Valley, Organic No Salt Added Lentil Soup

1 cup (240g)

Amount per serving	Amount per serving	Amount per serving
Calories 140	**Cholesterol** 0mg	**Total Carbohydrate** 27g
Total Fat 1.5g	**Sodium** 30mg	Dietary Fiber 8g
Saturated Fat 0g	**Protein** 9g	Sugars 5g

Health Valley, Organic No Salt Added Minestrone Soup

1 cup (240g)

Amount per serving	Amount per serving	Amount per serving
Calories 90	**Cholesterol** 0mg	**Total Carbohydrate** 16g
Total Fat 2g	**Sodium** 50mg	Dietary Fiber 3g
Saturated Fat 0g	**Protein** 4g	Sugars 5g

Health Valley, Organic No Salt Added Mushroom Barley Soup

1 cup (240g)

Amount per serving	Amount per serving	Amount per serving
Calories 90	**Cholesterol** 0mg	**Total Carbohydrate** 15g
Total Fat 2.5g	**Sodium** 60mg	Dietary Fiber 3g
Saturated Fat 0g	**Protein** 2g	Sugars 2g

Health Valley, Organic No Salt Added Pasta Fagioli Soup

1 cup (240g)

Amount per serving	Amount per serving	Amount per serving
Calories 130	**Cholesterol** 0mg	**Total Carbohydrate** 21g
Total Fat 3g	**Sodium** 90mg	Dietary Fiber 6g
Saturated Fat 0g	**Protein** 6g	Sugars 4g

Health Valley, Organic No Salt Added Potato Leek Soup

1 cup (240g)

Amount per serving	Amount per serving	Amount per serving
Calories 100	**Cholesterol** 0mg	**Total Carbohydrate** 20g
Total Fat 2g	**Sodium** 30mg	Dietary Fiber 3g
Saturated Fat 0g	**Protein** 2g	Sugars 2g

Health Valley, Organic No Salt Added Rice Primavera Soup

1 cup (240g)

Amount per serving	Amount per serving	Amount per serving
Calories 110	**Cholesterol** 0mg	**Total Carbohydrate** 17g
Total Fat 3g	**Sodium** 135mg	Dietary Fiber 3g
Saturated Fat 0g	**Protein** 3g	Sugars 3g

Health Valley, Organic No Salt Added Split Pea Soup

1 cup (240g)

Amount per serving	Amount per serving	Amount per serving
Calories 140	**Cholesterol** 0mg	**Total Carbohydrate** 26g
Total Fat 2.5g	**Sodium** 85mg	Dietary Fiber 8g
Saturated Fat 1g	**Protein** 8g	Sugars 4g

Health Valley, Organic No Salt Added Tomato Soup

1 cup (240g)

Amount per serving	Amount per serving	Amount per serving
Calories 100	**Cholesterol** 5mg	**Total Carbohydrate** 19g
Total Fat 2.5g	**Sodium** 60mg	Dietary Fiber 3g
Saturated Fat 1g	**Protein** 1g	Sugars 13g

Health Valley, Organic No Salt Added Vegetable Soup

1 cup (240g)

Amount per serving	Amount per serving	Amount per serving
Calories 100	**Cholesterol** 0mg	**Total Carbohydrate** 18g
Total Fat 2.5g	**Sodium** 50mg	Dietary Fiber 4g
Saturated Fat 0g	**Protein** 3g	Sugars 4g

Imagine®, Natural Creations, Creamy Portobello Mushroom Soup

1 cup (240 ml)

Amount per serving	Amount per serving	Amount per serving
Calories 70	**Cholesterol** 0mg	**Total Carbohydrate** 12g
Total Fat 2.5g	**Sodium** 420mg	Dietary Fiber 1g
Saturated Fat 0g	**Protein** 2g	Sugars 1g

Imagine®, Natural Creations, Low Sodium Kosher Chicken Broth

1 cup (240 ml)

Amount per serving	Amount per serving	Amount per serving
Calories 5	**Cholesterol** >5mg	**Total Carbohydrate** 0g
Total Fat 0g	**Sodium** 140mg	Dietary Fiber 0g
Saturated Fat 0g	**Protein** <1g	Sugars 0g

Imagine®, Natural Creations, Natural Cream of Mushroom Soup

1 cup (245g)

Amount per serving	Amount per serving	Amount per serving
Calories 100	**Cholesterol** 10mg	**Total Carbohydrate** 15g
Total Fat 3.5g	**Sodium** 510mg	Dietary Fiber <1g
Saturated Fat 1.5g	**Protein** 1g	Sugars 0g

Imagine®, Natural Creations, Organic Beef Flavored Broth

1 cup (240 ml)

Amount per serving	Amount per serving	Amount per serving
Calories 20	**Cholesterol** >5mg	**Total Carbohydrate** 2g
Total Fat 1g	**Sodium** 670mg	Dietary Fiber 0g
Saturated Fat 0g	**Protein** 1g	Sugars >1g

Imagine®, Natural Creations, Organic Beef Flavored Cooking Stock

1 cup (240 ml)

Amount per serving	Amount per serving	Amount per serving
Calories 15	**Cholesterol** 0mg	**Total Carbohydrate** 1g
Total Fat 0g	**Sodium** 620mg	Dietary Fiber 0g
Saturated Fat 0g	**Protein** 2g	Sugars 0g

Imagine®, Natural Creations, Organic Beef Low Sodium Cooking Stock

1 cup (240 ml)

Amount per serving	Amount per serving	Amount per serving
Calories 10	**Cholesterol** 0mg	**Total Carbohydrate** <1g
Total Fat 0g	**Sodium** 140mg	Dietary Fiber 0g
Saturated Fat 0g	**Protein** 2g	Sugars <1g

Imagine®, Natural Creations, Organic Broccoli Soup

1 cup (240 ml)

Amount per serving	Amount per serving	Amount per serving
Calories 70	**Cholesterol** 0mg	**Total Carbohydrate** 12g
Total Fat 1.5g	**Sodium** 550mg	Dietary Fiber 2g
Saturated Fat 0g	**Protein** 2g	Sugars 1g

Imagine®, Natural Creations, Organic Chicken & Dumplings Soup

1 cup (245g)

Amount per serving	Amount per serving	Amount per serving
Calories 130	**Cholesterol** 20mg	**Total Carbohydrate** 18g
Total Fat 4.5g	**Sodium** 530mg	Dietary Fiber 1g
Saturated Fat 2g	**Protein** 5g	Sugars 1g

Imagine®, Natural Creations, Organic Chicken Cooking Stock

1 cup (240 ml)

Amount per serving	Amount per serving	Amount per serving
Calories 10	**Cholesterol** 0mg	**Total Carbohydrate** <1g
Total Fat 0g	**Sodium** 500mg	Dietary Fiber 0g
Saturated Fat 0g	**Protein** <1g	Sugars <1g

Imagine®, Natural Creations, Organic Chicken Corn Tortilla Soup

1 cup (245g)

Amount per serving	Amount per serving	Amount per serving
Calories 130	**Cholesterol** 5mg	**Total Carbohydrate** 18g
Total Fat 3g	**Sodium** 480mg	Dietary Fiber 3g
Saturated Fat 1g	**Protein** 7g	Sugars 2g

Imagine®, Natural Creations, Organic Chicken Low Sodium Cooking Stock

1 cup (240 ml)

Amount per serving	Amount per serving	Amount per serving
Calories 10	**Cholesterol** 0mg	**Total Carbohydrate** <1g
Total Fat 0g	**Sodium** 140mg	Dietary Fiber 0g
Saturated Fat 0g	**Protein** <1g	Sugars <1g

Imagine®, Natural Creations, Organic Classic Corn Chowder Soup

1 cup (245g)

Amount per serving	Amount per serving	Amount per serving
Calories 130	**Cholesterol** 15mg	**Total Carbohydrate** 20g
Total Fat 5g	**Sodium** 650mg	Dietary Fiber 2g
Saturated Fat 2g	**Protein** 3g	Sugars 3g

Imagine®, Natural Creations, Organic Creamy Acorn Squash & Mango Soup

1 cup (240 ml)

Amount per serving	Amount per serving	Amount per serving
Calories 70	**Cholesterol** 0mg	**Total Carbohydrate** 15g
Total Fat 1g	**Sodium** 450mg	Dietary Fiber 2g
Saturated Fat 0g	**Protein** 1g	Sugars 6g

Imagine®, Natural Creations, Organic Creamy Butternut Squash Soup

1 cup (240 ml)

Amount per serving	Amount per serving	Amount per serving
Calories 100	**Cholesterol** 0mg	**Total Carbohydrate** 20g
Total Fat 1.5g	**Sodium** 440mg	Dietary Fiber 2g
Saturated Fat 0g	**Protein** 1g	Sugars 7g

Imagine®, Natural Creations, Organic Creamy Carrot Almond Soup

1 cup (240 ml)

Amount per serving	Amount per serving	Amount per serving
Calories 90	**Cholesterol** 0mg	**Total Carbohydrate** 13g
Total Fat 4g	**Sodium** 600mg	Dietary Fiber 3g
Saturated Fat 0g	**Protein** 2g	Sugars 4g

Imagine®, Natural Creations, Organic Creamy Celery Soup

1 cup (240 ml)

Amount per serving	Amount per serving	Amount per serving
Calories 70	**Cholesterol** 0mg	**Total Carbohydrate** 11g
Total Fat 1.5g	**Sodium** 480mg	Dietary Fiber 2g
Saturated Fat 0g	**Protein** 3g	Sugars <1g

Imagine®, Natural Creations, Organic Creamy Golden Beet Soup

1 cup (240 ml)

Amount per serving	Amount per serving	Amount per serving
Calories 50	**Cholesterol** 0mg	**Total Carbohydrate** 11g
Total Fat 0g	**Sodium** 540mg	Dietary Fiber 2g
Saturated Fat 0g	**Protein** 1g	Sugars 3g

Imagine®, Natural Creations, Organic Creamy Potato Leek Soup

1 cup (40 ml)

Amount per serving	Amount per serving	Amount per serving
Calories 80	**Cholesterol** 0mg	**Total Carbohydrate** 13g
Total Fat 2.5g	**Sodium** 440mg	Dietary Fiber 2g
Saturated Fat 0g	**Protein** 2g	Sugars 1g

Imagine®, Natural Creations, Organic Creamy Pumpkin Soup

1 cup (240 ml)

Amount per serving	Amount per serving	Amount per serving
Calories 60	**Cholesterol** 0mg	**Total Carbohydrate** 14g
Total Fat 0.5g	**Sodium** 590mg	Dietary Fiber NA
Saturated Fat 0g	**Protein** <1g	Sugars 5g

Imagine®, Natural Creations, Organic Creamy Red Bliss Potato & Roasted Garlic Soup

1 cup (240 ml)

Amount per serving	Amount per serving	Amount per serving
Calories 90	**Cholesterol** 0mg	**Total Carbohydrate** 17g
Total Fat 2.5g	**Sodium** 220mg	Dietary Fiber 2g
Saturated Fat 0g	**Protein** 2g	Sugars 2g

Imagine®, Natural Creations, Organic Creamy Sweet Corn Soup

1 cup (240 ml)

Amount per serving	Amount per serving	Amount per serving
Calories 110	**Cholesterol** 0mg	**Total Carbohydrate** 23g
Total Fat 1.5g	**Sodium** 510mg	Dietary Fiber 3g
Saturated Fat 1g	**Protein** 3g	Sugars 3g

Imagine®, Natural Creations, Organic Creamy Sweet Potato Soup

1 cup (240 ml)

Amount per serving	Amount per serving	Amount per serving
Calories 110	**Cholesterol** 0mg	**Total Carbohydrate** 23g
Total Fat 1.5g	**Sodium** 400mg	Dietary Fiber 1g
Saturated Fat 0g	**Protein** 2g	Sugars 2g

Imagine®, Natural Creations, Organic Creamy Sweet Potato Soup

1 cup (240 ml)

Amount per serving	Amount per serving	Amount per serving
Calories 110	**Cholesterol** 0mg	**Total Carbohydrate** 23g
Total Fat 1.5g	**Sodium** 400mg	Dietary Fiber 1g
Saturated Fat 0g	**Protein** 2g	Sugars 2g

Imagine®, Natural Creations, Organic Creamy Tomato Basil Soup

1 cup (240 ml)

Amount per serving	Amount per serving	Amount per serving
Calories 110	**Cholesterol** 0mg	**Total Carbohydrate** 21g
Total Fat 2g	**Sodium** 410mg	Dietary Fiber 2g
Saturated Fat 0g	**Protein** 3g	Sugars 10g

Imagine®, Natural Creations, Organic Creamy Tomato Soup

1 cup (240 ml)

Amount per serving	Amount per serving	Amount per serving
Calories 100	**Cholesterol** 0mg	**Total Carbohydrate** 20g
Total Fat 1.5g	**Sodium** 440mg	Dietary Fiber 2g
Saturated Fat 0g	**Protein** 1g	Sugars 7g

Imagine®, Natural Creations, Organic Free Range Chicken Broth

1 cup (240 ml)

Amount per serving	Amount per serving	Amount per serving
Calories 20	**Cholesterol** <5mg	**Total Carbohydrate** 2g
Total Fat 0.5g	**Sodium** 740mg	Dietary Fiber 0g
Saturated Fat 0g	**Protein** 1g	Sugars <1g

Imagine®, Natural Creations, Organic Hearty Beef Barley Soup

1 cup (245g)

Amount per serving	Amount per serving	Amount per serving
Calories 110	**Cholesterol** 10mg	**Total Carbohydrate** 19g
Total Fat 1.5g	**Sodium** 480mg	Dietary Fiber 2g
Saturated Fat 0.5g	**Protein** 5g	Sugars 2g

Imagine®, Natural Creations, Organic Homestyle Chicken Noodle Soup
1 cup (250g)

Amount per serving | Amount per serving | Amount per serving

Calories 90
Total Fat 2g
 Saturated Fat 0g

Cholesterol 15mg
Sodium 730mg
Protein NA

Total Carbohydrate 12g
 Dietary Fiber <1g
 Sugars <1g

Imagine®, Natural Creations, Organic Italian Style Wedding Soup
1 cup (245g)

Amount per serving | Amount per serving | Amount per serving

Calories 150
Total Fat 4.5g
 Saturated Fat 2g

Cholesterol 10mg
Sodium 480mg
Protein 7g

Total Carbohydrate 20g
 Dietary Fiber 4g
 Sugars 3g

Imagine®, Natural Creations, Organic Italian Vegetables and Beans Soup
1 cup (245g)

Amount per serving | Amount per serving | Amount per serving

Calories 120
Total Fat 1.5g
 Saturated Fat 0g

Cholesterol 0mg
Sodium 590mg
Protein 5g

Total Carbohydrate 24g
 Dietary Fiber 7g
 Sugars 5g

Imagine®, Natural Creations, Organic Kosher Chicken Broth
1 cup (240 ml)

Amount per serving | Amount per serving | Amount per serving

Calories 5
Total Fat 0g
 Saturated Fat 0g

Cholesterol 0mg
Sodium NA
Protein <1g

Total Carbohydrate 0g
 Dietary Fiber 0g
 Sugars 0g

Imagine®, Natural Creations, Organic Light in Sodium Creamy Butternut Squash Soup
1 cup (240 ml)

Amount per serving | Amount per serving | Amount per serving

Calories 100
Total Fat 1.5g
 Saturated Fat 0g

Cholesterol 0mg
Sodium 440mg
Protein 1g

Total Carbohydrate 20g
 Dietary Fiber 2g
 Sugars 7g

Imagine®, Natural Creations, Organic Light in Sodium Creamy Garden Broccoli Soup
1 cup (240 ml)

Amount per serving | Amount per serving | Amount per serving

Calories 70
Total Fat 1.5g
 Saturated Fat 0g

Cholesterol 0mg
Sodium 190mg
Protein 2g

Total Carbohydrate 12g
 Dietary Fiber 2g
 Sugars 1g

Imagine®, Natural Creations, Organic Light in Sodium Creamy Harvest Corn Soup

1 cup (240 ml)

Amount per serving	Amount per serving	Amount per serving
Calories 90	**Cholesterol** 0mg	**Total Carbohydrate** 17g
Total Fat 2.5g	**Sodium** 190mg	Dietary Fiber 2g
Saturated Fat 0g	**Protein** 2g	Sugars 3g

Imagine®, Natural Creations, Organic Light in Sodium Creamy Sweet Potato Soup

1 cup (240 ml)

Amount per serving	Amount per serving	Amount per serving
Calories 110	**Cholesterol** 0mg	**Total Carbohydrate** 23g
Total Fat 1g	**Sodium** 140mg	Dietary Fiber 3g
Saturated Fat 0g	**Protein** 2g	Sugars 7g

Imagine®, Natural Creations, Organic Light in Sodium Creamy Tomato Soup

1 cup (240 ml)

Amount per serving	Amount per serving	Amount per serving
Calories 90	**Cholesterol** 0mg	**Total Carbohydrate** 17g
Total Fat 1.5g	**Sodium** 310mg	Dietary Fiber 2g
Saturated Fat 0g	**Protein** 2g	Sugars 10g

Imagine®, Natural Creations, Organic Loaded Baked Potato Soup

1 cup (245g)

Amount per serving	Amount per serving	Amount per serving
Calories 120	**Cholesterol** 15mg	**Total Carbohydrate** 18g
Total Fat 5g	**Sodium** 610mg	Dietary Fiber 1g
Saturated Fat 2.5g	**Protein** 3g	Sugars <1g

Imagine®, Natural Creations, Organic Low Sodium Beef Flavored Broth

1 cup (240 ml)

Amount per serving	Amount per serving	Amount per serving
Calories 20	**Cholesterol** <5mg	**Total Carbohydrate** 2g
Total Fat 1g	**Sodium** 125mg	Dietary Fiber 0g
Saturated Fat 0g	**Protein** 1g	Sugars <1g

Imagine®, Natural Creations, Organic Low Sodium Free Range Chicken Broth

1 cup (240 ml)

Amount per serving	Amount per serving	Amount per serving
Calories 20	**Cholesterol** <5mg	**Total Carbohydrate** 2g
Total Fat 0.5g	**Sodium** 115mg	Dietary Fiber 0g
Saturated Fat 0g	**Protein** 1g	Sugars <1g

Imagine®, Natural Creations, Organic Low Sodium Vegetable Broth

1 cup (240 ml)

Amount per serving	Amount per serving	Amount per serving
Calories 20	Cholesterol 0mg	Total Carbohydrate 4g
Total Fat 0g	Sodium 140mg	Dietary Fiber <1g
Saturated Fat NA	Protein <1g	Sugars 2g

Imagine®, Natural Creations, Organic Low Sodium Vegetarian No-Chicken Broth

1 cup (240 ml)

Amount per serving	Amount per serving	Amount per serving
Calories 10	Cholesterol 0mg	Total Carbohydrate 2g
Total Fat 0g	Sodium 140mg	Dietary Fiber 0g
Saturated Fat 0g	Protein 0g	Sugars <1g

Imagine®, Natural Creations, Organic Moroccan Chickpea & Carrot Soup

1 cup (245g)

Amount per serving	Amount per serving	Amount per serving
Calories 100	Cholesterol 0mg	Total Carbohydrate 21g
Total Fat 1g	Sodium 480mg	Dietary Fiber 3g
Saturated Fat 0g	Protein 2g	Sugars 7g

Imagine®, Natural Creations, Organic Potato Quinoa and Spinach Soup

1 cup (245g)

Amount per serving	Amount per serving	Amount per serving
Calories 100	Cholesterol 10mg	Total Carbohydrate 16g
Total Fat 3.5g	Sodium 600mg	Dietary Fiber 1g
Saturated Fat 1.5g	Protein 2g	Sugars <1g

Imagine®, Natural Creations, Organic Savory Black Bean Soup

1 cup (245g)

Amount per serving	Amount per serving	Amount per serving
Calories 140	Cholesterol 0mg	Total Carbohydrate 29g
Total Fat 0g	Sodium 570mg	Dietary Fiber 8g
Saturated Fat 0g	Protein 7g	Sugars 6g

Imagine®, Natural Creations, Organic Split Pea Soup

1 cup (250g)

Amount per serving	Amount per serving	Amount per serving
Calories 180	Cholesterol 5mg	Total Carbohydrate 30g
Total Fat 2.5g	Sodium 760mg	Dietary Fiber 9g
Saturated Fat 1g	Protein 9g	Sugars 5g

Imagine®, Natural Creations, Organic Sweet Pea Soup

1 cup (240 ml)

Amount per serving	Amount per serving	Amount per serving
Calories 80	Cholesterol 0mg	Total Carbohydrate 14g
Total Fat 1.5g	Sodium 570mg	Dietary Fiber 3g
Saturated Fat 0g	Protein 4g	Sugars 4g

Imagine®, Natural Creations, Organic Tomato Bisque Soup

1 cup (245g)

Amount per serving	Amount per serving	Amount per serving
Calories 80	Cholesterol 10mg	Total Carbohydrate 15g
Total Fat 2.5g	Sodium 630mg	Dietary Fiber 1g
Saturated Fat 1.5g	Protein 2g	Sugars 8g

Imagine®, Natural Creations, Organic Vegetable Broth

1 cup (240 ml)

Amount per serving	Amount per serving	Amount per serving
Calories 20	Cholesterol 0mg	Total Carbohydrate 4g
Total Fat 0g	Sodium 640mg	Dietary Fiber >1g
Saturated Fat 0g	Protein >1g	Sugars 2g

Imagine®, Natural Creations, Organic Vegetable Cooking Stock

1 cup (240 ml)

Amount per serving	Amount per serving	Amount per serving
Calories 20	Cholesterol 0mg	Total Carbohydrate 4g
Total Fat 0g	Sodium 490mg	Dietary Fiber <1g
Saturated Fat 0g	Protein <1g	Sugars 3g

Imagine®, Natural Creations, Organic Vegetarian No-Chicken Broth

1 cup (240 ml)

Amount per serving	Amount per serving	Amount per serving
Calories 15	Cholesterol 0mg	Total Carbohydrate 2g
Total Fat 0g	Sodium 520mg	Dietary Fiber 0g
Saturated Fat 0g	Protein 0g	Sugars <1g

Imagine®, Natural Creations, Organic White Bean & Kale Soup

1 cup (245g)

Amount per serving	Amount per serving	Amount per serving
Calories 110	Cholesterol 0mg	Total Carbohydrate 20g
Total Fat 1g	Sodium 480mg	Dietary Fiber 4g
Saturated Fat 0g	Protein 4g	Sugars 1g

Muir Glen Organic, Chicken & Wild Rice Soup

1 cup (243g)

Amount per serving	Amount per serving	Amount per serving
Calories 70	**Cholesterol** 10mg	**Total Carbohydrate** 10g
Total Fat 1.5g	**Sodium** 710mg	Dietary Fiber 1g
Saturated Fat 0.5g	**Protein** 4g	Sugars 1g

Muir Glen Organic, Chicken Noodle Soup

1 cup (244g)

Amount per serving	Amount per serving	Amount per serving
Calories 70	**Cholesterol** 10mg	**Total Carbohydrate** 10g
Total Fat 1.5g	**Sodium** 800mg	Dietary Fiber 1g
Saturated Fat 0.5g	**Protein** 4g	Sugars 1g

Muir Glen Organic, Chicken Tortilla Soup

1 cup

Amount per serving	Amount per serving	Amount per serving
Calories 120	**Cholesterol** 10mg	**Total Carbohydrate** 17g
Total Fat 1.5g	**Sodium** 830mg	Dietary Fiber 3g
Saturated Fat 0.5g	**Protein** 6g	Sugars 2g

Muir Glen Organic, Classic Minestrone Soup

1 cup (245g)

Amount per serving	Amount per serving	Amount per serving
Calories 110	**Cholesterol** 0mg	**Total Carbohydrate** 19g
Total Fat 1.5g	**Sodium** 960mg	Dietary Fiber 5g
Saturated Fat 0.5g	**Protein** 4g	Sugars 3g

Muir Glen Organic, Creamy Tomato Bisque Soup

1 cup (253g)

Amount per serving	Amount per serving	Amount per serving
Calories 170	**Cholesterol** 15mg	**Total Carbohydrate** 26g
Total Fat 6g	**Sodium** 840mg	Dietary Fiber 2g
Saturated Fat 2g	**Protein** 4g	Sugars 16g

Muir Glen Organic, Garden Vegetable Soup

1 cup (245g)

Amount per serving	Amount per serving	Amount per serving
Calories 80	**Cholesterol** 0mg	**Total Carbohydrate** 14g
Total Fat 0.5g	**Sodium** 960mg	Dietary Fiber 3g
Saturated Fat 0g	**Protein** 3g	Sugars 5g

Muir Glen Organic, Homestyle Split Pea Soup

1 cup (248g)

Amount per serving	Amount per serving	Amount per serving
Calories 170	**Cholesterol** 0mg	**Total Carbohydrate** 35g
Total Fat 0.5g	**Sodium** 900mg	Dietary Fiber 5g
Saturated Fat 0g	**Protein** 10g	Sugars 4g

Muir Glen Organic, Reduced Sodium Chicken Noodle Soup

1 cup (246g)

Amount per serving	Amount per serving	Amount per serving
Calories 90	**Cholesterol** 15mg	**Total Carbohydrate** 11g
Total Fat 2g	**Sodium** 480mg	Dietary Fiber 1g
Saturated Fat 0.5g	**Protein** 7g	Sugars 1g

Muir Glen Organic, Reduced Sodium Garden Vegetable Soup

1 cup (246g)

Amount per serving	Amount per serving	Amount per serving
Calories 80	**Cholesterol** 0mg	**Total Carbohydrate** 17g
Total Fat 0.5g	**Sodium** 480mg	Dietary Fiber 3g
Saturated Fat 0g	**Protein** 3g	Sugars 5g

Muir Glen Organic, Savory Lentil Soup

1 cup (249g)

Amount per serving	Amount per serving	Amount per serving
Calories 130	**Cholesterol** 0mg	**Total Carbohydrate** 23g
Total Fat 1.5g	**Sodium** 950mg	Dietary Fiber 3g
Saturated Fat 0.5g	**Protein** 6g	Sugars 2g

Muir Glen Organic, Southwest Black Bean Soup

1 cup (250g)

Amount per serving	Amount per serving	Amount per serving
Calories 130	**Cholesterol** 0mg	**Total Carbohydrate** 25g
Total Fat 0.5g	**Sodium** 680mg	Dietary Fiber 8g
Saturated Fat 0g	**Protein** 7g	Sugars 4g

Muir Glen Organic, Tomato Basil Soup

1 cup (250g)

Amount per serving	Amount per serving	Amount per serving
Calories 130	**Cholesterol** 0mg	**Total Carbohydrate** 25g
Total Fat 1.5g	**Sodium** 880mg	Dietary Fiber 2g
Saturated Fat 0.5g	**Protein** 5g	Sugars 19g

Pacific, Organic Beef Broth

8 fl oz

Amount per serving	Amount per serving	Amount per serving
Calories 20	Cholesterol 5mg	Total Carbohydrate 1g
Total Fat 1g	Sodium 570mg	Dietary Fiber 0g
Saturated Fat 0g	Protein 2g	Sugars 1g

Pacific, Organic Butternut Squash Bisque

1 cup

Amount per serving	Amount per serving	Amount per serving
Calories 110	Cholesterol 10mg	Total Carbohydrate 18g
Total Fat 3.5g	Sodium 510mg	Dietary Fiber 4g
Saturated Fat 1.5g	Protein 2g	Sugars 5g

Pacific, Organic Chicken and Wild Rice Soup

1 cup

Amount per serving	Amount per serving	Amount per serving
Calories 220	Cholesterol 10mg	Total Carbohydrate 13g
Total Fat 4g	Sodium 660mg	Dietary Fiber 2g
Saturated Fat 1g	Protein 5g	Sugars 1g

Pacific, Organic Cream of Chicken Condensed Soup

1/2 cup

Amount per serving	Amount per serving	Amount per serving
Calories 90	Cholesterol 15mg	Total Carbohydrate 10g
Total Fat 3.5g	Sodium 850mg	Dietary Fiber NA
Saturated Fat 2g	Protein 4g	Sugars NA

Pacific, Organic Cream of Mushroom Condensed Soup

1/2 cup

Amount per serving	Amount per serving	Amount per serving
Calories 100	Cholesterol 10mg	Total Carbohydrate 18g
Total Fat 2.5g	Sodium 740mg	Dietary Fiber 1g
Saturated Fat 1.5g	Protein 2g	Sugars 2.9g

Pacific, Organic Creamy Butternut Squash Soup

8 fl oz

Amount per serving	Amount per serving	Amount per serving
Calories 90	Cholesterol 0mg	Total Carbohydrate 17g
Total Fat 2g	Sodium 550mg	Dietary Fiber 3g
Saturated Fat 0g	Protein 2g	Sugars 4g

Pacific, Organic Creamy Tomato Soup

8 fl oz

Amount per serving	Amount per serving	Amount per serving
Calories 100	**Cholesterol** 10mg	**Total Carbohydrate** 16g
Total Fat 2g	**Sodium** 750mg	Dietary Fiber 1g
Saturated Fat 1.5g	**Protein** 5g	Sugars 12g

Pacific, Organic Free Range Chicken Broth

8 fl oz

Amount per serving	Amount per serving	Amount per serving
Calories 10	**Cholesterol** 0mg	**Total Carbohydrate** 1g
Total Fat 0g	**Sodium** 570mg	Dietary Fiber 0g
Saturated Fat 0g	**Protein** 1g	Sugars 1g

Pacific, Organic Free Range Low Sodium Chicken Broth

8 fl oz

Amount per serving	Amount per serving	Amount per serving
Calories 15	**Cholesterol** 0mg	**Total Carbohydrate** 1g
Total Fat 0g	**Sodium** 70mg	Dietary Fiber 0g
Saturated Fat 0g	**Protein** 2g	Sugars 0g

Pacific, Organic French Onion Soup

8 fl oz

Amount per serving	Amount per serving	Amount per serving
Calories 30	**Cholesterol** 0mg	**Total Carbohydrate** 5g
Total Fat 1g	**Sodium** 720mg	Dietary Fiber 0g
Saturated Fat 0.5g	**Protein** 1g	Sugars 3g

Pacific, Organic Hearty Tomato Bisque

1 cup

Amount per serving	Amount per serving	Amount per serving
Calories 150	**Cholesterol** 30mg	**Total Carbohydrate** 17g
Total Fat 9g	**Sodium** 750mg	Dietary Fiber 2g
Saturated Fat 5g	**Protein** 2g	Sugars 10g

Pacific, Organic Light Sodium Creamy Butternut Squash Soup

8 fl oz

Amount per serving	Amount per serving	Amount per serving
Calories 90	**Cholesterol** 0mg	**Total Carbohydrate** 17g
Total Fat 2g	**Sodium** 280mg	Dietary Fiber 3g
Saturated Fat 0g	**Protein** 2g	Sugars 4g

Pacific, Organic Light Sodium Creamy Tomato Soup

8 fl oz

Amount per serving	Amount per serving	Amount per serving
Calories 100	**Cholesterol** 10mg	**Total Carbohydrate** 16g
Total Fat 2g	**Sodium** 380mg	Dietary Fiber 1g
Saturated Fat 1.5g	**Protein** 5g	Sugars 12g

Pacific, Organic Light Sodium Roasted Red Pepper & Tomato Soup

8 fl oz

Amount per serving	Amount per serving	Amount per serving
Calories 110	**Cholesterol** 10mg	**Total Carbohydrate** 16g
Total Fat 0g	**Sodium** 360mg	Dietary Fiber 1g
Saturated Fat 1.5g	**Protein** 5g	Sugars 12g

Pacific, Organic Low Sodium Vegetable Broth

0 fl oz

Amount per serving	Amount per serving	Amount per serving
Calories 15	**Cholesterol** 0mg	**Total Carbohydrate** 3g
Total Fat 0g	**Sodium** 530mg	Dietary Fiber 1g
Saturated Fat 0g	**Protein** 0g	Sugars 2g

Pacific, Organic Mushroom Broth

8 fl oz

Amount per serving	Amount per serving	Amount per serving
Calories 5	**Cholesterol** 0mg	**Total Carbohydrate** 1g
Total Fat 0g	**Sodium** 530mg	Dietary Fiber 0g
Saturated Fat 0g	**Protein** 0g	Sugars 0g

Pacific, Organic Roasted Red Pepper & Tomato Bisque

1 cup

Amount per serving	Amount per serving	Amount per serving
Calories 110	**Cholesterol** 10mg	**Total Carbohydrate** 16g
Total Fat 2g	**Sodium** 720mg	Dietary Fiber 1g
Saturated Fat 1.5g	**Protein** 5g	Sugars 12g

Pacific, Organic Roasted Red Pepper & Tomato Soup

8 fl oz

Amount per serving	Amount per serving	Amount per serving
Calories 110	**Cholesterol** 10mg	**Total Carbohydrate** 16g
Total Fat 2g	**Sodium** 720mg	Dietary Fiber 1g
Saturated Fat 1.5g	**Protein** 5g	Sugars 12g

Pacific, Organic Vegetable Broth

8 fl oz

Amount per serving	Amount per serving	Amount per serving
Calories 15	**Cholesterol** 0mg	**Total Carbohydrate** 3g
Total Fat 0g	**Sodium** 530mg	Dietary Fiber 1g
Saturated Fat 0g	**Protein** 0g	Sugars 2g

Swanson®, Certified Organic Chicken Broth

1 cup

Amount per serving	Amount per serving	Amount per serving
Calories 15	**Cholesterol** 0mg	**Total Carbohydrate** 1g
Total Fat 0.5g	**Sodium** 550mg	Dietary Fiber 0g
Saturated Fat 0g	**Protein** 1g	Sugars 1g

Swanson®, Certified Organic Vegetable Broth

1 cup

Amount per serving	Amount per serving	Amount per serving
Calories 15	**Cholesterol** 0mg	**Total Carbohydrate** 3g
Total Fat 0g	**Sodium** 530mg	Dietary Fiber 0g
Saturated Fat 0g	**Protein** 0g	Sugars 2g

Appendix

Organic Organizations and Associations

CCOF Foundation
2155 Delaware Avenue, Suite 150
Santa Cruz, CA 95060
Phone: (831) 423-2263
Fax: (831) 423-4528
Email: *ccof@ccof.org*
Website: *www.ccof.org*

Certified Naturally Grown
540 President Street, Third Floor
Brooklyn, NY 11215
Phone: (845) 687-2058
Email: *info@naturallygrown.org*
Website: *www.naturallygrown.org*

Demeter Certified Biodynamic
Demeter Association, Inc.
P.O. Box 1390
Philomath, OR 97370
Phone: (541) 929-7148
Website *www.demeter-usa.org*

Environmental Working Group
1436 U Street NW, Suite 100
Washington, DC 20009
Phone: (202) 667-6982
Website: *www.ewg.org*

Fairtrade International (FLO)
Bonner Talweg 177
53129 Bonn, Germany
Phone: +49 228 949230
Fax: +49 228 2421713
Email: *info@fairtrade.net*
Website: *www.fairtrade.net*

Fair Trade USA
1500 Broadway, Suite 400
Oakland, CA 94612
Phone: (510) 663-5260
Fax: (510) 663-5264
Website: *www.fairtradeusa.org*

Food Alliance
P.O. Box 86457
Portland, OR 97286
Email: *info@foodalliance.org*
Website: *www.foodalliance.org*

Humane Farm Animal Care
P.O. Box 727
Herndon, VA 20172
Phone: (703) 435-3883
Email: *info@certifiedhumane.org*
Website: *www.certifiedhumane.org*

International Federation of Organic Agriculture Movements (IFOAM)
Head Office
Charles-de-Gaulle-Str. 5
53113 Bonn, Germany
Phone: +49-228-92650-10
Fax: +49-228-92650-99
Email: *headoffice@ifoam.org*
Website: *www.ifoam.org*

Marine Stewardship Council
MSC Regional Office – Americas
2110 North Pacific Street, Suite 102
Seattle, WA 98103
Website: *www.msc.org*

Non GMO Project
1200 Harris Avenue, Suite #305
Bellingham, WA 98225
Phone: (877) 358-9240
Fax: (866) 272-8710
Email: *info@nongmoproject.org*
Website: *www.nongmoproject.org*

Northeast Organic Farming Association
168 Fairview Lane
Portsmouth, RI 02871
Email: *web@nofa.org*
Website: *www.nofa.org*

Oregon Tilth
2525 SE 3rd Street
Corvallis, OR 97333
(503) 378-0690
1-877-378-0690
Farmer Hotline: (503) 581-8102
Email: *organic@tilth.org*
Website: *www.tilth.org*

The Organic Center
The Hall of the States
444 North Capitol Street NW,
Suite 445A
Washington, D.C. 20001
Phone: (802) 275-3897
Email: *info@organic-center.org*
Website: *www.organic-center.org*

Organic.org
Email: *info@organic.org*
Website: *www.organic.org*

Organic Consumers Association (OCA)
6771 South Silver Hill Drive
Finland, MN 55603
Phone: (218) 226-4164
Fax: 218-353-7652
Website: *www.organicconsumers.org*

Organic Trade Association
28 Vernon Street, Suite 413
Brattleboro, VT 05301
Phone: (802) 275-3800
Fax: (802) 275-3801
Website: *www.ota.com*

Quality Assurance International (QAI) Certified Organic
9191 Towne Centre Drive, Suite 200
San Diego, CA 92122
Email: *consumer@qai-inc.com*
Website: *www.qai-inc.com*

Rainforest Alliance
233 Broadway, 28th Floor
New York, NY 10279
Phone: (212) 677-1900
Fax: (212) 677-2187
Email: *info@ra.org*
Website: *www.rainforest-alliance.org*

SCS Global Services
2000 Powell Street, Suite 600
Emeryville, CA 94608
Toll Free: 1 (800) 326-3228
Email: info@SCSglobalservices.com
Website: www.scsglobalservi ces.com

USDA Organic
U.S. Department of Agriculture
1400 Independence Avenue, S.W.
Washington, DC 20250
Information Hotline: (202) 720-2791
Website: www.usda.gov/wps/portal/usda/
usdahome?navid=organic-agriculture

US Department of Agriculture
Economic Research Service
355 E Street SW
Washington, DC 20024-3221
Information Hotline: (202) 720-2791
Website: www.www.usda.gov/wps/por
tal/usda/usdahome

The Whole Grains Council
Oldways
266 Beacon Street
Boston, MA 02116 USA
Phone: (617) 421-5500
Fax: (617) 421-5511
Email: cynthia@oldwayspt.org
Website: www.wholegrainscouncil.org

Online Resources

Healthy Eating on the Run
www.healthyeatingontherun.com/
natural-and-organic-food.html

Local Harvest
www.localharvest.org

Living Green Magazine
www.livinggreenmag.com/2012/01/13/
food-health/organic-food-coupons-
online-resources-help-you-eat-healthy-on-
the-cheap-by-richard-kujawski

**Midwest Organic & Sustainable
Education Service (MOSES)**
www.mosesorganic.org

Natural and Organic Choices
www.natural-and-organic-
choices.com/organic-food.html

Organic Eating.com
www.organiceating.com

OrganicFoodDirectory.com
www.organicfooddirectory.org

Organic Food for Everyone
www.organic-food-for-everyone.com/
organic-food-store.html

Organic Guide
www.organicguide.com

Organic.org
www.organic.org

The Organic Pages.com
www.theorganicpages.com/topo/index.html

**United States Department of
Agriculture National Agricultural
Library**
www.nal.usda.gov/afsic/pubs/ofp/
orgfind.shtml

Organic Food Companies

365 Organics
P.O. Box 1337
Zephyr Cove, NV 89448
Phone: (805) 669-7266
Email: info@365-organics.com
Website: *www.wholefoodsmarket.com/
about-our-products/product-lines/365-
everyday-value*

Allegro Coffee Company
12799 Claude Court
Thornton, CO 80241
Phone: (303) 444-4844
Toll Free: (800) 666-4869
Customer Service: (800) 530-3995
Fax: (303) 920-5468
Fax (Toll Free): (800) 530-3993
Websites: *www.allegrocoffee.com;
www.allegrocoffee.com/shop/tea*

Alter Eco
2339 Third Street, Suite 70
San Francisco, CA 94107
Phone: (415) 701-1212
Fax: (415) 701-1213
Company has an online contact form
Website: *www.alterecofoods.com*

Arora Creations, Inc.
469 Clinton Avenue, Suite 1
Brooklyn, NY 11238
Phone: (347) 335-0972
Email: *info@aroracreations.com*
Website: *www.aroracreations.com*

**Maurice A. Aueberbach, Inc.
(Auerpak)**
117 Seaview Drive
Secaucus, NJ 07094
Phone: (201) 807-9292
Fax: (201) 807-9596
Website: *www.auerpak.com*

B&M, Inc. (Red Monkey Products)
Brinkhoff & Monoson, Inc.
1206 Industrial Park Drive
Mount Veron, MO 65712
Phone: (417) 466-9109
Website: *www.redmonkeyfoods.com*

Barbara's Bakery
300 Nickerson Road
Marlboro, MA 01752
Phone: (800) 343-0590
Website: *www.barbara.com*

Baugher Ranch Organics
7030 County Road 25
Orland, CA 95963
Email: *brorganics@msn.com*
Website: *www.bro-almonds.com*

Best Organics, Inc.
Phone: (303) 499-6742
(Monday–Friday, 9am–5pm MT)
Website: *www.americabestorganics.com*

Beretta Organic Farms, Inc.
Etobicoke, Ontario, Canada
Phone: (416) 674-5609, ext. 230
Email: *lho@berettafarms.com*
Website: *www.berettafamilyfarms.com*

Betty Lou's Just Great Stuff
750 SE Booth Bend Road
McMinnville, OR 97128
Phone: (503) 434-5205
Toll Free: (800) 242-5205
Company has an online contact form
Website: www.bettylousinc.com

Bioitalia Distribuzione S.r.l.
Via Giuseppe Garibaldi
Pollena Trocchia
Napoli
+39 081 5302305
Company has an online contact form
Website: www.bioitalia.it/en/organic

Bionatura
P.O. Box 98
North Franklin, CT 06254
Phone: (860) 642-6996
Fax: (860) 642-6990
Email: info@bionaturae.com
Website: www.bionaturae.com

Blake's All Natural Food
178 Silk Farm Road
Concord, NH 03301
Phone: (603) 225-3532
Email: info@blakesallnatural.com
Website: www.blakesallnatural.com

Blue Marble
196 Court Street
Brooklyn NY 11201
Phone: (347) 384-2100
World Headquarters:
Phone: (718) 858-5551
Email: thescoop@bluemarbleicecream.com
Website: www.bluemarbleicecream.com

Bragg Live Food, Inc.
Box 7
Santa Barbara, CA 93102
Phone: (800) 446-1990
Phone (Local): (805) 968-1020
Fax: (805) 968-1001
Email: info@bragg.com
Website: www.bragg.com

Cal Naturale Svelte
Customer Service
Phone: (877) 941-9311
Email: contactus@sveltebrand.com
Website: www.drinksvelte.com

Campomar Natura
Produced by **Campomar Nature**
Ctra. de Madrid, 69, 03007 Alicante
(Spain)
Ctra. Puente Genil s/n, Pol. Ind.
El Bujeo,
41567 Herrera - Sevilla (Spain)
Websites: www.campomarnature.com
www.organicpaellafromspain.com

Captain Jeff's Premium Spices, LLC
Company has an online contact form
Website: www.captainjeffs.com

Cedar's Mediterranean Foods, Inc.
50 Foundation Avenue
Ward Hill, MA 01835
Phone: (978) 372-8010
Email: info@cedarsfoods.com
Website: www.cedarsfoods.com

Chameleon Cold Brew
P.O. Box 4518
Austin, TX 78765-4518
Email: *info@chameleoncoldbrew.com*
Website: *www.chameleoncoldbrew.com*

Chia Star
Denville, NJ
Phone: (862) 209-1343
Company has an online contact form
Website: *www.chiastar.com*

Choice Organic Teas
c/o WorldPantry.com, Inc.
1192 Illinois Street
San Francisco, CA 94107
Phone (Toll Free): (866) 972-6879
(Monday–Friday, 6am–5pm PT)
Fax: (415) 401-0087
Email: *customerservice@worldpantry.com*
Website: *www.choiceorganicteas.com*

Christopher Ranch
305 Bloomfield Avenue
Gilroy, CA 95020
Company has an online contact form
Website: *www.christopherranch.com*

Clif Bar & Company / (Clif Kid Z Bar)
1451 66th Street
Emeryville, CA 94608-1004
Phone: (510) 596-6300
Phone (Toll Free): (800) 254-3227
(Monday–Friday, 8am–5pm PST)
Company has an online contact form
Website: *www.clifbar.ca*

Cocoa Mill Chocolatier
Phone: (800) 421-6220
(540) 464-8400 in Lexington, VA
(540) 460-1555 in Staunton, VA

Email: *info@cocoamill.com*
Website: *chocolate.cocoamill.com*

Columbia Gorge Organic
3610 Central Vale Road
Hood River, OR 97031
Phone: (541) 354-1066
Fax: (541) 354-1369
Email: *info@cogojuice.com*
Website: *www.cogojuice.com*

Country Choice Organics
P.O. Box 44247
Eden Prairie, MN 55344
Phone: (952) 829-8824
Fax: (952) 833-2090
Email: *sales@countrychoiceorganic.com*
Website: *www.countrychoiceorganic.com*

Country Sweet Products
5060 B Street
Bakersfield, CA
Phone: (661) 858-1075
Fax: (661) 858-0306
Company has an online contact form
Website: *www.countrysweetproduce.com*

Crofter's Food Ltd.
7 Great North Road
Parry Sound
Ontario, Canada P2A 2X8
Company has an online contact form
Website: *www.croftersorganic.com*

George E. Delallo Co. Inc.
6390 Route 30
Jeannette, PA 15644
Phone: 1-877-DELALLO
Company has an online contact form
Website: *www.delallo.com*

Devonsheer
Company has an online contact form
Website: *www.devonsheer.com*

Dream Foods International, LLC
1223 Wilshire Blvd., Suite 355
Santa Monica, CA 90403
Phone: (310) 315-5739
Fax: (310) 388-1322
Website: *www.dreamfoods.com*

Earth Mama Angel Baby
9866 SE Empire Court
Clackmas, OR 97015
Phone: (503) 607-0607
Fax: (503) 607-0067
Website: *www.earthmamaangelbaby.com*

Earth Circle Organics
355 Crown Point Circle, Suite D
Grass Valley, CA 95945
Phone: (877) 922-FOOD
Email: *info@earthcircleorganics.com*
Website: *www.earthcircleorganics.com*

Earth's Best Organic
The Hain Celestial Group, Inc.
4600 Sleepytime Drive
Boulder, CO 80301
Phone: (800) 442-4221
(Monday–Friday, 9–6pm ET)
Website: *www.earthsbest.com*

Egg Innovations, LLC
4811 West 100N
Warsaw, IN 46580
Phone: (574) 267-7545
Company has an online contact form
Website: *www.egginnovations.com*

Earthbound Farm
1721 San Juan Highway
San Juan Beutista, CA 95045
Phone: (831) 623-7880
Phone (Toll Free): 1 (800) 690-3200
Website: *www.ebfarm.com*

Emerald Cove
Great Eastern Sun
92 McIntosh Road
Ashville, NC 28806
Phone (Toll Free): (800) 334-5809
Company has an online contact form
Website: *www.great-eastern-sun.com*

Engine2 Plant Strong
(a division of Whole Foods Market)
Company has an online contact form
Website: *www.wholefoodsmarket.com/
healthy-eating/engine-2*

Equal Exchange
50 United Drive
West Bridgewater, MA 02379
Phone: (774) 776-7333
Fax: (508) 587-3833
Email: *orders@equalexchange.coop*
Website: *equalexchange.coop*

Evergreen Juices, Inc.
P.O. Box 1
Don Mills ON, Canada
Phone: (877) 915-8423
Fax: (905) 866-5633
Company has an online contact form
Website: *www.evergreenjuices.com*

Evolution Fresh
Phone: (800) 794-9986
Email: *info@evolutionfresh.com*
Website: *www.evolutionfresh.com*

Explore Asian Authentic Cusine
Email: *info@explore-asian.com*
Website: *www.explore-asian.com*

Farmer's Market Foods, Inc.
P.O. Box 817
Corvallis, OR 97339-0817
Phone: (541) 757-1497
Email: *information@farmersmarketfoods.com*
Website: *www.farmersmarketfoods.com*

Farmhouse Culture
303 Potrero Street, #40F
Santa Cruz, CA 95060
Phone: (831) 466-0499
Email: *info@farmhouseculture.com*
Website: *www.farmhouseculture.com*

Fig Food Company, LLC
Phone: (855) FIG-FOOD
Website: *www.figfood.com*

Fior di Frutta
168 Court Street
Woodland, CA 95695
Fax: (530) 662-0929
Website: *www.nuggetmarket.com*

Food for Life Baking Company
Toll Free: 1 (800) 797-5090
Customer Service: (951) 279-5090
Website: *www.foodforlife.com*

Food Source
Robinson Fresh
14701 Charlson Road
Eden Prairie, MN 55347
Phone: (855) 350-0014
Website: *www.robinsonfresh.com*

Follow Your Heart
21825 Sherman Way
Canoga Park, CA 91303
Phone: 1 (888) 394-3949
Email: *info@followyourheart.com*
Website: *www.followyourheart.com*

The Ginger People
North American Headquarters
Royal Pacific Foods/The Ginger People
215 Reindollar Avenue
Marina, CA 93933
Phone: (831) 582-2494
Fax: (831) 582-2495
Email: *info@gingerpeople.com*
Website: *www.gingerpeople.com.au*

Go Go Squeez
20 West 22nd Street, 12th floor
New York, NY 10010
Phone: 1 (888) 288-7148
Company has an online contact form
Website: *www.gogosqueez.com*

Go Hunza
Company has an online contact form
Website: *www.gohunza.com*

Go Raw Organics
San Jose, CA
Phone: (650) 962-9299
Fax: (650) 962-9000
Company has an online contact form
Website: *www.goraw.com*

Good Belly
Team Goodbelly
P.O. Box 17460
Boulder, CO 80308
Phone: (303) 443-3631
Email: *info@goodbelly.com*
Website: *www.goodbelly.com*

Good Neighbor Organics
9825 Engles Road
Northport, MI 49670
Phone: (231) 386-5636
Website: *goodneighbororganics.com*

Good Water Farms
Phone: (631) 907-4345
Company has an online contact form
Website: *www.goodwaterfarms.com*

Great River Organic Milling
P.O. Box 185
Fountain City, WI 54629
Phone: (608) 687-9580
Email: *contact@greatrivermilling.com*
Website: *www.greatrivermilling.com*

Green Valley Organics
Phone: (707) 823-8250
Fax: (707) 823-6976
Company has an online contact form
Email: *contact@GreenValleyLactoseFree.com*

Guayaki Tea
6782 Sebastopol Avenue, Suite 100
Sebastopol, CA 95472
Phone: (888) 482-9254
(Monday–Friday, 8am–5pm)
Website: *guayaki.com*

Haiku Tea
Great Eastern Sun
92 McIntosh Road
Asheville, NC 28806
Toll Free: 1-800-334-5809
Company has an online contact form
Website: *www.great-eastern-sun.com/
shop/haiku-organic-japanese-teas*

Handsome Brook Farms
Betsy & Bryan Babcock
4132 East Handsome Brook Road
Franklin, NY 13775
Phone: (607) 829-2587
Email: *bbabcock@handsomebrookfarm.com*
Website: *www.handsomebrookfarm.com*

Happy Tree
Bismarck, AZ
Email: *hello@drinkhappytree.com*
Website: *www.drinkhappytree.com*

Harmless Harvest
Phone: (347) 467-0733
Company has an online contact form
Email: *info@harmlessharvest.com*
Website: *www.harmlessharvest.com*

Healthy Beverage, LLC
200 South Clinton Street, Suite 202
Doylestown, PA 18901
Phone: (800) 295-1388
Fax: (866) 642-9179
Email: *info@steaz.com*
Website: *www.steaz.com*

Health Valley Company
Phone: 1 (866) 595-8917
(Monday–Friday, 8am–5pm CT)
The Hain Celestial Group, Inc.
Company has an online contact form
Website: *www.healthvalley.com*

High Quality Organics
12101 Moya Blvd.
Reno, Nevada 8950
Phone: (775) 971-8550
Website: *www.hqorganics.com*

Himalayan Harvest Organics
International Harvest
606 Franklin Avenue
Mount Vernon, NY 10550
Phone (Office): (914) 699-5600
Toll Free: (800) 277-4268
Fax: (914) 699-5626
Email: info@internationalharvest.com
Website: www.internationalharvest.com

Hope Hummus LLC
1850 Dogwood Street
Louisville, CO 80027
Phone: (303) 248-7019
Fax: (303) 265-9522
Company has an online contact form
Website: www.hopehummus.com

I Love Produce, LLC.
P.O. Box 140
Kelton, PA 19346-0140
Phone: (610) 869-4664
Email: sales@iloveproduce.com
Website: www.iloveproduce.com

Imagine Foods
Imagine Consumer Relations
The Hain Celestial Group, Inc.
4600 Sleepytime Drive
Boulder, CO 80301
Phone: 1 (800) 434-4246
(Monday–Friday, 7am–5pm MT)
Company has an online contact form
Website: www.imaginefoods.com

In/Fusion
Infusion Company
28 rue Hamelin
75116 Paris, France
Email: info@infusion-company.com
Website: www.infusion-company.com/
herbal-tea-organic.html

Irving Farms Coffee
27 West 20th Street, Suite 1100
New York, NY 10011
Phone: (212) 206-0707
Company has an online contact form
Email: holler@irvingfarm.com
Website: shop.irvingfarm.com

Julie's Organic Ice Cream
Company has an online contact form
Website: www.juliesorganic.com

Ke Vita Inc.
2220 Celsius Avenue, Suite A
Oxnard, CA 93030
Phone: (888) 310-6106
Website: kevita.com

Kiju Organic
1440-2 King Street, North, Box 555
St. Jacobs, Ontario (Canada) N0B 2N0
Phone: (519) 664-1664
1 (866) 494-KIJU (5458)
Email: info@kijuorganic.com
Website: www.kijuorganic.com/en

Kikkoman
Customer Service Department
W-S PO Box 420784
San Francisco, CA 94142-0784
Company has an online contact form
Website: www.kikkomanusa.com

King Soba
Fabulous Foods
Unit B409 The Chocolate Factory
5 Clarendon Road
London N22 6Xj
Company has an online contact form
Email: info@kingsoba.co.uk
Website: www.kingsoba.com

Koyo Organic
Aliments Koyo Inc.
4605 Hickmore
Montreal QC H4T1S5
Koyo Foods Inc.
51 Scottfield Drive
Scarborough ON M1S 5R4
Website: *www.koyofoods.com*

Organic Kombucha
Phone: (231) 360-7043
Email: *info@organic-kombucha.com*
Website: *www.organic-kombucha.com*

La Preferida Organics
3400 West 35th Street
Chicago, IL 60632
Toll Free: (800) 621-5422
Website: *www.lapreferida.com*

Lake Champlain Chocolates
750 Pine Street
Burlington, VT 05401
Toll Free: (800) 465-5909
(Monday–Friday, 8:30am–5pm)
Company has an online contact form
Email: *info@lakechamplainchocolates.com*
Website: *www.lakechamplainchocolates.com*

Lakewood Juice Company
Phone: (866) 324-5900
Company has an online contact form
Website: *www.lakewoodjuices.com*

Late July Organics Snacks
3166 Main Street
Barnstable, MA 02630
Phone: (508) 362-5859
Fax: (508) 362-5868
Email: *info@latejuly.com*
Website: *www.latejuly.com*

Life Glow Organic Farm
Phone: (305) 989-1551
Email: *LifeGlowOrganiFarm@Gmail.com*
Website: *www.lifegloworganics.com*

Lightlife
Company has an online contact form
Toll Free: (800) 769-3279
(Monday–Friday, 9am–5pm)
Website: *www.lightlife.com*

Little Duck Organics
55-C 9th Street
Brooklyn, NY 11215
Website: *www.littleduckorganics.com*

Los Chileros de Nuevo Mexico
Gourmet Southwestern Cuisine
309 Industrial Avenue NE
Albuquerque, NM 87107
Phone: (505) 242-7513
Company has an online contact form
Website: *www.loschileros.com*

Lotus Foods
Toll Free: (866) 972-6879
Monday–Friday, 6am–5pm PT
Saturday–Sunday, 9am–5pm PT
Website: *www.lotusfoods.com*

Lundberg Family Farm
5311 Midway
P.O. Box 369
Richvale, CA 95974
Phone: (530) 538-3500
(Monday–Friday, 8:30am–5pm PT)
Company has an online contact form
Website: *www.lundberg.com*

Made in Nature
1708 13th Street
Boulder, CO 80302
Phone: 1 (800) 906-7426
(Monday–Friday, 9am–5pm ET)
Company has an online contact form
Website: www.madeinnature.com

Madhava Organics
14300 E I-25 Frontage Road
Longmont, CO 80504-9626
Phone: (800) 530-2900
Email: hello@madsweets.com
Website: www.madhavasweeteners.com

Mama Chia
5205 Avenue Encinas, Suite E
Carlsbad, CA 92008
Company has an online contact form
Website: www.mammachia.com

McGeary Organics
P.O. Box 299
Lancaster, PA 17608-0299
Toll Free: 1 (800) 624-3279
Phone: (717) 394-6843
Fax: (717) 394-6931
Email: sales@mcgearyorganics.com
Website: www.mcgearyorganics.com

Mediterranean Organic
Company has an online contact form
Website: www.mediterraneanorganic.com

Melissa's World Variety Produce, Inc.
P.O. Box 14599
Los Angeles, CA 90051
Phone: (800) 588-0151
Email: hotline@melissas.com
Website: www.melissas.com

Melt Organic
Prosperity Organic Foods, Inc.
475 West Main Street
Boise, ID 83702
Phone: (208) 429-9800
Phone: 1 (888) 557-5741
Fax: (208) 854-0907
Website: www.meltorganic.com

Mestemacher
Am Anger 29
D-33332 Gutersloh
Germany
Phone: + 49 52 41 / 87 09 - 71
Email: export@mestemacher.de
Website: www.mestemacher-gmbh.com

Middle Earth Olive Oil Co.
737 Broadway
Dunedin, FL 34698
Phone: (727) 797-1300
Website: www.middleeartholiveoil.com

Miline Fruit Products, Inc.
804 Bennett Avenue
P.O. Box 111
Prosser, WA 99350
Phone: (509) 786-2611
Fax: (509) 786-1724
Website: www.milnefruit.com

Mumm's Sprouting Seeds
Box 80
Parkside, SK SOJ2A0 Canada
Phone: 1 (306) 747-2935
Company has an online contact form
Website: www.sprouting.com

Missouri Northern Pecans
Toll Free: 1 (866) PECANS8
Website: www.mopecans.com

Moo Organic
The Cow Shed
Crediton Dairy
Church Lane
Crediton EX17 2AH
Email: *moo.milk@creditondairy.co.uk*
Website: *www.moomilk.co.uk*

Mushroom Harvest, Inc.
P.O. Box 584
Athens, OH 45701
Phone: (740) 448-7376
Fax: (740) 448-8007
Email: *info@mushroomharvest.com*
Website: *www.mushroomharvest.com*

Nasoya
Vitasoy USA Inc.
One New England Way
Ayer, MA 01432
Toll Free: (800) 848-2769
 (Monday-Friday, 10am-2pm EST)
Email: *info@vitasoy-usa.com*
Website: www.nasoya.com

Nature's All Foods
Company has an online contact form
Website: *naturesallfoods.com*

Nature's Path Organics
Consumer Services
9100 Van Horne Way
Richmond, BC Canada
V6X 1W3
Phone: (866) 880-7284
Website: *us.naturespath.com*

Nature's SunGrown Foods
700 Irwin Street, Suite 103
San Rafael, CA 94901
Phone: (415) 491-4944
Fax: (415) 532-2233
Email: *sales@naturesungrown.com*

Newman's Own
246 Post Road East
Westport, CT 06880
Company has an online contact form
Website: *www.newmansownorganics.com*

Next Organics
Tropical Valley Foods
P.O. Box 2994
Plattsburgh, NY 12901
Phone: 1 (866) 595-8917
Company has an online contact form
Email: *customerservice1@eyelevel
solutions.com*
Website: *www.nextorganicschocolate.com*

Numi Organic Tea
P.O. Box 20420
Oakland, CA 94620
Phone: (888) 404-6864
Fax: (510) 536-6864
Email: *info@numitea.com*
Website: *www.numitea.com*

Nutiva
213 West Cutting Blvd.
Richmond, CA 94804
Phone: (800) 993-4367
Email: *help@nutiva.com*
Website: *nutiva.com/contact*

NutraSun Foods
P.O. Box 30059
Regina, Saskatchewan, Canada
S4N 4N0
Phone: (306) 751-2040
Fax: (306) 751-2047
Email: *info@nutrasunfoods.com*
Website: *www.nutrasunfoods.com*

Nuttzo Organic
Phone: (888) 325-0553
Company has an online contact form
Website: *gonuttzo.com*

Ocho Organic
Five Star Organics LLC
P.O. Box 934
Lafayette, CA 94549-0934
Website: *www.ochocandy.com*

Olivia's Organics
P.O. Box 6277
Chelsea, MA 02150
Email: *olivia@oliviasorganics.org*
Website: *www.oliviasorganics.org*

Once Again Nut Butter Collective, Inc.
12 South State Place
P.O. Box 429
Nunda, NY 14517
Phone: (585) 468-2535
Toll Free: (888) 800-8075
Fax: (585) 468-5995
Website: *www.onceagainnutbutter.com*

Oregon Chai
Phone: (888) 874-CHAI (2424)
Email: *nirvana@oregonchai.com*
Website: *www.oregonchai.com*

Orgain, Inc.
P.O. Box 4918
Irvine, CA 92616
Email: *info@drinkorgain.com*
Website: *www.shop.orgain.com*

Organica Fresh
255 West Julian Street, Suite 502
San Jose, CA 95110
Phone: (408) 297-9797

Company has an online contact form
Website: *www.organicafresh.com*

Organic Girl
900 Work Street
Salinas, CA 93901
Phone: (866) 782-7096
Company has an online contact form
Website: *www.iloveorganicgirl.com*

Organicville Brand
Sky Valley Organics
878 Firetower Road
Yanceyville, NC 27379
Company has an online contact form
Website: *organicvillefoods.com*

Pacific Grain & Foods
4067 West Shaw Avenue
Fresne, CA 93722
Phone: (559) 276-2580
Fax: (559) 276-2936
Website: *www.pacificgrainandfoods.com*

Panorama Meats, Inc.
Organic Grass-Fed Meats
Phone: (530) 668-8920
Website: *www.panoramameats.com*

Paromi Tea
Phone: (877) 727-6648
(Monday–Friday, 8am–6pm)
Website: *paromi.com*

Peak Organic Brewing Co.
110 Marginal Way, #802
Portland, ME 04101
Phone: (207) 586-5586
Email: *info@peakbrewing.com*

Peeled Snacks
65 15th Street, FL 1
Brooklyn, NY 11215
Phone: (212) 706-2001
Fax: (646) 478-9518
Website: *www.peeledsnacks.com*

Pero Family Farms
Company has an online contact form
Website: *perofamilyfarms.com*

Pete and Gerry's
140 Buffum Road
Monroe, NH 03771
Phone: (603) 344-3276
Website: *peteandgerrys.com*

Premier Japan
Edward and Sons Trading Co., Inc.
P.O. Box 1326
Carpinteria, CA 93014
Phone: (805) 684-8500
Fax: (805) 684-8220
Website: *www.edwardandsons.com*

Prince of Peace Enterprises, Inc.
3536 Arden Road
Haywood, CA 94545-3908
Phone: (510) 887-1899
Fax: (510) 887-1799
Website: *www.popus.com*

Pro Bugs Lifeway Foods Inc.
6431 West Oakton Street
Morton Grove, IL 60053
Phone: (877) 281-3874
Fax: (847) 967-6556
Website: *www.lifeway.net*

Purity Organics
14900 West Belmont Avenue
Kerman, CA 93630
Phone: (555) 842-5601
Website: *www.purityorganics.com*

Pyure
Company has an online contact form
Website: *www.pyuresweet.com*

Riding Moon Organics
Website: *www.bluemarblebrands.com*

Rigoni di Asiago USA
3449 NE 1st Avenue, Suite L32
Miami, FL 33137
Phone: (305) 470-7583
Company has an online contact form
Email: *info@rigonidiasiago-usa.com*
Website: *rigonidiasiago-usa.com*

Road's End Organics
Edward and Sons Trading Co., Inc.
P.O. Box 1326
Carpinteria, CA 93014
Phone: (805) 684-8500
Website: *www.roadsendorganics.com*

Rudi's Organic
4600 Sleepytime Drive
Boulder, CO 80301
Phone: (877) 293-0876
Company has an online contact form
Website: *www.rudisbakery.com*

Runa
33 Flatbush Avenue, Suite 505
Brooklyn, NY 11217
Toll Free: (800) 485-3803
Email: *info@runa.org*

Rustic Crust
Phone: (603) 435-5119
Fax: (603) 435-5141
Email: info@crusticcrust.com
Website: www.rusticcrust.com

RW Knudsen
Phone: (888) 569-6993
(Monday–Friday, 9am–7pm)
Company has an online contact form
Website: www.rwknudsenfamily.com

Santa Cruz Organics
Phone: 1 (888) 569-6993
(Monday–Friday, 9am–7pm)
Company has an online contact form
Website: www.santacruzorganic.com

Seeds of Change
P.O. Box 4908
Rancho Dominquez, CA 90220
Phone: (888) 762-7333
(Monday–Friday, 7am–11pm CT)
Website: www.seedsofchange.com

Shasha Bread Company
20 Plastics Avenue
Toronto, ON, M8Z 4B7
Phone: (416) 255-0416
Fax: (416) 255-9672
Email: info@sgasgabread.com
Website: www.shashabread.com

Severino Pasta Co.
110 Haddon Avenue
Westmont, NJ 08108
Phone: (856) 854-7666
Fax: (856) 854-6098
Email: info@severinopasta.com
Website: www.severinopasta.com

Shady Maple Farms
1324 Main Street
East End, PA 17519
Website: www.shady-maple.com

Sky Valley Organics
878 Firetower Road
Yanceyville, NC 27379
Company has an online contact form
Website: www.organicvillefoods.com

Smart Juice LLC
Bethleham, PA
Phone: (610) 625-1531
Fax: (888) 625-0295
Email: info@smartjuice.us
Website: www.smartjuice.us

So Delicious Dairy Free
P.O. Box 21938
Eugene, OR 97402
Phone: (541) 338-9400
Fax: (541) 743-4333
Website: sodeliciousdairyfree.com

Straus Family Creamery
1105 Industrial Avenue, Suite 200
Petaluma, CA 94952
Phone: (707) 776-2887
Fax: (707) 776-2888
Company has an online contact form
Email: sfc@strausmilk.com
Website: www.strausfamilycreamery.com

Suja Juice
8380 Camino Santa Fe, Suite 200
San Diego, CA 92121
Phone: (855) 879-7852
Website: www.sujajuice.com

Sunset Valley Organic
31567 Highway 99 West
Corvallis, OR 97333
Phone: (541) 752-0460
Call only between 8am and 6pm PST
Website: www.sunsetvalleyorganics.com

Suzanne's Specialties, Inc.
421 Jersey Avenue, Suite B
New Brunswick, NJ 08901
Toll Free: (800) 762-2135
Phone: (732) 828-8500
Fax: (732) 828-8563
Email: info@suzannes-specialties.com
Website: www.suzannes-specialties.com

Sweet Leaf Iced Tea
Phone: (877) 291-6793
Company has an online contact form
Website: www.sweetleaftea.com

Taylor Farms Organic
947 B Blanco Circle
Salinas, CA 93901
Company has an online contact form
Website: www.taylorfarms.com

Tazo
Toll Free: (855) 829-6832
(Monday–Friday, 5am–8pm;
Saturday–Sunday, 6am–4pm)

The Sprout Man
Phone: 1 (800) SPROUT1 (777-6881)
Website: www.sproutman.com

Theo
3400 Phinney Avenue North
Seattle, WA 98103
Phone: (206) 632-5100
Fax: (206) 632-0413
Website: www.theochocolate.com

Third Street Chai
408 South Pierce Avenue
Louisville, CO 80027
Phone: (800) 636-3790
Email: info@3rfstreetchai.com
Website: www.thirdstreetchai.com

Three Twins Ice Cream
419 1st Street
Petaluma, CA 94952
Phone: (707) 763-8946
Website: www.threetwinicecream.com

Thunder Island
Company has an online contact form
Phone: (631) 204-1110
Website: www.thunderislandcoffee.com

Tolerant
Company has an online contact form
Website: www.tolerantfoods.com

Tom's Roasting Company
Phone: (855) 333-1584
(Monday–Friday, 8am–5pm)
Website: www.toms.com

Traditional Medicinals
4515 Ross Road
Sebastopol, CA 95472
Toll Free: (800) 543-4372
Company has an online contact form
Website: www.traditionalmedicinals.com

Tres Agaves Products
P.O. Box 5205
Berkeley, CA 94705
Phone: (510) 900-8009
Fax: (510) 900-8010
Website: www.tresagaves.com

Trickling Springs Creamery
Company has an online contact form
Website: *www.tricklingspringscreamery.com*

TruJoy Sweets
648 Wheeling Road
Wheeling, IL 60090
Phone: (224) 676-1070
Email: *info@trusweets.com*

Tru Roots
Enray Inc., home of Truroots
6999 Southfront Road
Livermore, CA 94551
Phone: (800) 288-3637
Company has an online contact form
Website: *truroots.com*

Tulsi Organic
Organic India, USA
5311 Western Avenue, Suite 110
Boulder, CO 80301
Phone: (888) 550-8332
(Monday–Friday, 9am–5pm)
Website: *organicindianausa.com*

Two Leaves
Phone: (855) 282-5450
Website: *www.twoleavestea.com*

Uncle Matt's Organic
P.O. Box 120187
Clermont, FL 34712
Phone: (352) 394-8737
Toll Free: (877) 364–2028
Fax: (352) 394–1003
Company has an online contact form
Email: *info@unclematts.com*

Vermont Bread Company (The Baker)
P.O. Box 1217
Brattleboro, VT 05302
Phone: (800) 721-4057
Company has an online contact form
Email: *askus@the-baker.com*
Website: *www.the-baker.com*

Vermont Organic Bread
Phone: (800) 721-4057
Email: *info@vermontbread.com*
Website: *www.vermontbread.com*

Vidal Fresh, Inc. Corporate
P.O. Box 1808
Morro Bay, CA 93443
Company has an online contact form
Website: *www.vidafresh.com*

Vital Farms
3913 Todd Lane, Suite 505
Austin, TX 78744
Phone: (877) 455–3063
Email: *info@vitalfarms.com*
Website: *vitalfarms.com*

Wan Ja Shan
Wanjashan International
4 Sands Station Road
Middletown, NY 10940
Phone: (845) 343-1515
Website: *www.wanjashan.com*

Westbrae Natural
Westbrae Customer Care
The Hain Celestial Group, Inc.
4600 Sleepytime Drive
Boulder, CO 80301
Phone: (800) 434-4246
(Monday–Friday, 9am–7pm)

Whole Foods Organics
Website: *www.wholefoodsmarket.com/ about-our-products/our-product-lines*

Wholesome Sweeteners
Company has an online contact form
Phone: (800) 680-1896
(Monday–Friday, 8am–6pm CT)
Email: *wholeearth@teamsweetener.com*
Website: *www.wholesweetners.com*

Wilcox Farms, Inc.
Phone: (360) 458-7774
Company has an online contact form
Website: *www.wilcoxfarms.com*

Wildwood Organics
Phone: (800) 588-7782
Company has an online contact form
Website: *www.wildwoodfoods.com*

Wolaver's Ale
793 Exchange Street
Middlebury, VT
Phone: (802) 388-0727
Website: *www.wolaversorganic.com*

Xochitl, Inc.
6020 Colwell Blvd.
Irving, TX 75039
Phone: (214) 800-3551
Fax: (214) 800-3547
Email: *info@salsaxochitl.com*
Website: *salsaxochitl.com*

Yogavive Organics
6 Neach Road, #863
Tiburon, CA 94920
Phone: (415) 366-6226
Fax: (415) 366-1750
Email: *info@yogavive.com*
Website: *www.yogavive.com*

Yogi Tea
1192 Illinois Street
San Francisco, CA 94107
Phone: (866) 972-6879
(Monday–Friday, 6am–5pm)
Fax: (415) 401-0087
Email: *yogitea.customerservice @yogiproducts.com*
Website: *shop.yogiproducts.com*

YummyEarth Inc.
79 North Franklin Turnpike, Suite 200
Ramsey, NJ 07446
Phone: (201) 857-8489
Fax: (201) 606-8215
Email: *support@yumearth.com*
Website: *www.yummyearth.com*

Zen Pudding
Company has an online contact form
Website: *www.zenzoy.com*

Zook Molasses Company
P.O. Box 160
4960 Horseshoe Pike
Honey Brook, PA 19344
Phone: (800) 327-4406
Website: *www.zookmolasses.com*

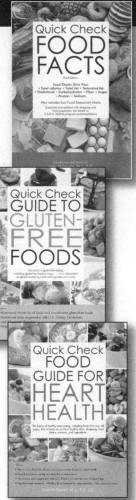